PAYMENT IN PRACTICE

2025 OB/GYN Coding Manual

ACOG
The American College of Obstetricians and Gynecologists

Payment in Practice: *2025 OB/GYN Coding Manual*

American College of Obstetricians and Gynecologists

Washington, DC : American College of Obstetricians and Gynecologists, [2025]
Identifiers: LCCN 2024049621 (print) | LCCN 2024049622 (ebook)
ISBN 9781948258920 (trade paperback) | ISBN 9781948258913 (ebook)

Printed in the United States of America
1 2 3 4 5 / 9 8 7 6 5
American College of Obstetricians and Gynecologists
409 12th Street SW
Washington, DC 20024-2188

Cover and interior design: Kathleen Dyson

ACOG has selected certain surgical CPT codes and descriptions that are commonly reported by obstetrician-gynecologists. The listing of a CPT procedure description and its code number in this publication does not restrict its use to a particular specialty group. Any procedure in this publication may be used to designate the services rendered by any qualified physician or other qualified health care professional (QHP).

This book was prepared by the American College of Obstetricians and Gynecologists for educational purposes only. It is not intended to represent the only, or necessarily the best, coding format or methods for the situations discussed, but rather represents an approach or opinion that may be helpful to persons responsible for diagnostic and procedural coding. The statements made in this publication should not be construed as ACOG policies or procedures, nor as standards of care. ACOG makes no representation or warranties, express or implied, regarding the accuracy of the information contained in this book and disclaims any liability or responsibility for any consequences resulting from or otherwise related to any use of, or reliance on, this book.

Suggestions and comments are welcome; submit your comments to https://acogcoding.freshdesk.com.

BIBLIOGRAPHY

The information in the *2025 OB/GYN Coding Manual* is a compilation of the following resources:

- The American Medical Association webpage on CPT® (Current Procedural Terminology) found at https://www.ama-assn.org/amaone/cpt-current-procedural-terminology
- The Centers for Medicare & Medicaid Services (CMS) internet-only manuals, including the Medicare Benefit Policy Manual and Medicare Claims Processing Manual, found at https://www.cms.gov/Regulations-and-Guidance/Guidance/Manuals/Internet-Only-Manuals-IOMs
- CMS Medicare Physician Fee Schedule, found at https://www.cms.gov/Medicare/Medicare-Fee-for-Service-Payment/PhysicianFeeSched
- CMS Medicare Learning Network educational tool, Medicare Preventative Services, found at https://www.cms.gov/Medicare/Prevention/PrevntionGenInfo/medicare-preventive-services/MPS-QuickReferenceChart-1.html
- The Centers for Disease Control and Prevention National Center for Health Statistics International Classification of Diseases, 10th Revision, Clinical Modification (ICD-10-CM), found at https://www.cdc.gov/nchs/icd/icd10cm.htm
- The American College of Surgeons' *Physicians as Assistants at Surgery: 2018 Study*. This resource was relied on for information concerning the need for a physician as an assistant surgeon. The American College of Surgeons conducted a survey of 16 surgical specialty organizations, including ACOG, to determine whether an operation as described by a CPT surgical code requires the use of a physician as an assistant at surgery: 1) almost always, 2) almost never, or 3) sometimes.

Scenarios and notes on documentation were adapted from case examples and CPT vignettes. They do not represent specific individuals or medical cases and are intended to be examples only.

ACKNOWLEDGMENTS

The American College of Obstetricians and Gynecologists (ACOG) gratefully acknowledges the contributions of the ACOG Committee on Health Economics and Coding (CHEC):

Members

Eilean L. Attwood, MD, MPH, Chair

John Patrick Horton, MD, Vice Chair

Jennifer E. Dietrich, MD

Coy Aiden Flowers, MD

Cecilia Bonaduce Leggett, MD

Lauren MacAfee, MD

Emily Boevers Solverson, MD

Adrienne D. Zertuche, MD, MPH

CPT Delegates and Advisors

Kathy Y. Jones, MD, Delegate

Judith K. Volkar, MD, Advisor

Lisa Hofer, MD, MPH, MBA, Advisor

Nichole Mahnert, MD, Advisor

Relative Value Scale Update Committee Delegates and Advisors

Gregory W. DeMeo, DO, Delegate

Gwenn Jackson, MD, Delegate

John Kent Hathaway, MD, PhD, Advisor

Eilean L. Attwood, MD, MPH, Advisor

John Patrick Horton, MD, Advisor

David O. Holtz, MD, Advisor

ACOG Staff

Sandra E. Brooks, MD, MBA
Chief Executive Officer

Christopher M. Zahn, MD
Chief, Clinical Practice and Health Equity and Quality

Jennifer Walsh
Chief Product and Marketing Officer

Lisa Satterfield, MS, MPH, CAE, CPH
Senior Director, Health and Payment Policy

Kehinde Taiwo, MS, CPPM, COC, CPC
Clinical Coding and Health Informatics Manager

Elizabeth Frey
Project Manager, Products

Martha Hawley-Bertsch
Director, Product Management

Jennifer Hicks, MS
Director, Editorial Development

William Howard, MA, ELS
Copyeditor/Proofreader

Taskin Monjur
Product Manager, Clinical and Patient Resources

Consultant

Brad Hart, MBA, MS, CMPE, CPC, CPMA, COBGC
Coding Consultant

INTRODUCTION

Thank you for your interest in ACOG's Payment in Practice: *2025 OB/GYN Coding Manual!*

Please note that we have consolidated all of our coding resources under the title "Payment in Practice," so when you encounter this phrase, you will know it refers to an ACOG coding product. Our ultimate aim is to seamlessly connect all of our resources across the organization. For instance, if you are focused on labor management, you will be able to find our most recent clinical guidance, along with instructions on how to document, code, and bill insurance—all accessible with minimal clicks!

That said, we are also working with the American Medical Association to update codes for obstetric care. We are hopeful that new codes will be developed that include all of the services provided—and time spent—by obstetrician–gynecologists throughout the pregnancy. Watch for updates on our News page and in the weekly *ACOG Rounds*.

Also of importance, please note that the ACOG Board of Directors recently issued a Statement of Policy titled Payment for Obstetricians and Gynecologists, reaffirming ACOG's commitment to ensuring fair and equitable payment for obstetric and gynecologic practices. Notably, the statement provides specific guidelines for appropriate billing of obstetric services, and we are actively advocating for their adoption by public and private payers.

We trust that you will find ACOG's Payment in Practice: *2025 OB/GYN Coding Manual* to be a valuable resource. For 2025, the most significant coding change is the creation of telehealth codes, which are outlined in Chapter 3 and Appendix CC of this manual.

Additionally, as with the previous edition, the 2025 manual does not include the ever-changing National Correct Coding Initiative (NCCI) edits. These edits are revised quarterly, and the current format of the coding manual does not allow for easy modification. You can find the NCCI Policy Manual for Medicare Services, along with quarterly updates for procedure-to-procedure (PTP) edits and medically unlikely edits (MUEs), at https://www.cms.gov/Medicare/Coding/NCCI-Coding-Edits. More information on how to use NCCI edits can be found in Chapter 1.

For this edition, the relative value units (RVUs) have been pulled from the 2025 Medicare Physician Fee Schedule, as published by the Centers for Medicare & Medicaid Services on November 1, 2024. While values could change slightly if there is legislative action, you can stay informed. To receive updates about changes to RVUs, the fee schedule, or payment policies, please visit https://acogcoding.Freshdesk.com.

Lastly, we encourage you to connect with us through our Payment in Practice: Knowledge Base portal. This resource offers updates specific to coding and policy, articles, and technical assistance for ACOG members and their billing and administrative staff. Staff can set up their own account, search articles, and submit questions or comments. We also provide assistance with denials and prior authorizations. Please use this free resource to improve your payment outcomes, and let us know how we are doing!

CONTENTS

Part I: Coding in Obstetrics and Gynecology

Part II: Components of Correct Coding

Part III: Appendices

PART I
Coding in Obstetrics and Gynecology

CHAPTER 1
Code Development

The first Current Procedural Terminology (CPT) codes were developed in 1966 by the American Medical Association (AMA) and included surgery procedures, medicine, radiology, and laboratory procedures. The publication was updated 3 times between 1970 and 1977, and in 1983, the Health Care Finance Administration (HCFA) adopted CPT as a part of the Healthcare Common Procedure Coding System (HCPCS) and mandated their use for the Medicare Part B (medical insurance) physician and outpatient reimbursement. Beginning in 1986 and 1987, HCFA required that state Medicaid agencies and facilities use CPT to report outpatient hospital surgical procedures. The Health Insurance Portability and Accountability Act of 1996 finalized the requirement that the Department of Health and Human Services name national standards for electronic transaction of health care information, including HCPCS and CPT, as code sets for billing and reimbursement.

STEPS IN CODE DEVELOPMENT

The Committee for Health Economics and Coding (CHEC) of the American College of Obstetricians and Gynecologists (ACOG) is charged with representing ACOG Fellows at the AMA CPT Editorial Panel, the AMA Relative Value Update Committee (RUC), and the Centers for Disease Control and Prevention (CDC) National Center for Health Statistics (NCHS) for International Classification of Diseases (ICD) diagnosis codes. Code proposals are brought forward by ACOG members, government agencies, industry, Centers for Medicare & Medicaid Services (CMS), or the AMA for development and review. ACOG supports the work of the CHEC to ensure ACOG Fellows and members receive fair and equitable payment for obstetric and gynecologic services.

Stakeholders interested in soliciting ACOG's support, partnership, or leadership for coding applications are welcome to submit their proposals for consideration by the CHEC through ACOG's Payment in Practice: Knowledge Base Portal (https://acogcoding.freshdesk.com). To start the process, users must:

- Register as a user of the portal (registration is free)
- Verify the account through the link sent via email
- Submit a ticket. Select "Request for a new diagnosis code" or "Request for a new procedure code"
- Include a brief summary of your interest (not the full proposal at this step, please)
- An email acknowledging your ticket with further instructions on what is necessary to submit a proposal will be sent. Of importance, proposals must include 3 peer-reviewed articles directly related to the request. Proposals without at least 3 peer-reviewed articles will not be considered.
- The applications are reviewed by ACOG staff for completeness and added to the CHEC meeting agenda according to the following schedule:
  - Proposals submitted November 2 to February 1:
    - Reviewed by CHEC at the February meeting
  - Proposals submitted February 2 to May 1:
    - Reviewed by CHEC at the May meeting
  - Proposals submitted May 2 to November 1:
    - Reviewed by CHEC at the November meeting

The CHEC will discuss the proposals based on the requirements of the CPT Editorial panel, the ability to support a strong RUC application, or the clinical needs for the ICD-10-CM codes. The CHEC may ask for additional information or require more data before a decision can be rendered. Applicants can resubmit their proposals if there are changes to the literature or data.

ICD-10-CM Codes

ICD-10-CM diagnostic code applications are submitted to the CDC NCHS Coordination and Maintenance Committee. There is not a specific form; however, code applications must be written and include the following:

- A description of the code(s)/change(s) being requested
- The rationale for why the new code/change is needed (including clinical relevancy)
- Supporting clinical references and literature

Anyone may submit an application. ACOG works closely with the CDC and will be contacted if a coding application for obstetric–gynecologic conditions are submitted. The CDC will consider ACOG's position on the application, so alerting ACOG through the CHEC provides more time for discussion and determination.

Additional instructions and timelines for the ICD-10-CM application are available at https://www.cdc.gov/nchs/icd/icd10_maintenance.htm.

More information about using ICD-10-CM codes can be found in Chapter 9, "Coding Basics for Reporting Diagnoses of Obstetric–Gynecologic Conditions."

CPT Codes

CPT codes can also be submitted by anyone. Because ACOG is the "umbrella" organization for all obstetric and gynecologic services, ACOG CPT Advisors will have an opportunity to Support, Oppose, or remain Neutral on all CPT applications. Again, codes submitted for consideration can be submitted ahead of time to the CHEC for review, advice, and input. However, unlike ICD-10-CM, once the coding application is submitted to the CPT Editorial Panel, ACOG can no longer engage in discussions with the applicants (unless, of course, ACOG is one of the applicants).

The CPT Editorial Panel meets 3 times a year to discuss and vote on CPT applications. The panel may determine that more information is needed and request the applicant to modify or change their application; in that case, the application will go on the next meeting agenda. If the application is denied, the applicant can resubmit for consideration at subsequent meetings. There is not a limit, per se, of how many times an application may be submitted. However, resubmitting applications without new information is generally not a good practice.

The CPT Editorial Panel develops the code description and determines the specific services that are included in or excluded from the procedure. That information is then used to create a clinical vignette. If the code description is later modified, the vignette is also modified.

If the panel accepts the code proposal, it is the responsibility of ACOG to provide the information necessary for the AMA RUC to assign a relative value to the code. This responsibility derives from the role ACOG plays at the AMA as an umbrella organization and is independent of who submitted the coding application.

The AMA RUC has very specific requirements and rules for valuing a procedure code that ACOG must follow. One important piece is the randomized member survey—which is developed by the AMA RUC and managed by ACOG. The survey is used to determine the physician work and time. Using the survey data, ACOG calculates relative value units (RVUs) for recommendation to the AMA RUC. The RUC debates the proposed RVUs and may vote to adopt or modify ACOG's proposal, or require a re-survey if there were not enough respondents or if the standard deviation is too large.

Once the RVUs are determined by the RUC, they are submitted to CMS, which makes the final determination through their annual fee schedules. CMS sends representatives to CPT and RUC so that they are aware of all of the discussions and the reasons for the determinations. CMS may accept or modify the RVUs and publish their decision in the Medicare Physician Fee Schedule Proposed Rule in July of each year. Stakeholders, including ACOG, meet with CMS and provide comments to any changes of concern, and the final fee schedule is published in November for implementation for services provided on or after January 1 of the following year.

CPT CODE CATEGORIES

CPT consists of Category I, Category II, and Category III codes.

Category I Codes

Category I codes are 5-character alphanumeric codes developed and copyrighted by the AMA. They comprise the primary set of codes used to describe the cognitive, procedural, and material services provided by a physician's practice to patients and are the primary focus of this coding manual.

Category I codes consist of 6 sections, each divided into subsections, headings and subheadings, and an index. The 6 sections are as follows:

- Evaluation and Management (E/M) Services (99202-99499)
- Anesthesia (00100-01999, 99100-99140)
- Surgery (10021-69990)
- Radiology, including Nuclear Medicine and Diagnostic Ultrasound (70010-79999)
- Pathology and Laboratory, including Reproductive Medicine Procedures (codes 80047-89398, 0001U-0222U)
- Medicine (also known as diagnostics), except Anesthesiology (90281-99199 and 99500-99607)

Category II Codes

These codes are used to collect information about the quality of care being provided, using nationally established performance measures. These optional codes are updated biannually in January and July and do not have RVUs associated with them. Generally, Category II codes should not be used as a substitute for existing Category I codes.

Category III Codes

These codes are used to collect specific data to assess the clinical efficacy, utilization, and outcomes for emerging technology, services, and procedures. Typically, new procedures will be first used as a Category III code to collect the data needed for the Category I application. They may be used by payers for billing and reimbursement; however, the payers will determine the payment amount.

CPT CODING CONVENTIONS

Coding conventions, terms, and punctuation in CPT assist in the selection of the most appropriate code.

Semicolons

CPT uses the semicolon as a kind of shorthand to avoid repeating words and phrases. For example, CPT lists:

57510	Cautery of cervix; electro or thermal
57511	Cryocautery; initial or repeat
57513	Laser ablation

Codes 57511 and 57513 both include the part of code 57510 that precedes the semicolon: "cautery of cervix." Therefore:

- The full description for code 57511 is "Cautery of cervix; cryocautery, initial or repeat."
- The full description for code 57513 is "Cautery of cervix; laser ablation."

Parentheses

Parentheses enclose parenthetical statements. Parenthetical statements either 1) provide additional guidance to help the user select the correct code, or 2) indicate that some codes from previous editions of CPT have been deleted. For example, these statements follow code 57556:

(For insertion of intrauterine device, use 58300)

(For insertion of any hemostatic agent or pack for control of spontaneous non-obstetrical hemorrhage, see 57180)

SYMBOLS

Many of the code numbers or phrases use symbols to provide additional information to the coder. In most cases, these symbols precede a code number.

● A bullet means that the code is new for the current year. Appendix B of the CPT book provides a summary of new code additions, deletions, and revisions.

▲ A triangle or delta sign means that the code description has been revised in the current year. See Appendix B of the CPT book for a summary of revised changes.

+ A plus sign means that the code is an "add-on" code and therefore does not require modifier 51 (multiple procedure). Add-on codes are reported only with other codes. They are never reported alone. A summary of CPT add-on codes is listed in Appendix D of the CPT book.

⦸ This symbol means that the code is a "modifier 51 exempt" code, and therefore the modifier is not required even when multiple procedures were performed. Appendix E lists a summary of CPT codes exempt from modifier 51.

▸◂ Arrows may be found before and after phrases, sentences, or whole paragraphs. The arrows enclose wording that is either new or has been revised in the current year.

⚡ This symbol means that the vaccine product code had not been approved by the FDA at the time the latest CPT book was published. Refer to Appendix K of the CPT book for a summary of these codes.

The hash symbol represents resequenced codes that do not appear in numeric order within the CPT book.

★ The star indicates a designated telehealth service.

CODING GUIDELINES

There are some general guidelines physicians should use when selecting a procedure code:

- Codes submitted to payers should reflect the most accurate code for the service and follow CPT's coding guidelines.
- Select the most specific code. The code must be the most accurate description of the service provided and be consistent with coding conventions and guidelines.
- Read any notes, instructions, or other explanatory statements printed under subsections, headings, or subheadings, and before and after codes.
- Know the bundling and unbundling rules used by CPT, your commercial payers, and CMS.

MEDICARE'S CORRECT CODING INITIATIVE

Both CPT and Medicare guidelines consider some smaller component services to be included or bundled into another more comprehensive service performed during the same session. CMS manages the bundled services through an extensive list known as the Correct Coding Initiative (CCI).

The CCI lists each CPT code and the codes that are bundled into it (and therefore not reported separately). CCI bundles are based on the following:

- Coding conventions in the CPT manual
- Medicare national and local policies and edits
- Analysis of standard medical and surgical practice
- Review of current coding practices using claims submitted to Medicare

The CCI lists "code pairs" in 2 columns. There are 2 kinds of code pairs: mutually exclusive and column 1/column 2 pairs. Column 1/column 2 code pairs include a comprehensive code (column 1) and codes that are considered components of that code (column 2). These pairs may be based on the following:

- Medicare's surgical package definition. For example, code 64435 (paracervical nerve block) is bundled into gynecologic surgical procedures since Medicare's global package includes any anesthesia provided by the surgeon.
- Standards of medical/surgical practice. A service may be considered "generic," that is, commonly part of all similar comprehensive procedures and necessary for the successful completion of the surgical procedure. For example, lysis of adhesions and surgical closure are bundled into open surgical procedures.
- A surgical approach and the surgical service. The exploration of the surgical field is included in the surgical code. For example, code 49000 (exploratory laparotomy) is bundled into 58150 (total abdominal hysterectomy).
- Components of a more comprehensive service. Many CPT code descriptions include a number of smaller, related procedures within a single code. For example, codes 57455 (colposcopy with biopsy) and 57456 (colposcopy with endocervical curettage) are bundled into 57454 (cervical colposcopy with biopsy and endocervical curettage).
- Families of codes. For example, comprehensive code 59400 (routine obstetric care including antepartum care, vaginal delivery, and postpartum care) includes these component codes in its family: 59050 and 59051 (fetal monitoring during labor), 59200 (insertion of a cervical dilator), 59300 (episiotomy, by other than attending), and 59414 (delivery of placenta). All of these component services are bundled into 59400.
- Mutually exclusive code pairs are bundled because they cannot reasonably be done in the same session on the same patient. For example, codes 58550-58554 (laparoscopic hysterectomy) are bundled into 58150 (total abdominal hysterectomy), and code 49520 (repair of inguinal hernia, recurrent) is bundled into 49505 (repair of inguinal hernia, initial).

Under some circumstances, it may be possible to report procedure codes that are bundled under CCI rules. A separate procedure can be reported with other procedures only if it "is performed on the same day but at a different session, or at an anatomically unrelated site." For example, code 57268 (repair of enterocele, separate procedure) is bundled into code 57284 (paravaginal defect repair). In order to bill as a separate procedure, a modifier must be added to the lesser, bundled code. Medicare accepts only these modifiers:

- 59 (distinct procedural service)
- HCPCS anatomic modifiers (eg, LT and RT)

- CPT modifiers 58 (staged or related procedure)
- Appropriate X{EPSU} sub-modifiers

Note that some CCI code pairs can never be reported together, even if a modifier is used and documentation is submitted with the claim.

MODIFIERS

As mentioned previously, modifiers are often necessary to separate a service or provide more information to the payer. Modifiers are 2-character appendages that are added to the end of either an E/M code or a procedure code. Correct use of modifiers can significantly affect physician reimbursement for services.

Unrelated Procedures - Modifier 59

A physician performs the following 2 procedures during the same surgical session:

Salpingo-oophorectomy (separate procedure code 58720) for benign ovarian neoplasms

Excision of Meckel's diverticulum (CPT code 44800)

The salpingo-oophorectomy is clearly not related to the excision procedure. Therefore, code 44800 and code 58720-59 are reported. The physician must document that the procedures were independent and unrelated to each other and link each code to a distinct ICD-10-CM diagnosis code.

Procedure Performed on Same or Different Sides of the Body - Modifiers LT/RT

Code 58805 (drainage of the cyst) is performed on the right ovary, and code 58940 (oophorectomy) is performed on the left ovary. Report both codes using modifiers LT and RT.

Using Modifier 59 or Modifier 51

Many physicians perform 2 procedures during the same session and are confused about whether to report modifier 59 (distinct procedural service) or modifier 51 (multiple procedures). The differences between these modifiers are as follows.

Modifier 59 indicates that:

- There is a CCI edit that indicates the services may be performed on the same day.
- Two procedures have been performed during this session.
- The procedures are usually bundled under either CPT or Medicare rules.
- Both procedures can be reported in this specific case because they are distinct and unrelated to each other.
- The bundled procedure should be reimbursed in this case.

Modifier 51 indicates that:

- There is not a CCI edit.
- Two procedures have been performed during this session.
- The procedures are not bundled under either CPT or Medicare rules.
- Both procedures can be reported and should be reimbursed.

An example of modifier 51 would be:

A physician performs multiple procedures with different CPT codes during the same surgical session. There are no CCI edits for these 2 procedures.

Vaginal hysterectomy, for uterus 250 g or less; with removal of tube(s) and/or ovary(s) (58262)

Combined anteroposterior colporrhaphy w/Cystoscopy (57260)

In this case, the services are reported on the claim form as follows:

- List the highest valued or most significant procedure first. No modifier is used. The highest valued procedure has the greatest number of RVUs.
- List the lesser-valued procedures in descending order of value with modifier 51.

Only those services that are not typically performed during the procedure should be listed separately. If a lesser procedure is almost always performed at the time of another procedure, it is generally included in the surgical CPT code. Modifier 59 would not be appropriate as these codes are not considered bundled per CCI rules.

CHAPTER 2
Evaluation and Management Services

Encounters with patients that are not procedure or surgery based are reported using Evaluation and Management codes (known as E/M codes). E/M services are either:

- Problem-oriented visits (eg, for the diagnosis and treatment of illness, disease, and symptoms); or
- Preventive visits (eg, when the patient has no current symptoms or diagnosed illness).

Reporting and documenting these services correctly can greatly affect practice income and also help protect the practice in the event of a claims review by Medicare or a commercial payer.

Outpatient or Inpatient

CPT defines these terms as follows:

- A patient is an outpatient until they are admitted to a health care facility as an inpatient. Outpatient areas include physicians' offices, emergency departments, observation areas, and outpatient surgical centers.
- A patient is an inpatient if she has been admitted to inpatient status at a health care facility.

Note that, in the updated E/M codes, CPT has moved observation services from outpatient to inpatient codes, for the purpose of coding. However, physicians should confirm if the patient has been admitted as an inpatient or is remaining and outpatient under the Centers for Medicare & Medicaid Services (CMS) classifications.

New or Established Patients

CPT defines these terms as follows:

- A new patient has not received any professional services from the physician/qualified health care professional (QHP) or another physician/QHP of the exact same specialty and subspecialty who belongs to the same group practice within the past 3 years.
- An established patient has received professional services from the physician/QHP or another physician/QHP of the exact same specialty and subspecialty who belongs to the same group practice within the past 3 years.

DETERMINING THE LEVEL OF E/M VISIT

Physicians choose whether their code selection will be based on medical decision making (MDM) or time. This determination may vary per each individual patient.

For code selection primarily based on time, the time used is total time on the date of service, which consists of total physician or QHP time on the date of service. This includes both face-to-face and non–face-to-face time.

Specifically, the AMA defines this for the E/M codes as follows:

> The total time on the date of the encounter including both face-to-face and non–face-to-face time personally spent by the physician and/or other QHP(s) on the date of the encounter (includes time in activities that require the physician or other QHP and does not include time in activities normally performed by clinical staff).

Activities for total time may include the following:

- Preparing to see the patient (eg, review of tests)
- Obtaining and/or reviewing separately obtained history
- Performing a medically appropriate examination and/or evaluation
- Counseling and educating the patient/family/caregiver
- Ordering medications, tests, or procedures

- Referring and communicating with other health care professionals (when not separately reported)
- Documenting clinical information in the electronic or other health record
- Independently interpreting results (not separately reported) and communicating results to the patient/family/caregiver
- Care coordination (not separately reported)

If using MDM, CPT, and CMS, include 3 elements for consideration of which level to select:

- number of diagnoses or management options;
- amount and/or complexity of data to be reviewed; and
- risk of complications and/or morbidity or mortality.

Appendix C provides more detail regarding MDM categories. Note that in order to select the MDM level, at least 2 of the 3 categories must meet or exceed that level.

E/M SERVICES

On February 9, 2019, the CPT Editorial Panel approved revisions to the E/M office visit CPT codes to address some of the issues related to administrative burden for physicians in the United States. These changes were implemented January 1, 2021. The E/M codes, their descriptors, and coding policies are in Part II, and Appendices B and C include tables for easy reference.

- Beginning with calendar year 2022, the AMA CPT Editorial Panel revised all E/M categories (except critical care services) to reflect the MDM and time framework outpatient E/M codes. History and physical exam will no longer be used to determine the visit level of the following E/M code families: Outpatient and office visits
- Hospital inpatient and observation services (consolidated)
- Consultations
- Emergency department services
- Nursing facility services
- Home health and Domiciliary (all facilities, consolidated)

The service times within the descriptors were also revised, and several codes consolidated a considerable number of the Other E/M CPT codes, with inpatient and observation visits being combined into a single code set, and home and domiciliary visits being combined into a single code set. Because of these changes, the 75 codes represented by the categories above are reduced to approximately 50 codes.

Appendix D outlines the inpatient and observation care codes in detail. Appendix E outlines in detail the hospital inpatient or observation care services provided to patients admitted and discharged on the same date of service. Appendix F reports consultations that are provided in the office or other outpatient site, including the home or residence, or emergency department. Appendix G describes the evaluation and management services provided in the emergency department.

Initial, Subsequent and Discharge Hospital Inpatient or Observation Services

The initial service codes (99221-99223) are used when the patient has not received services from a physician or other qualified health care professional in the exact same specialty or subspecialty who belongs to the same group practice.

If the patient is transferred from another site of service to inpatient or observation status, the service at the initial site may be separately reported. For example, a visit at the hospital emergency department, office, or nursing facility may be an initial visit, and the distinct, separately identifiable service by the same physician on the same date when the patient is inpatient or observation status may be reported with the modifier -25. If the service is not a separate service, the subsequent visit is a consultation visit and uses 99231, 99232, or 99233.

A transfer from observation status to inpatient status is not a new stay, and the initial inpatient or observation service codes are not appropriate.

The discharge hospital inpatient or observation codes (99238, 99239) are used to report the time on activities specifically related to the discharge, including the final examination, instructions for care upon discharge, and the preparations of records, prescriptions, and referrals. These codes should be used on a different date of service than the initial hospital inpatient or observations discharge services. For same-day admission and discharge, use 99234-99236.

(Same Day) Hospital Inpatient or Observation Care Services (including Admission and Discharge Services)

Codes 99234, 99235, and 99236 are used for inpatient or observation care services when the patient is admitted and discharged on the same date of service and the physician or other qualified health care provider visits the patient at least twice on the same date, one visit being an admission encounter and the other being a discharge encounter. If a patient is admitted and discharged during the same encounter, 99221, 99222, or 99223 is appropriate. If the admission and discharge spans multiple dates, 99221, 9922, 99223, 99232, 99233, 99238, or 99239 should be used.

Consultations

Consultations are a type of E/M service provided at the request of another physician or other appropriate source to provide an opinion/services for a specific condition or problem. The consultation must include a report to the requesting physician, other qualified health care professional, or other appropriate sources (lawyer, insurance company).

A consultation initiated by a patient or family member is not reported using consultation codes.

Consultation codes (99242-99245, 99252-99255) are defined as outpatient (office, clinic, home or residence, or emergency department) or inpatient or observation (inpatient, observation, nursing facilities). Only one consultation can be reported per admission, and follow-up services are reported using the appropriate E/M codes for established patients or subsequent visits.

Emergency Department

Emergency department codes (99281-99285, 99288) are used for care in hospital-based facility for patients seeking immediate medical care. However, a patient seen in the emergency department for the convenience of the physician or other qualified health care professional should be billed with the outpatient codes (99202-99215). There is no difference between new or established patients.

Unlike the other E/M codes, time is not a component of the emergency department E/M levels. The levels are based solely on the medical decision making.

E/M Services Modifiers

Appendix I summarizes the modifiers used with E/M services.

CHAPTER 3
Telehealth

Post-pandemic, some health insurers have rolled back telehealth coverage; however, it has not lessened for physicians and patients. The landscape of telehealth policy remains dynamic, varying from state to state and payer to payer.

The key points for 2025 are as follows:

- During the public health emergency, Medicare, several Medicaid programs, and most private payers allowed for the updated descriptions for 2021 Outpatient Evaluation and Management (E/M) to be the standard by which to select the appropriate E/M code to be billed with a –95 modifier. In addition, Medicare reimbursed the telephone codes (99441–99443) at the same rate as the in-person office visit.
- In response to the changes, the American Medical Association convened a work group to develop permanent codes for office visits performed by telehealth. The codes, available January 1, 2025, represent months of effort by ACOG and other specialty societies. Many of you may have participated in the valuation survey, and we thank you!
- The 17 codes consist of eight codes for synchronous audio-video (AV) services, eight codes for synchronous audio-only services, and a code for a brief virtual check-in encounter to determine whether a more extensive visit is required. Both sets of eight codes include four codes for new patients and four codes for established patients.
- The telephone codes (99441–99443) have been deleted from the CPT code book.
- The two AV and audio-only code sets mirror the format of the outpatient E/M codes, with the option to select medical decision making (MDM) or total time on the date of the encounter. Similar to the E/M codes, there are codes for straightforward, low, moderate, and high levels of MDM. All of the telehealth codes require the presence of a physician or qualified health care professional (QHP).
- All of the telehealth codes are synchronous, real-time, interactive encounters. Asynchronous services (those without real-time interaction between the physician/QHP and patient) are reported with the online digital E/M codes 99421–99423.
- Telehealth services must be performed on a separate date of service than another E/M service. If telehealth is performed on the same day as an E/M code, the time should be totaled and reported with one code.
- If, during an AV encounter, the connection is lost and only audio can be restored, select the code that represents the majority of the time of the interactive portion. Keep in mind that 10 minutes of medical discussion and/or patient observation must be exceeded in order to report these codes.

Audio-Video: New Patient

98000: *Synchronous audio-video visit for the evaluation and management of a new patient, which requires a medically appropriate history and/or examination and straightforward medical decision making. When using total time on the date of the encounter for code selection, 15 minutes must be met or exceeded.*

98001: *Synchronous audio-video visit for the evaluation and management of a new patient, which requires a medically appropriate history and/or examination and low medical decision making. When using total time on the date of the encounter for code selection, 30 minutes must be met or exceeded.*

98002: *Synchronous audio-video visit for the evaluation and management of a new patient, which requires a medically appropriate history and/or examination and moderate medical decision making. When using total time on the date of the encounter for code selection, 45 minutes must be met or exceeded.*

98003: *Synchronous audio-video visit for the evaluation and management of a new patient, which requires a medically appropriate history and/or examination and high medical decision making. When using total time on the date of the encounter for code selection, 60 minutes must be met or exceeded. (For services 75 minutes or longer, use prolonged services code 99417.)*

As with the outpatient E/M services, a new patient is defined by CPT as one who has not received any professional services from the physician or a QHP or another physician/QHP of the exact same specialty and subspecialty who belongs to the same group practice within the past 3 years.

Audio-Video: Established Patient

98004: *Synchronous audio-video visit for the evaluation and management of an established patient, which requires a medically appropriate history and/or examination and straightforward medical decision making. When using total time on the date of the encounter for code selection, 10 minutes must be met or exceeded.*

98005: *Synchronous audio-video visit for the evaluation and management of an established patient, which requires a medically appropriate history and/or examination and low medical decision making. When using total time on the date of the encounter for code selection, 20 minutes must be met or exceeded.*

98006: *Synchronous audio-video visit for the evaluation and management of an established patient, which requires a medically appropriate history and/or examination and moderate medical decision making. When using total time on the date of the encounter for code selection, 30 minutes must be met or exceeded.*

98007: *Synchronous audio-video visit for the evaluation and management of an established patient, which requires a medically appropriate history and/or examination and high medical decision making. When using total time on the date of the encounter for code selection, 40 minutes must be met or exceeded.*

As with the outpatient E/M services, an established patient is defined by CPT as one who has received professional services from the physician or a QHP or another physician/QHP of the exact same specialty and subspecialty who belongs to the same group practice within the past 3 years.

Audio-Only: New Patient

98008: *Synchronous audio-only visit for the evaluation and management of a new patient, which requires a medically appropriate history and/or examination, straightforward medical decision making, and more than 10 minutes of medical discussion. When using total time on the date of the encounter for code selection, 15 minutes must be met or exceeded.*

98009: *Synchronous audio-only visit for the evaluation and management of a new patient, which requires a medically appropriate history and/or examination, low medical decision making, and more than 10 minutes of medical discussion. When using total time on the date of the encounter for code selection, 30 minutes must be met or exceeded.*

98010: *Synchronous audio-only visit for the evaluation and management of a new patient, which requires a medically appropriate history and/or examination, moderate medical decision making, and more than 10 minutes of medical discussion. When using total time on the date of the encounter for code selection, 45 minutes must be met or exceeded.*

98011: *Synchronous audio-only visit for the evaluation and management of a new patient, which requires a medically appropriate history and/or examination, high medical decision making, and more than 10 minutes of medical discussion. When using total time on the date of the encounter for code selection, 60 minutes must be met or exceeded. (For services 75 minutes or longer, use prolonged services code 99417.)*

Audio-only visits are synchronous, interactive, verbal medical discussions. Except when communicating with digital communication technology for the deaf, audio-only does not include written messaging such as emails or online chats.

Audio-Only: Established Patient

98012: *Synchronous audio-only visit for the evaluation and management of an established patient, which requires a medically appropriate history and/or examination, straightforward medical decision making, and more than 10 minutes of medical discussion. When using total time on the date of the encounter for code selection, 10 minutes must be exceeded.*

98013: *Synchronous audio-only visit for the evaluation and management of an established patient, which requires a medically appropriate history and/or examination, low medical decision making, and more than 10 minutes of medical discussion. When using total time on the date of the encounter for code selection, 20 minutes must be met or exceeded.*

98014: *Synchronous audio-only visit for the evaluation and management of an established patient, which requires a medically appropriate history and/or examination, moderate medical decision making, and more than 10 minutes of medical discussion. When using total time on the date of the encounter for code selection, 30 minutes must be met or exceeded.*

98015: *Synchronous audio-only visit for the evaluation and management of an established patient, which requires a medically appropriate history and/or examination, high medical decision making, and more than 10 minutes of medical discussion. When using total time on the date of the encounter for code selection, 40 minutes must be met or exceeded. (For services 55 minutes or longer, use prolonged services code 99417.)*

Audio-only visits are synchronous, interactive, verbal medical discussions. Except when communicating with digital communication technology for the deaf, audio-only does not include written messaging such as emails or online chats.

Virtual Check-in

98016: *Brief communication technology-based service (eg, virtual check-in) by a physician or other qualified health care professional who can report evaluation and management services, provided to an established patient, not originating from a related evaluation and management service provided within the previous 7 days nor leading to an evaluation and management service or procedure within the next 24 hours or soonest available appointment, 5–10 minutes of medical discussion.*

The virtual check-in code 98016 replaces HCPCS code G2012 and involves 5-1- omits of medical discussion. It is anticipated that this is patient initiated (through electronic messaging or a phone call) and it does not require video technology. The virtual check-in may NOT be billed if it is related to an E/M service furnished within the previous 7 days or if it results in an E/M visit or procedure within 24 hours or the soonest available appointment. If the virtual check-in is an E/M in the next 24 hours, and if that E/M visit is reported based on time, then time from the virtual check-in may be added to the E/M visit time for the total time. The date of encounter for that situation is the date of the E/M visit.

Digital E/M Services

Asynchronous, digital online E/M codes are for established patients (99421–99423). These codes can be billed once a week and cannot be billed within a 7-day period of a separately reported E/M service, unless the patient is initiating an online inquiry for a new problem not addressed in the separately reported E/M visit. These services must be initiated by the patient (eg, patient portal, secure email) and should not include time spent by clinical staff for performing chronic (99437, 99491) or principal care management services (99424, 99425).

CHAPTER 4
Preventive Medicine and Medicare Screening Services

Preventive medicine services are reported for comprehensive E/M services provided to patients who have no current symptoms or diagnosed illness. Preventive codes are used to report annual "well-woman" examinations and include the following:

- Counseling/anticipatory guidance/risk factor reduction interventions
- Age- and gender-appropriate comprehensive history
- Age- and gender-appropriate comprehensive physical examination including in most cases but not limited to

  — gynecological (pelvic) examination
  — breast examination
  — collection of a Pap smear specimen

- Discussions about the status of previously diagnosed stable conditions
- Ordering of appropriate laboratory/diagnostic procedures and immunizations
- Discussions about issues related to the patient's age or lifestyle

Preventive medicine codes (Appendix J) differ in several ways from problem-oriented E/M services. Preventive codes:

- do not require a chief complaint, history of present illness, or medical decision making;
- cannot be reported using time; and
- may be performed in any setting.

Centers for Medicare & Medicaid Services (CMS) E/M Documentation Guidelines do not apply to preventive services codes.

Medicare and other payers have different rules for reporting and reimbursing for these services. As always, physicians should check with their specific commercial carrier about their rules.

INITIAL PREVENTIVE PHYSICAL EXAMINATION — MEDICARE

This examination (referred to as the IPPE or "Welcome to Medicare Exam") covers specific services for new Medicare beneficiaries. The examination is payable once in a lifetime, and only if provided within the first 12 months of the beneficiary's first Part B coverage period. The deductible and copay/coinsurance are waived.

The service may be provided by a physician or qualified health professional (eg, physician assistants [PAs], nurse practitioners [NPs], and clinical nurse specialists [CNSs]) and includes the following:

- **Medical and Social History:** Review of patient's history with particular attention to modifiable risk factors for disease.
- **Depression Risk Assessment:** Review of the patient's risk factors for depression, including current or past experience with depression or other mood disorders. Patients cannot have a current diagnosis of depression. The physician may use one of the standardized screening tests designed for this purpose and recognized by national medical professional organizations.
- **Functional Ability and Level of Safety:** The physician may select from screening questions or standardized questionnaires designed for the purpose of reviewing, at a minimum, hearing impairment, daily living, fall risk, and home safety. The screening tools provided for the IPPE should be recognized by national medical professional organizations.

- **Examination:** Measurements and tests including measurement of the patient's height, weight, body mass index (BMI), blood pressure, a visual acuity screen, and other factors as deemed appropriate, based on her medical and social history and current clinical standards.
- **End-of-Life Planning (Upon an Individual's Consent):** End-of-life planning is defined as verbal or written information regarding: 1) an individual's ability to prepare an advance directive (AD) in the case that an injury or illness causes the individual to be unable to make health care decisions, and 2) whether or not the physician is willing to follow the individual's wishes as expressed in the AD.
- **Education, Counseling, and Referral Based on Previous 5 Components:** Provided as appropriate, based on the results of the first 5 elements of the IPPE.
- **Education, Counseling, and Referral Based on Other Preventive Services:**
  - Brief written plan such as a checklist should be provided to the patient for obtaining appropriate screening and other preventive services that are separately covered under Medicare Part B benefits (eg, screening services described above, vaccinations, diabetes self-management, glaucoma screening, and medical nutrition therapy).
  - Optional Electrocardiogram: Performance and interpretation by physician or by referral physician. This is a once-in-a-lifetime benefit for a screening electrocardiogram (EKG/ECG), as appropriate.

  NOTE: Although the EKG is an optional service, if the physician or qualified health care professional (QHP) cannot perform the EKG in the office suite, alternative arrangements can be made with an outside entity. However, if performed, the primary care physician must incorporate the results of the EKG into the beneficiary's medical record.

For the purposes of the IPPE benefit, "medical history" is defined as:

- Past medical and surgical history, including experiences with illnesses, hospital stays, operations, allergies, injuries, and treatment
- Current medications and supplements, including calcium and vitamins
- Family history, including a review of medical events in the patient's family, including diseases that may be hereditary or place the individual at risk

For the purposes of this benefit, "social history" is defined as:

- History of alcohol, tobacco, and illicit drug use
- Diet
- Physical activities

HCPCS codes are used to report preventive care for Medicare patients and are available in Appendix K.

Other covered preventive, screening, or problem-oriented services may be performed at the same encounter as the IPPE. These are reported using the appropriate codes. If reporting an E/M service, add a modifier 25 to the problem E/M code. The documentation for the problem-oriented portion of the encounter must support the level of service reported.

ANNUAL WELLNESS VISITS — MEDICARE

In addition to the IPPE, CMS reimburses for 2 wellness services:

- The patient's first annual wellness visit (AWV), which is distinct from and must occur at least 12 months after the patient's "Welcome to Medicare" physical AND
- Subsequent annual wellness visits

Personalized Prevention Plan Services (PPPS) are an essential part of the AWV service and include the following components:

- Establish or update the individual's medical and family history
- List the individual's current medical physicians and suppliers and all prescribed medications
- Record measurements of height, weight, BMI, blood pressure, and other routine measurements
- Detect any cognitive impairment
- Establish or update a screening schedule for the next 5-10 years including screenings appropriate for the general population, and any additional screenings that may be appropriate because of the individual patient's risk factors
- Furnish personalized health advice and appropriate referrals to health education or preventive services

Appendix K includes codes for the AWV.

Per CMS, practitioners furnishing a preventive medicine E/M service that does not meet the requirements for the IPPE or the AWV should continue to report one of the preventive medicine E/M services CPT codes (99381-99397) if required and as appropriate to the patient's circumstances. These codes continue to be noncovered by Medicare.

Reporting, as always, will depend upon the services actually performed. However, it is suggested not to report these multiple services at the same visit since CMS has indicated that, typically, preventive service codes are not billed on the same date as the AWV.

MEDICARE SCREENING SERVICES AND THE ADVANCED BENEFICIARY NOTICE

Medicare screening services are limited to a specific frequency (eg, once every 2 years, once every year). A physician may not know whether a patient is eligible for a screening service in a given year. If they are not eligible, the service will be denied. Therefore, the physician should ask the patient to sign an advance beneficiary notice of noncoverage (ABN) using the form provided by Medicare. For more information on Medicare's ABN form instructions and requirements, go to https://www.cms.gov/Medicare/Medicare-General-Information/BNI/ABN.

When a Medicare beneficiary signs an ABN, claims for Medicare patients should be submitted with the appropriate modifier:

- GA modifier indicates that a required ABN form has been signed and is on file. (Waiver of liability statement issued as required by payer policy, individual case)
- GZ modifier indicates that an ABN form has not been signed. (Item or service expected to be denied as not reasonable and necessary)
- GX modifier indicates that a voluntary ABN has been signed for a noncovered service. This modifier may be reported for services formerly reported with the Notice of Exclusion from Medicare Benefits (NEMB) form. The NEMB form has been discontinued. (Notice of liability issued, voluntary under payer policy)
- GY modifier indicates that the service provided is not a covered Medicare benefit. The service is being reported to Medicare in order to receive a denial. (Item or service statutorily excluded; does not meet the definition of a Medicare benefit)

Using the appropriate modifier ensures that the patient will receive the correct information on her Explanation of Benefits (EOB). For example, when a service is reported with a GY modifier, the EOB will state that it is not covered and therefore the patient's responsibility.

Medicare Screening Service at the Time of Covered E/M Services

Medicare will reimburse separately for covered screening services (eg, G0101, Q0091) when performed at the same encounter as a covered E/M service, such as a problem-oriented visit (codes 99202-99215). The level of E/M service reported is based solely on the evaluation of the problem.

Collection of Screening Pap Smear Specimen

Medicare reimburses for collection of a screening Pap smear every 2 years (in most cases). This service is reported using HCPCS code Q0091 (Screening Papanicolaou smear; obtaining, preparing, and conveyance of cervical or vaginal smear to laboratory). Both the deductible and copay/coinsurance are waived for the laboratory's interpretation of the test.

The Pap collection is reimbursed every year if the patient meets Medicare's criteria for high risk. Following are the only criteria that are accepted by Medicare to indicate a high-risk patient:

- Woman is of childbearing age AND
  - Cervical or vaginal cancer is present (or was present) OR
  - Abnormalities were found within last 3 years OR
  - Is considered high risk (as described below) for developing cervical or vaginal cancer.
- Woman is not of childbearing age AND she has at least one of the following:
  - High-risk factors for cervical and vaginal cancer
  - Onset of sexual activity under 16 years of age
  - Five or more sexual partners in a lifetime
  - History of sexually transmitted diseases (including human papillomavirus and/or HIV infection)
  - Fewer than 3 negative or any Pap smears within previous 7 years
  - DES (diethylstilbestrol)-exposed daughters of women who took DES during pregnancy.

Screening Pelvic Examination

Medicare reimburses for a screening pelvic examination every 2 years (in most cases).

The screening pelvic exam is reported using HCPCS code G0101 (Cervical or vaginal cancer screening; pelvic and clinical breast examination). If the patient meets Medicare's criteria for high risk, the examination is reimbursed every year. These criteria are the same as the ones listed above for the collection of screening Pap smear specimen. The diagnosis codes for Pap smear collection and screening pelvic examination are listed below.

A screening pelvic examination (HCPCS code G0101) should include documentation of at least 7 of the following 11 elements:

- Inspection and palpation of breasts for masses or lumps, tenderness, symmetry, or nipple discharge
- Digital rectal examination including sphincter tone, presence of hemorrhoids, and rectal masses
- External genitalia (for example, general appearance, hair distribution, or lesions)
- Urethral meatus (for example, size, location, lesions, or prolapse)
- Urethra (for example, masses, tenderness, or scarring)
- Bladder (for example, fullness, masses, or tenderness)
- Vagina (for example, general appearance, estrogen effect, discharge, lesions, pelvic support, cystocele, or rectocele)
- Cervix (for example, general appearance, lesions, or discharge)
- Uterus (for example, size, contour, position, mobility, tenderness, consistency, descent, or support)
- Adnexa/parametria (for example, masses, tenderness, organomegaly, or nodularity)
- Anus and perineum

If an organ is documented as surgically absent, it can be counted as 1 of the 7 elements.

HCPCS code G0101 includes only the above examination elements. It does not include the many other services normally included in a comprehensive preventive visit as reported with CPT codes 99384-99397.

Information about the screening Pap smear and the screening pelvic examination is found in Appendix L.

OTHER MEDICARE PREVENTIVE SERVICES

Appendices M-Q include CPT codes, ICD-10 codes, indications, and frequency for the following Medicare Screening Services.

Mammogram (Appendix M)

Medicare covers one baseline screening mammogram for women aged 35-39 years and annual mammograms for women 40 years or older. Both the Medicare deductible and copay/coinsurance are waived for this service. A diagnostic mammogram (when the patient has an illness, disease, or symptoms that indicate the need for a mammogram) is covered whenever it is medically necessary. When it is appropriate to report a screening and a diagnostic mammogram on the same day, use modifier -GG to show that a screening mammography became a diagnostic mammography. When reporting dual diagnosis codes, report for specific quadrants instead of unspecified quadrants, if feasible.

Bone Mass (Appendix M)

Medicare covers bone mass measurements every 2 years for qualified individuals. Both the deductible and copay/coinsurance are waived.

A "qualified individual" meets at least one of these medical indications:

- Estrogen-deficient and at clinical risk for osteoporosis
- Vertebral abnormalities
- Receiving (or expecting to receive) glucocorticoid (steroid) therapy for more than 3 months
- Has a diagnosis of primary hyperparathyroidism
- Being monitored to assess the response to or efficacy of a Food and Drug Administration (FDA)-approved osteoporosis drug therapy

Medicare may pay for more frequent screenings when medically necessary. Examples include, but are not limited to, the following medical circumstances:

- Monitoring beneficiaries on long-term (more than 3 months) glucocorticoid (steroid) therapy
- Confirming baseline bone mass measurements to permit monitoring of beneficiaries in the future

Hepatitis B and C, Sexually Transmitted Disease, Human Immunodeficiency Virus, and Human Papillomavirus (Appendices N, O, and P)

Medicare will cover screening for sexually transmitted infections (STIs)—specifically chlamydia, gonorrhea, syphilis, hepatitis B and C, and screening for human immunodeficiency virus (HIV) and human papillomavirus (HPV).

The high/increased-risk individual sexual behaviors, based on the U.S. Preventive Services Task Force (USPSTF) guidelines, include any of the following:

- Multiple sex partners
- Using barrier protection inconsistently
- Having sex under the influence of alcohol or drugs

- Having sex in exchange for money or drugs
- Sexually active women aged 24 years or younger
- Having an STI within the past year
- IV drug use (hepatitis B only)

HIV screening is recommended for all adolescents and adults at risk for HIV infection, as well as all pregnant women. Typically, an annual voluntary HIV screening for beneficiaries between the ages of 15 and 65 is a covered benefit. An annual screening for Medicare beneficiaries younger than 15 years and adults older than 65 who are at increased risk for HIV infection is also covered. CMS covers both standard and FDA-approved HIV rapid screening tests for Medicare beneficiaries at increased risk for HIV infection per USPSTF guidelines.

For HIV screening in women who are pregnant, a maximum of 3 tests will be covered for each pregnancy beginning with the date of the first test. Patients with any known prior diagnosis of HIV-related illness are not eligible for this screening test.

CMS will cover screening for cervical cancer with HPV co-testing under the following conditions:

- HPV testing once every 5 years for asymptomatic beneficiaries aged 30 to 65 years;
- Use of a Pap smear test with the appropriate FDA-approved/cleared laboratory tests;
- Consistent with FDA-approved labeling; and
- Compliance with the Clinical Laboratory Improvement Act (CLIA) regulations.

Both the deductible and copay/coinsurance are waived for this type of screening if conditions of coverage are met.

Cardiovascular Screening Blood Tests (Appendix P)

This benefit provides a blood test for the early detection of cardiovascular disease or abnormalities associated with an elevated risk for this disease. Three clinical laboratory tests are covered:

- total cholesterol
- high-density lipoprotein (HDL)
- triglycerides.

These tests are covered once every 5 years and can be ordered as one of each individual test or combination as a panel. Medicare covers cardiovascular disease screening for all beneficiaries without apparent signs and symptoms of the disease. Both the deductible and copay/coinsurance are waived.

The tests must be ordered by a treating physician and used in the management of the patient. Laboratories must offer physicians the ability to order a lipid panel without the direct low-density lipoprotein (LDL) measurement. However, if the screening lipid panel results illustrate a triglycerides level that indicates the need for a direct LDL measurement, the physician may order this test.

Colorectal Cancer Screening (Appendix P)

For colorectal cancer screening using multitarget SDNA test, Medicare covers beneficiaries who meet ALL of the following 3 requirements:

- Aged 50 to 85 years
- Asymptomatic
- At average risk of developing colorectal cancer

For screening colonoscopies, fecal occult blood tests (FOBTs), flexible sigmoidoscopies, and barium enemas, Medicare covers all beneficiaries who are:

- 50 years and older and at normal risk for developing colorectal cancer, AND/OR
- At high risk for developing colorectal cancer.

There is no age limitation for coverage of screening colonoscopies.

Unless the beneficiary does not meet the criteria for high risk for developing colorectal cancer and has had a screening colonoscopy within the last 10 years, a screening flexible sigmoidoscopy may be covered only after at least 119 months have passed since the month the beneficiary received the previous screening colonoscopy.

For all surgical procedures (CPT 10000-69999) provided on the same date and during the same encounter with a screening colonoscopy initiated as flexible sigmoidoscopy or barium enema for colorectal cancer screening purposes, no deductible is paid. In this scenario, modifier -PT (Colorectal cancer screening test; converted to diagnostic test or other procedure) should be applied to the surgical procedure code in CPT range of 10000 to 69999.

To waive Medicare beneficiary copayment/coinsurance and deductible when providing a separately payable anesthesia in conjunction with a screening colonoscopy (G0105 and G0121), the anesthesia code 00812 should be used with modifier -33, Preventive services. Append modifier -PT (Colorectal cancer screening test converted to diagnostic test or other procedure) to the anesthesia code when a screening colonoscopy becomes a diagnostic colonoscopy.

Both the deductible and copay/coinsurance are waived for this service except for codes G0106 and G0120. For G0106 and G0120, only the deductible is waived, but the copayment/coinsurance still applies.

Diabetes Screening (Appendix P)

The diabetes screening tests include a fasting blood glucose test, post-glucose challenge tests, and either an oral glucose tolerance test with a glucose challenge of 75 grams of glucose for nonpregnant adults or a 2-hour post-glucose challenge test alone.

Individuals are eligible for the benefit if they have one or more of the following risk factors:

- Hypertension (high blood pressure)
- Dyslipidemia (history of abnormal cholesterol and triglyceride levels)
- Obesity (BMI of 30 kg/m^2 or more)
- Previous identification of an elevated impaired fasting glucose or glucose tolerance OR
- Have at least 2 of the following risk factors:
  - Overweight (BMI greater than 25 kg/m^2, but less than 30)
  - A family history of diabetes
  - A history of gestational diabetes mellitus or delivery of a baby weighing greater than 9 pounds
  - 65 years of age or older
  - Two screening tests per year are covered for individuals who have been diagnosed with pre-diabetes or one screening per year if previously tested but not diagnosed with pre-diabetes or if never tested. Pre-diabetes is defined as a fasting glucose level of 100-125 mg/dL, or a 2-hour post-glucose challenge of 140-199 mg/dL.

Patients previously diagnosed with diabetes are not covered for this screening service.

Modifier -TS (Follow-up service) should be appended when submitting claims for Medicare beneficiaries with pre-diabetes.

Alcohol Reduction and Misuse (Appendix P)

All Medicare beneficiaries are eligible for alcohol screening. Medicare beneficiaries who test positive (those who misuse alcohol but whose levels or patterns of alcohol consumption do not meet criteria for alcohol dependence) are eligible for counseling if:

- They are competent and alert at the time that counseling is provided; and
- Counseling is furnished by qualified primary care physicians or other primary care practitioner in a primary care setting.

Alcohol dependence is defined by at least 3 of the following:

- Tolerance
- Withdrawal symptoms
- Impaired control
- Preoccupations with acquisition and/or use
- Persistent desire or unsuccessful efforts to quit
- Sustains social, occupational, or recreational disability, OR
- Use continues despite adverse consequences AND
- Who are competent and alert at the time that counseling is provided AND
- Whose counseling is furnished by a qualified primary care physician or other primary care practitioner in a primary care setting

Tobacco Use Cessation Counseling (Appendix P)

Cessation counseling benefits are for individuals who:

- Use tobacco, regardless of whether they exhibit signs or symptoms of tobacco-related disease;
- Are competent and alert at the time of counseling; and
- Receive counseling furnished by a qualified or other Medicare-recognized practitioner.

Medicare covers counseling for tobacco cessation for outpatients and for inpatients. Inpatients are covered only if counseling for tobacco use is not the primary reason for the patient's hospital stay. The counseling during an E/M service must be either intermediate or intensive. Intermediate counseling is 2-3 sessions of 3-10 minutes each.

Intensive counseling is 4 sessions of more than 10 minutes each. Minimal counseling involving sessions lasting less than 3 minutes is considered part of an E/M service and is not reimbursed separately. Each attempt may include a maximum of 4 intermediate or intensive counseling sessions. The total annual benefit is for 8 sessions in a 12-month period. Services may be provided by a physician, physician assistant, nurse practitioner, clinical nurse specialist, qualified psychologist, or clinical social worker.

Obesity (Appendix P)

Certain screening services are considered reasonable and necessary for the prevention or early detection of an illness or disability. Obesity is directly or indirectly associated with many chronic diseases, such as cardiovascular disease, musculoskeletal conditions, and diabetes. Due to those risk factors, Medicare covers beneficiaries diagnosed with obesity, defined as a BMI of 30 kg/m^2 or higher.

Medicare beneficiaries with obesity, who are competent and alert at the time that counseling is provided and whose counseling is furnished by a qualified primary care physician or other primary care practitioner and in a primary care setting, are allowed:

- One face-to-face visit every week for the first month
- One face-to-face visit every other week for months 2-6
- One face-to-face visit every month for months 7-12, if certain requirements are met.

A reassessment of obesity and a determination of the amount of weight loss must be provided at the 6-month visit. To be eligible for additional face-to-face visits occurring once a month for an additional 6 months, beneficiaries must have lost at least 3 kg. For beneficiaries who do not achieve a weight loss of at least 3 kg during the first 6 months, a reassessment of their readiness to change and BMI is appropriate after an additional 6-month period.

Depression (Appendix P)

The USPSTF and CMS have determined that, for the prevention and early detection of depression, Medicare beneficiaries should be screened annually in primary care settings that have staff-assisted depression care supports in place to ensure accurate diagnosis, effective treatment, and follow-up.

In the *Diagnostic and Statistical Manual of Mental Disorders*, Fifth Edition, Text Revision (DSM-5-TR), the criteria for a major depressive episode include 5 or more of the following symptoms in the same 2-week period:

- Depressed mood most of the day, nearly every day, as indicated either by subjective report (eg, feels sad or empty) or observation made by others (eg, appears tearful);
- Markedly diminished interest or pleasure in all, or almost all, activities most of the day, nearly every day (as indicated either by subjective account or observation made by others);
- Significant weight loss when not dieting or weight gain (eg, a change of more than 5% of body weight in a month), or decrease or increase in appetite nearly every day;
- Insomnia or hypersomnia nearly every day;
- Psychomotor agitation or retardation nearly every day (observable by others, not merely subjective feelings of restlessness or being slowed down);
- Fatigue or loss of energy nearly every day;
- Feelings of worthlessness or excessive or inappropriate guilt (which may be delusional) nearly every day (not merely self-reproach or guilt about being sick);
- Diminished ability to think or concentrate, or indecisiveness, nearly every day (either by subjective account or as observed by others);
- Recurrent thoughts of death (not just fear of dying), recurrent suicidal ideation without a specific plan, or a suicide attempt or specific plan for committing suicide.

Modifier 33

Modifier 33 was created to allow physicians to identify preventive services that are not subject to cost sharing. Only specific screening services require modifier 33, and those services require the modifier only when they are provided during a visit whose primary purpose is not preventive. If the primary purpose of the visit is preventive and screening services are provided, no cost sharing is required for the services provided during the visit. In this case, the modifier is not required.

For separately reported services specifically identified as preventive, the modifier should not be used.

CHAPTER 5
Global Surgical Package

Medicare and CPT have differing definitions concerning which services are included in a global surgical package. In addition, some commercial payers create their own definitions, sometimes encompassing elements of CPT's and/or Medicare's surgical package rules. One of the more significant variances is that the CPT and Medicare global packages have different rules for reporting the treatment of intraoperative complications:

- Under Medicare rules, intraoperative treatment of complications performed by the primary surgeon is not reported separately; however, treatment performed by another physician of a different specialty can be reported and reimbursed.
- Under CPT rules, intraoperative treatment of complications can be reported and reimbursed separately whether performed by the primary surgeon or another physician. It is not required that the other physician be from a different specialty. Whether a practice chooses to bill payers and patients for intraoperative complications is a practice management and, possibly, a public relations decision. However, it is not a billing/coding decision.

On the other hand, CPT and Medicare global package rules are the same when reporting the treatment of postoperative complications requiring a return to the operating room. Under both CPT and Medicare rules, these services will be separately reimbursed, with an appropriate modifier attached.

In order to be effective in reporting surgical services and obtaining appropriate payment, physicians and their staff should endeavor to clearly understand which definition is used by their respective payers.

MEDICARE GLOBAL SURGICAL PACKAGES

Medicare defines 2 distinct surgical packages: one for major procedures and another for minor procedures.

	MINOR PROCEDURES	MAJOR PROCEDURES
Global (Postoperative) Period	0 or 10 days	90 days
Included Preoperative Services	Same-day visits (unless a separately identifiable E/M service is furnished)	All preoperative E/M services beginning 1 day before the procedure (unless the decision for surgery was made at that visit)
Intraoperative Services	The procedure and all integral procedures (including anesthesia provided by the surgery) and supplies usually included in the procedure	Services that are usual and necessary parts of the surgical procedure, as well as anesthesia administered by the surgeon
Included Postoperative Services	0 days—related visits on the date of service 10 days—follow-up visits for 10 days following the service that are related to recovery from the surgery	Medical or surgical services, performed by the surgeon for complications which do not require a return trip to the OR or procedure room Follow-up visits during the 90-day period following the procedure that are related to recover from the surgery

The global periods for codes that are commonly reported by obstetricians and gynecologists are included for each code in Part II.

Postoperative services are typically the same for every surgical procedure, are valued into the surgical procedure, and include the following:

- In the operating room:
    - Application of dressings and packings
    - Removal of manipulators, probes, and packs
    - Securing, removal, or replacement of catheters and drains
    - Completion of operating room record
- In the recovery room:
    - Patient evaluation and stabilization
    - Postoperative orders
    - Dictation of operative report
    - Consultation with family
- Included postoperative services before discharge:
    - Hospital visit(s) to assess patient status
    - Removal of packs, drains, catheters, sutures, staples
    - Discharge care
        - Review of pathology and laboratory reports
        - Patient instructions
        - Complete discharge summary/medical record
- In the office:
    - Follow-up visit(s) as clinically indicated during the global period
    - Review of pathology and laboratory reports
    - Removal of drains, catheters, sutures, staples
    - Continue postoperative assessment and care during the expected recovery period
    - Wound care/pain management (if applicable)

PHYSICIANS PERFORMING ONLY PART OF THE SURGICAL PACKAGE

In some instances, one physician may perform a portion of the services included in the global surgical package (pre-, intra-, or postoperative services only) while another physician performs the remaining portion(s).

Include one of the following modifiers:

- 54 (surgical care only)
- 55 (postoperative management only)
- 56 (preoperative management only). Modifier 56 is rarely reported by ob-gyns.

Most commercial insurance companies do not recognize CPT modifiers 54, 55, and 56. Some payers may follow the Medicare rules. In Medicare, payment depends on whether the first physician has formally transferred care of the patient to the second physician.

Formal transfer of care requires that the first physician document that the patient's care was transferred to a second physician. Each physician is then paid a percentage of the total RVUs designated for the code according to the assigned percentage of the total RVUs for the preoperative, intraoperative, or postoperative portions. For example, suppose code 58925 (ovarian cystectomy) is valued at 22.95 RVUs. The RVUs are divided as follows: 12% (about 2.75 RVUs) for preoperative services; 74% (about 16.98 RVUs) for intraoperative services; and 14% (about 3.21 RVUs) for postoperative services. When each physician reports the same surgical code with a modifier (54 or 55), each receives the assigned percentage. The payment to each physician providing a portion of the global package may not exceed the total amount Medicare would have paid if a single physician had provided the global services.

If no formal transfer of care was documented, payment depends on 2 factors: whether the physicians belong to the same physician group and same specialty, and whether they have a reciprocal billing (covering) arrangement.

- Physicians within the same group practice:
  - Physicians of the same specialty. The group practice bills for the entire global package. No modifiers are used.
  - Physicians of different specialties. Each physician reports the same surgical code with a modifier (54 or 55) indicating the services he or she provided and receives a percentage of the total RVUs.
- Physicians in different, unaffiliated practices:
  - Reciprocal billing (covering) arrangement. The primary physician bills for the entire global package.
    - No modifiers are used.
  - No reciprocal billing arrangement. Each physician reports the same surgical code with a modifier (54 or 55) indicating the services he or she provided and receives a percentage of the total RVUs.

SERVICES OUTSIDE THE GLOBAL SURGICAL PACKAGE

The above rules apply only to the routine preoperative, intraoperative, or postoperative services included in the global package. If one of the physicians provided services that are not routine, they may report them separately. This premise applies under both CPT and Medicare rules.

As an example, suppose a surgeon provides all the services included in a global surgical package. Subsequently, another physician of a different specialty treats a problem or complication related to the surgery either during the intraoperative or postoperative period. In this case:

- The primary surgeon reports the appropriate surgical procedure code(s). They will be reimbursed for the full global package.
- The other physician reports an appropriate E/M service code and/or procedure code(s) for treatment of the problem or complication. They will be reimbursed separately for these services. No modifier is necessary.

Medicare and CPT rules are relatively clear concerning which preoperative and postoperative services are included in Medicare's and CPT's global surgical packages; however, the rules for intraoperative services are not as clear. As discussed in Chapter 1, Medicare's Correct Coding Initiative (CCI) edits affect how multiple surgical services are billed on the same date of service. The code edits are listed for each procedure code in the manual and should be referenced before submitting a claim. It is important to note that private payers may or may not adhere to CCI edits.

As a reminder, a service is considered bundled into another procedure when the service:

- Represents the standard of care in accomplishing the overall procedure;

- Is necessary to successfully accomplish the comprehensive procedure (that is, failure to perform the service may compromise the success of the procedure); and
- Is not separate and unrelated to the comprehensive procedure.

Of course, there may be an exception. Consider the following examples:

- A colposcopy with biopsy and endocervical curettage (code 57454) following an abnormal Pap smear result is performed. While performing the colposcopy, a vaginal polyp is noted and removed (57100, separate procedure code). Under CPT rules, these procedures can be reported together since they are independent and unrelated, even though code 57100 is a separate procedure code. However, under the CCI edit rules, code 57100 is listed as bundled into 57454, but may be reported under special circumstances. A different ICD-10-CM code is linked to each code and a modifier 59 is added to code 57100 to make it a separately payable service.
- A biopsy on the right ovary (code 58900, separate procedure) and removal of the left ovary (code 58940) are performed. Under CPT rules, these procedures can be reported together since they involved different ovaries, even though code 58900 is a separate procedure code. Under the CCI edit rules, these procedures are listed as bundled and never paid. No modifier is allowed to override the bundling edit. These services will not typically be reimbursed. Since the services were performed on different ovaries, however, modifiers LT and RT could be added (if your payer recognizes these modifiers) to indicate that different ovaries were involved. If both procedures had been performed on the same ovary, only code 58940 (the most extensive procedure) would be reported under either CPT or CCI rules.
- A paravaginal defect repair (57284) and enterocele repair (57268, separate procedure) are performed. Under CPT rules, these procedures may be reported together even though code 57268 is a separate procedure code. A different ICD-10-CM code is linked to each code and a modifier 59 (to indicate that the procedures are distinct) is added to code 57268. If the procedure is performed to prevent formation of an enterocele, then code 57268 is not reported. Under the CCI edit rules, these procedures are bundled and will never be reimbursed when performed at the same session, even with distinct diagnoses and a modifier 59.

Surgical Services Modifiers (Appendices S and T)

Modifiers used with surgical services may indicate circumstances that occurred during the procedure. Other modifiers indicate circumstances occurring before or after the surgery itself and relate to the global surgical package. These modifiers are summarized in Appendices S and T.

CHAPTER 6
Global Obstetric Package

The global obstetric codes include antepartum services, delivery, and postpartum care. Global services can be billed when one provider or practice supplies all of the patient's routine (scheduled) obstetric services. When global services cannot be billed (for a variety of reasons), there are codes found in the global obstetric section that allow for separate billing of the component parts of the global package (see Appendix U).

Antepartum care includes the services normally provided in uncomplicated pregnancies. Routine obstetric care typically includes approximately 13 antepartum visits, which include the following:

- Initial and subsequent history
- Physical examinations
- Recording of weight, blood pressures, fetal heart tones
- Routine dipstick analysis
- Monthly visits up to 28 weeks (5-6 visits)
- Biweekly visits up to 36 weeks (4 visits)
- Weekly visits from 36 weeks until delivery (3-4 visits)

The global obstetric code includes payment to the physician or other qualified health care professional for the delivery of services, including:

- Admission to the hospital (including the admitting history and physical examination)
- Management of uncomplicated labor
- Vaginal or cesarean delivery (with or without episiotomy, forceps, or vacuum extraction)
- Delivery of the placenta
- Routine inpatient care immediately after the delivery
- Induction of labor (unless the obstetrician personally starts the IV and sits with the patient during the infusion)
- Insertion of cervical dilator on day of delivery (CPT code 59200)
- Simple removal of cerclage (not under anesthesia)

Finally, postpartum services are included in the comprehensive code. CPT codes do not explicitly define the postpartum period. It is commonly accepted to be the first 6 weeks following delivery, although ACOG indicates that routine postpartum can be provided for up to 12 weeks post-delivery. Postpartum services include the following:

- Recovery room visit
- Uncomplicated inpatient hospital visits
- Uncomplicated outpatient visits
- Discussion of contraception
- Removal of sutures (if appropriate)

Providers will not be able to report the full obstetric package in these instances:

- More than 1 physician or qualified obstetric health professional (QOHP) (practice) provides routine obstetric care for a patient;
- Only 1 physician (practice) provides care for the patient, but the services provided are significantly less than the usual obstetric package; or,
- The patient changes insurers during her pregnancy
- The patient transfers out of or into the practice during the pregnancy
- The patient miscarries or terminates the pregnancy.

Services Outside the Global Obstetric Package

Certain services can be reported separately at the time of service during the pregnancy, including medically necessary diagnostic tests and procedures, facility-based E/M services, and services unrelated to the pregnancy, such as an upper respiratory infection or urinary tract infection.

If complications of pregnancy lead to additional antepartum visits in the office (ie, more than 13), they can be reported as E/M visits at the time of delivery. The additional visits for the complications must be linked to the appropriate diagnosis code(s), such as gestational diabetes or placenta previa. Any facility-based E/M service that occurs on the calendar date of delivery or the calendar date before delivery is included in the delivery and cannot be billed separately.

If a patient is seen more than 13 times because of their at-risk status, the additional visit(s) should be reported only if the complication occurs in the current pregnancy. For example, if the patient is being monitored closely because of a complication in a previous pregnancy, but no complications develop in this pregnancy, the additional visits are not reported separately and only a global obstetric package code is reported.

There are additional codes to bill along with the global obstetric code not included in the delivery. These codes are provided in this manual and include the following:

- External cephalic version
- Postpartum dilation and curettage
- Subtotal or total hysterectomy
- Insertion of cervical dilator by physician before day of delivery
- E/M services (eg, observation, inpatient services, critical care) if provided more than 1 calendar day before the delivery

These services must be linked to an appropriate diagnosis code and are reported at the same time as the global package code.

If additional services are required in the postpartum period, they are excluded from the global obstetric code if they are related to complications or are otherwise independent of the postpartum care. Services must be linked to an appropriate diagnosis code, and a 24 modifier is typically required for an E/M service and a 79 modifier is required for a procedural service. However, if the treatment is for a related condition and requires an unplanned return to the operating room, modifier 78 is added to the procedure code.

Multiple-Gestation Delivery Reporting

Multiple gestation creates potential complications for pregnancies, may involve more work, and often complicates the coding of some services.

Coding for twin or other multiple-gestation deliveries is relatively straightforward per CPT guidelines. Multiple-gestation deliveries should be reported as illustrated in the following chart:

Vaginal Delivery	Baby A	59400	Global service—vaginal
	Baby B	59409-59	Delivery only—vaginal
VBAC	Baby A	59610	Global service—VBAC
	Baby B	59612-59	Delivery only—VBAC
Cesarean Delivery	Baby A & Baby B	59510-22	Global service—cesarean
Failed TOLAC	Baby A & Baby B	59618-22	Global service—cesarean following attempted vaginal delivery after previous cesarean delivery
Vaginal Delivery + Cesarean Delivery	Baby B	59510	Global service—cesarean
	Baby A	59409-51	Delivery only—vaginal
Successful VBAC for Fetus 1 & Failed TOLAC for Additional Fetus	Baby B	59618	Global service—repeat cesarean
	Baby A	59612-51	Delivery only—VBAC

When both twins are delivered vaginally (global codes 59400 and 59610), a 59 modifier is required for the second fetus to "unbundle" the second "delivery only" service from the global package for the first fetus.

When one twin is delivered vaginally and the other is delivered by cesarean, the global charge should be associated with the cesarean delivery. A "delivery only" vaginal service is reported for the delivery of twin A. A 51 modifier is necessary because it is a secondary procedure that is not bundled into the primary procedure.

There is no protocol by which twins delivered by cesarean can be reported independently. If the twin delivery has complications, a 22 modifier can be added to the cesarean delivery code. It is typically not appropriate to add a modifier to an "uncomplicated" cesarean twin delivery.

There are no universal rules for billing procedures for multiple fetuses—especially when distinct work must be provided for each fetus, such as nonstress tests and amniocentesis. Most commonly, the procedure is billed with a unit quantity of "2." Some payers may require a 22 modifier on a single line item, while others may require the service for each fetus to be reported on a separate line.

Interruption of Pregnancy and Stillbirth

A spontaneous abortion after 20 weeks 0 days is reported using a delivery code. However, some state legislatures have legally defined the difference between a miscarriage and a stillbirth by the number of gestational weeks or by gram weight of the fetus. This legal definition may determine which CPT code is selected. In this case, it is important to know your payer policies and your state laws and regulations. Appendices V and W summarize coding for terminations of pregnancy.

CHAPTER 7
Ultrasound Coding

All ultrasound services, regardless of type, must include the elements listed in the table below:

ACTION	PERSON(S) INVOLVED	FOCUS
Testing	Sonographer/Physician	Performance of ultrasound exam
Results	Sonographer/Physician	Compiling of findings from ultrasound exam
Interpretation	Physician	Determination of the meaning of the findings with consideration of clinical circumstances
Report	Physician	Work product of the interpretation of test results. Permanent report (written or digital) of results and interpretation required.

GYNECOLOGIC ULTRASOUND EXAMINATIONS

The elements included in obstetric ultrasounds are specifically defined in the CPT code book; however, the required elements for gynecological ultrasounds are not detailed in the same fashion for all gynecologic codes. The codes selected depend on the approach used, extent of service, and documentation (eg, image documentation and written report).

CPT provides the following guidelines for reporting nonobstetrical ultrasounds:

> "Use of ultrasound, without thorough evaluation of organ(s) or anatomic region, image documentation, and final, written report, is not separately reportable."

This statement means that nonobstetrical ultrasound codes are not reported when:

- An ultrasound is used as a means to perform a component of a physical examination
- The ultrasound equipment does not produce a hard copy or permanent digital image
- There is only a brief summary of the ultrasound noted in the E/M service
- There is no formal ultrasound report, with physician interpretation

Further details about ACOG's recommendations concerning nonobstetric ultrasound examination codes are found in Appendix X.

OBSTETRIC ULTRASOUND EXAMINATIONS

Obstetric ultrasound codes are very specific about the services included. These services may be abdominal ultrasound, vaginal ultrasound, or biophysical profiles. Appendix Y includes the codes and classifies them by extent of evaluation, trimester, gestation, and approach (ie, transabdominal, transvaginal, or either).

All of the ultrasound codes include the supervision of the sonographer performing the examination and the preparation of the report for the medical record. In order to report an ultrasound code, there must be a separate, final written report with interpretation of the findings of the radiological procedure. A summary with an E/M service is insufficient as an ultrasound report. All diagnostic ultrasound examinations require permanently recorded images with measurements when such measurements are clinically indicated. The report and interpretations should be stored in the medical record.

ULTRASOUND GUIDANCE PROCEDURES

In certain circumstances, the physician may report both an ultrasound guidance code and a procedural service if they performed both and there is documentation of both services. A separate ultrasound report is not necessary for the guidance codes, but the use of the ultrasound must be documented in the procedure report and appropriate image documentation must be present in the record. The obstetrician can also report both services if the sonographer performed the ultrasound guidance while the obstetrician performed the ultrasound.

DESCRIPTION	PROCEDURE CODE	RADIOLOGICAL COMPONENT
Intrauterine fetal transfusion	36460	76941
Intrauterine cordocentesis	59012	76941
Chorionic villus sampling	59015	76945
Amniocentesis	59000	76946
Aspiration of ova	58970	76948
Sonohysterography	58340	76831
Hysterosalpingography	58340	74740
Transcervical catheterization of fallopian tube	58345	74742

If guidance is used but there is no specific ultrasound guidance code for the associated procedure, report 76998 (ultrasonic guidance, intraoperative) or 76999 (unlisted ultrasound procedure [eg, diagnostic, interventional]). For other procedures, the guidance is included in the ultrasound code and not reported separately. For example, all fetal surgery codes include ultrasound guidance.

MODIFIERS AND ULTRASOUND PROCEDURES

If an ultrasound procedure is performed in the physician's office, either by the physician or an employee, and the physician owns the equipment, the appropriate code is reported without a modifier.

If an ultrasound procedure is performed in a hospital or other facility setting, it may be appropriate to use a modifier. The modifiers are included in Appendix Y.

CHAPTER 8
Coding for COVID-19–Related Services

The COVID-19 public health emergency (PHE) has challenged the normal coding processes. In response to the PHE, the American Medical Association (AMA) CPT Editorial Panel, the AMA Relative Value Update Committee (RUC), and the Centers for Disease Control and Prevention (CDC) National Center for Health Statistics (NCHS) expedited codes for tracking the disease and the vaccinations. What would normally have taken multiple years was completed in a couple of months, thanks to the physician volunteers from ACOG and other physician societies that developed the codes.

DIAGNOSIS CODING

A new ICD-10-CM diagnosis code chapter, Chapter 22, Codes for Special Purposes (U00-U85), was created during the COVID-19 pandemic, and several new diagnosis codes were made available for reporting the coronavirus diagnosis.

COVID-19-Related Diagnosis Codes

U07.1: COVID-19

- U07.1 should be used only for confirmed cases of COVID-19 with positive or presumptive-positive test results
- U07.1 should be sequenced first, followed by the appropriate codes for associated manifestations, except in the case of obstetric patients
- For obstetric patients with confirmed COVID-19 during pregnancy, childbirth, or the puerperium, code O98.5, other viral diseases, should be reported as the primary diagnosis, followed by code U07.1 and any codes for associated manifestation(s).

U09.9: Post-COVID-19 condition, unspecified

- U09.9 should only be reported as a secondary diagnosis. The primary diagnosis(es) should be the condition(s) related to COVID-19, if known.

Z86.16: Personal history of COVID-19

- Z86.16 should only be reported when a patient has a history of COVID-19. Patients should not be receiving any active or have any manifestations documented as due to COVID-19.

If COVID-19 is not confirmed or if testing is negative, the following diagnosis encounter codes should be used:

- Z11.52: Encounter for screening for COVID-19
  - Asymptomatic, no known exposure, results unknown or negative
- Z20. 822: Contact with and (suspected) exposure to COVID-19
  - Possible exposure to COVID-19, infection ruled out or results unknown

For immunization status related to COVID-19, the following code has been created to report this status:

- Z28.31: Underimmunization for COVID-19 status

The following codes should not be used for individuals who are not eligible for the COVID-19 vaccines.

- Z28.310: Unvaccinated for COVID-19
- Z28.311: Partially vaccinated for COVID-19
- Z28.39: Other underimmunization status

According to the ICD-10 CM guidelines, the description of the new codes is:

- Unvaccinated is assigned when the patient has not received at least one dose of any COVID-19 vaccine.
- Partially vaccinated may be assigned when the patient has received at least one dose of a multidose COVID-19 vaccine series but has not received the full set of doses necessary to be considered "fully vaccinated "as defined by the Centers for Disease Control and Prevention (CDC).

For (extended) counseling related to COVID-19 and other vaccines, the following code has been created:

- Z71.85: Encounter for immunization safety counseling
  - Code also, if applicable, encounter for immunization (Z23)
  - Code also, if applicable, immunization not carried out (Z28.-)

SWAB COLLECTION

There is no specific procedure code for swabbing/sample collection for COVID-19. If a staff member performs the swab without the physician seeing the patient, 99211 can be billed for the collection. Swab collection is included in the E/M service billed by a physician or qualified health care professional (QHP). However, if the sample is collected in the office and transported to the laboratory, CPT code 99000 can be reported:

99000 Handling and/or conveyance of specimens for transfer from office to a laboratory

LABORATORY CODING

There are a variety of laboratory codes for COVID-19 testing. These codes are found in Appendix AA.

COVID-19 VACCINE ADMINISTRATION CODES

While there are CPT codes assigned for the various COVID-19 vaccines, they will not be reported to payers because there is no cost to the practice associated with obtaining these vaccines. During the COVID-19 public health emergency, the AMA has created a new code set for the administration of the COVID-19 vaccines. The codes are found in Appendix BB.

CHAPTER 9
Coding Basics for Reporting Diagnoses of Obstetric–Gynecologic Conditions

The International Classification of Diseases, 10th Revision, Clinical Modification (ICD-10-CM) implemented on October 1, 2015, is the national standard for reporting diagnosis codes in the United States. ICD-10-CM diagnosis codes identify diseases, related health problems, and other reasons for health care encounters. ICD-10-CM codes and their descriptive terminology are developed and maintained by the ICD-10-CM Coordination and Maintenance Committee, managed by the Centers for Disease Control and Prevention (CDC) National Center for Health Statistics (NCHS).

The origins of ICD-10-CM is the International Statistical Classification of Diseases and Related Health Problems (ICD) published by the World Health Organization (WHO). Although the use of ICD internationally is largely for the collection of statistical data and disease classification, it used in the United States for billing and reimbursement for health services. In 2000, the ICD Code Set was mandated by the Department of Health and Human Services as the national coding standard for diagnostic codes. All financial and administrative health care transactions sent electronically must use the ICD code set.

ICD-10-CM is not a static code set. Revisions, often significant ones, are made annually to keep pace with clinical changes in medicine and current medical practice. New code sets are published every year on October 1. Modifications to ICD-10-CM must be consistent with WHO conventions.

The CDC NCHS has an ICD-10-CM Browser Tool that is updated annually and includes the most current guidelines for using ICD-10-CM for billing and reimbursement. This chapter of the coding manual will provide highlights and general diagnostic coding conventions; for specific issues, please refer to the CDC NCHS tool.

ICD-10-CM CONTENTS

The ICD-10-CM diagnostic codes are organized by system and include 3-7 alphanumeric codes. The more digits used, the greater the specificity of the code. In general, it is best to select the most specific ICD-10-CM code possible.

The chapters in ICD-10-CM are typically consistent year to year and include the following:

CHAPTER	CODE RANGE	CHAPTER TITLE
1	A00-B99	Certain Infectious and Parasitic Diseases
2	C00-D49	Neoplasms
3	D50-D89	Diseases of the Blood and Blood-Forming Organs and Certain Disorders Involving the Immune Mechanism
4	E00-E89	Endocrine, Nutritional, and Metabolic Diseases
5	F01-F99	Mental and Behavioral Disorders
6	G00-G99	Diseases of the Nervous System
7	H00-H59	Diseases of the Eye and Adnexa
8	H60-H95	Diseases of the Ear and Mastoid Process
9	I00-I99	Diseases of the Circulatory System
10	J00-J99	Diseases of the Respiratory System
11	K00-K99	Diseases of the Digestive System
12	L00-L99	Diseases of the Skin and Subcutaneous Tissue
13	M00-M99	Diseases of the Musculoskeletal System and Connective Tissue

(continued)

ICD-10-CM Contents *(cont.)*

CHAPTER	CODE RANGE	CHAPTER TITLE
14	N00-N99	Diseases of the Genitourinary System
15	O00-O9A	Pregnancy, Childbirth, and the Puerperium
16	P00-P96	Certain Conditions Originating in the Perinatal Period
17	Q00-Q99	Congenital Malformations, Deformations, and Chromosomal Abnormalities
18	R00-R99	Symptoms, Signs, and Abnormal Clinical and Laboratory Findings, Not Elsewhere Classified
19	S00-T88	Injury, Poisoning, and Certain Other Consequences of External Causes
20	V00-Y99	External Causes of Morbidity
21	Z00-Z99	Factors Influencing Health Status and Contact with Health Services
22	U00-U85	Codes for Special Purposes

GENERAL CODING GUIDELINES

Diagnosis codes submitted to payers should reflect the most accurate and specific code for the service (medical necessity) and follow ICD-10 coding guidelines. This includes:

- Coding to the highest degree of specificity.
- Coding to the highest degree of certainty.
- Connecting the diagnosis code to the procedure code (CPT) on the claim.
- Sequencing the diagnoses, reporting the primary diagnosis first, followed by the secondary, etc.
- Coding only diagnoses relevant to the current encounter.

Codes titled "unspecified" are used when the information in the medical record is insufficient to assign a more specific code and should be avoided when possible. NOS stands for "Not otherwise specified" and is the equivalent of unspecified. A dash (-) following a code indicates that additional characters are required for an accurate and complete code.

It may be necessary to report an unspecified diagnosis until clinical information is available to support a more specific code. Unspecified codes should be reported when they most accurately reflect what is known about the patient's condition at the time of the encounter. For example, an ultrasound may indicate an ovarian cyst, but the specific nature of the cyst may not be readily apparent. ICD-10-CM offers specific codes for follicular cysts (N83.0-) and corpus luteum cysts (N83.1-). If the clinical information is not available to accurately select a code from one of these code sections, then the code for an unspecified ovarian cyst (N83.20-) could be selected. Note that the codes from section N83.29- (other ovarian cyst) are not reported since this code means that a specific condition is known but there is not an ICD-10-CM code for the condition.

Up to 12 diagnoses can be submitted on an electronic claim. Some practice management programs may limit the number of diagnoses that can be reported on each claim. Each diagnosis must be linked to the appropriate procedure to establish medical necessity for each service. Some payer software reads only the first diagnosis linked to an individual CPT code when processing the claim. It is therefore important to prioritize and link diagnosis codes accurately.

Do not code conditions that were either previously treated or no longer exist. Additionally, do not report codes for risk factors (eg, family history of a disease), if the patient has not been diagnosed with the condition. Instead, report codes for personal or family history as a secondary diagnosis only if the history has an impact on the current care or influences treatment. Personal and family history codes in ICD-10 are found in Chapter 21 (Factors Influencing Health Status and Contact With Health Services).

It is always inappropriate to select a code that is not supported by the medical record. The documentation in the medical record should support the ICD code reported to the payer. Under ICD guidelines, the entire record may be used to determine the appropriate ICD code.

INCLUSION AND EXCLUSION NOTES

ICD-10-CM includes notes to further define or give examples of the content of the category. Inclusion notes are a list of synonyms or various conditions covered by that code; however, the list should not be considered an exhaustive list. Additional terms may also be found in the Alphabetic Index.

Similarly, exclusion notes define conditions that should not be coded using the listed code (NOT INCLUDED HERE) or codes that should not be coded simultaneously (NOT CODED HERE). There are some exceptions that may be further defined by payers.

MULTIPLE CODES FOR A SINGLE CONDITION

Some conditions have both an underlying etiology (cause) and multiple body system manifestations (signs/symptoms) due to the underlying condition. For these conditions, the ICD-10-CM convention requires that the underlying condition be reported first followed by the manifestations. In these instances, there is a "use additional code" note at the etiology code and a "code first" at the manifestation code. Generally, the manifestation code will have "in diseases classified elsewhere" in the code title.

Example:

N72 Inflammatory disease of the cervix uteri

Use additional code (B95-B97) to identify the infectious agent

There are instances other than the etiology/manifestation convention that require more than one code to describe a single condition. ICD-10-CM uses the same "code first" and "use additional code" instructions for these conditions as for etiology/manifestation codes. Multiple codes may be needed for sequela, complication codes, and obstetric codes to more fully describe a condition.

Example:

O22.3 Deep phlebothrombosis in pregnancy
Deep vein thrombosis, antepartum

Use additional code to identify the deep vein thrombosis (I82.4-, I82.5-, I82.62-, I82.72-)

Use additional code, if applicable, for associated long-term use of anticoagulants (Z79.01)

ACUTE AND CHRONIC CONDITIONS

If the same condition is described as both acute (subacute) and chronic, separate ICD-10-CM codes should be reported when available. The acute condition is always reported first.

For example, a patient may have chronic pelvic peritonitis but is treated for an acute exacerbation. This should be coded as follows:

N73.3 Female acute pelvic peritonitis

N73.4 Female chronic pelvic peritonitis

LATERALITY

Some ICD-10-CM codes specify whether the condition occurs on the right, on the left, or bilaterally. If no bilateral code exists and the condition is bilateral, then both the code for the right and left side must be reported. If the side is not identified in the medical record, then the code for unspecified site should be reported.

Conditions that may be classified to a particular code are listed beneath the code description. Note also that in ICD-10, the word "and" should be interpreted to mean either "and" or "or" when it appears in a title. The word "with" should be interpreted to mean "associated with" or "due to" when it appears in a title, the Alphabetic Index, or an instructional note.

DIFFERENCES FOR INPATIENT AND OUTPATIENT SERVICES

ICD-10-CM conventions and general guidelines apply to all settings. However, there are differences between inpatient and outpatient ICD-10-CM coding in 2 main areas:

- The Uniform Hospital Discharge Data Set (UHDDS) definition of principle diagnosis applies only to inpatients in acute, short-term, and long-term care, and psychiatric hospitals.
- Coding guidelines for inconclusive diagnoses are for inpatient reporting and do not apply to outpatients.

The UHDDS definitions are used by hospitals to report inpatient data elements in a standardized manner. The Guidelines for Outpatient Services apply to hospitals and providers when coding and reporting hospital-based outpatient services and provider-based office visits.

The selection of the first-listed diagnosis (principal diagnosis in the inpatient setting) is based primarily on the general and disease-specific guidelines. Since diagnoses may not always be established at the time of the initial encounter, it may take 2 or more visits before a diagnosis can be confirmed.

UNCERTAIN DIAGNOSIS

The guideline for reporting to the highest degree of certainty applies when an uncertain diagnosis is documented. When a diagnosis is documented as probable, suspected, rule out, working diagnosis, or other similar term, it is inappropriate to code for that condition. In these instances, the code for the sign, symptom, or abnormal test results is reported.

If the diagnostic service is for routine laboratory or radiology testing and there are no signs, symptoms, or associated diagnosis, code Z01.89 (Encounter for other specified special examinations) should be reported.

SIGNS OR SYMPTOMS

Signs or symptoms that are associated routinely with a disease process should not be reported as additional codes unless instructed to do so by the specific code classification. For example, you would not report the code for dysuria (R30.0) if a urinary tract infection (N39.0) has been diagnosed since this commonly occurs with a urinary tract infection. However, you can report signs or symptoms in addition to a definitive diagnosis when the sign/symptom is not routinely associated with that diagnosis. This may often occur with complex syndromes. In this situation, the diagnosis code should be reported before the symptom code. For example, some patients with polycystic ovarian syndrome (E28.2) may have thickened or darkened areas on the skin. Since this is not routinely associated with the condition, code R23.4 (changes in skin texture) may be reported as a secondary diagnosis.

POSTOPERATIVE COMPLICATIONS

ICD-10 contains codes for postoperative complications in the specific body system chapters. For example, Chapter 14, category N99 (Intraoperative and postprocedural complications and disorders of genitourinary system, not elsewhere classified) has several subcategories for complications. Two subcategories distinguish between intraoperative (N99.6) and postprocedural (N99.8-) hemorrhage and hematoma of a genitourinary system organ. Subcategory N99.8 further divides the categories into specific subsections for postprocedural hemorrhage, hematoma, and seroma. The codes in these subcategories, along with subcategory N99.7 (Accidental puncture and laceration of a genitourinary system organ or structure during a procedure) differentiate between complications that occur during a genitourinary procedure and during "other" procedures.

REASON FOR ENCOUNTER CODES

Encounters for reasons other than a disease, injury, sign, or symptom are found in ICD-10-CM, Chapter 21, Factors Influencing Health Status and Contact with Health Services (Z00-Z99). The Reason for Encounter codes should be used when:

- there is not a clinical diagnosis when there are no signs or symptoms of a disease;
- for preventive services, counseling services, or routine visits;
- to document personal or family history; or
- for continued surveillance or observation of a resolved condition.

Chapter 21 also contains categories of codes for obstetrical and reproductive services (Z30- Z39). The Z codes for pregnancy are used when there are no complications or problems included in the codes from the Obstetrical Chapter. Routine prenatal and postpartum codes are included in Chapter 21. Routine prenatal codes for high-risk pregnancies are coded from the Obstetrical Chapter.

PREGNANCY AND OBSTETRICS

Codes for pregnancy and obstetric care have their own unique rules. It is important to note that the codes in Chapter 15 (Pregnancy, Childbirth, and the Puerperium) are assigned in the maternal condition, not the newborn record. Additionally, the Chapter 15 codes are always first in the order of diagnosis, the exception being if there are no complications and the encounter codes are used instead of Chapter 15 codes. A code from Chapter 15 should never be reported in conjunction with routine prenatal care. Codes from other chapters can be reported as appropriate, as additional diagnoses.

A code from category 009 (Supervision of high-risk pregnancy) should be listed first for routine prenatal visits for a patient with an at-risk pregnancy who has developed complications.

When a patient is seen for a complication of pregnancy, the complication chiefly responsible for the encounter should be listed first on the claim. If there are multiple complications, all that are treated or monitored should be reported.

Many codes in Chapter 15 have a final character indicating the trimester of pregnancy. Assignment of the trimester character is based on the provider's documentation of the trimester or the number of weeks for the current encounter. An additional code from category Z3A, Weeks of gestation, can be reported to identify the specific week of pregnancy. Category Z3A includes codes specifying the number of weeks of gestation at the time of the encounter.

Code Z34.0- (Encounter for supervision of normal first pregnancy) is only reported for the first pregnancy, regardless of the outcome-whether completed or aborted. All other pregnancies would be reported with Z34.8- (Encounter for supervision of other normal pregnancy). The "normal" refers to the pregnancy type (ie, normal versus "high-risk" pregnancy) and does not refer to the outcome. In the scenario described above, a second pregnancy with a previous history of miscarriage counts as "other normal pregnancy" and would be reported with diagnosis code Z34.8-.

Preexisting Conditions Versus Conditions Due to Pregnancy

Certain categories in Chapter 15 distinguish between conditions that the mother had prior to pregnancy and those that are a direct result of pregnancy. Proper code selection requires a determination of whether the condition was preexisting or occurred first during pregnancy. Two common examples include hypertension and diabetes. After coding the Chapter 15 preexisting condition, it is appropriate to select an additional code from the appropriate chapter (eg, Chapter 9 for hypertension, Chapter 4 for diabetes).

Consistent with general unspecified rules, unspecified maternal hypertension and unspecified diabetes should be avoided when additional clinical information is known and documented.

Patients who develop edema and protein in their urine, may progress to preeclampsia or eclampsia. These conditions are found in categories 014 and 015, respectively, and require designation of the trimester.

Multiple Gestation

Some codes require a seventh character extension to identify the fetus for which the complication applies. A code from O30.- (Multiple gestation) should also be reported. If a condition affects more than one fetus, then the code must be assigned for each fetus affected.

Possible seventh character extensions are as follows:

- 0 Not applicable
- 1-5 Fetus number
- 9 Other fetus

The seventh character extension "0" is assigned when:

- There is a single gestation.
- The documentation is insufficient to determine the affected fetus, and clarification is not possible.
- It is not possible to clinically determine which fetus is affected.

Delivery

In the event of a delivery, the primary diagnosis is the main circumstance or complication of the delivery. For a cesarean delivery, the primary diagnosis is the condition that was responsible for the patient's admission. If a particular condition resulted in the admission and the cesarean procedure, that condition should be listed first. If the patient was admitted to the hospital for a condition unrelated to the reason for the cesarean, the reason for the admission should be reported for the E/M service(s) and the reason the cesarean was required should be reported on the day of delivery.

The maternal record should include a code from category Z37 (Outcome of delivery) when a delivery occurs. The normal delivery code should be reported if the outcome is

- A full-term uncomplicated delivery.
- A single, healthy infant.
- The absence of complications during the antepartum, the delivery, or postpartum during the delivery episode.

Postpartum care

Routine postpartum care is reported using code Z39.2 (Encounter for routine postpartum care). Admissions for routine postpartum care following a delivery outside the hospital is reported using code Z39.0 (Encounter for care and examination of mother immediately after delivery).

ICD-10-CM defines the postpartum period as beginning immediately after delivery and continuing for 6 weeks. The peripartum period is defined by ICD-10-CM as the last month of pregnancy to 5 months postpartum. Even with these definitions, Chapter 15 codes can be used after the peripartum or postpartum periods if the documentation supports the condition as pregnancy related.

SOCIAL DETERMINANTS OF HEALTH

The American College of Obstetricians and Gynecologists recommends that obstetrician–gynecologists inquire about and document the patient's social determinants of health (SDOH) and health-related social needs (HRSN). Those findings should be taken into consideration when developing a patient-centered plan of care.

Social determinants of health, as defined by the World Health Organization, are nonmedical factors that influence health outcomes. They may include income and financial security, education, working conditions, food insecurity, housing, early childhood development, and access to affordable health care.

Increasingly, public and private payers are requesting or requiring ICD-10-CM codes on the claim that represent the SDOH and HRSN shared by the patient. The Agency for Healthcare Research and Quality has a list of tools to help physicians identify social needs, and the CMS Office of Minority Health has created a resource for using ICD-10-CM Z codes to capture SDOH. Codes that may be used by obstetrician–gynecologists include those under Z55–Z65 (Persons with potential health hazards related to socioeconomic and psychosocial circumstances). There are several options that may be used; however, those most commonly used by obstetrician–gynecologists are outlined in the table below.

Z56	**Problems related to employment and unemployment**	
	Z56.0	Unemployment, unspecified
	Z56.2	Threat of job loss
	Z56.3	Stressful work schedule
	Z56.6	Other physical and mental strain related to work
Z57	**Occupational exposure to risk factors**	
	Z57.1	Occupational exposure to radiation
	Z57.3	Occupational exposure to other air contaminants
	Z57.4	Occupational exposure to toxic agents in agriculture
	Z57.6	Occupational exposure to extreme temperature
Z59.0	**Problems related to housing and economic circumstances: Homelessness**	
	Z59.00	Homelessness...unspecified
	Z59.01	Sheltered homelessness
	Z59.02	Unsheltered homelessness
Z59.1	**Inadequate housing**	
	Z59.10	Inadequate housing...unspecified
	Z59.11	Inadequate housing...environmental temperature
	Z59.12	Inadequate housing...utilities
Z59.4	**Lack of adequate food**	
	Z59.41	Food insecurity
Z59.5	**Extreme poverty**	
Z59.6	**Low income**	

Z59.7	**Insufficient social insurance and welfare support**		
Z59.8	**Other problems related to housing and economic circumstances**		
	Z59.81	Housing instability, housed	
		Z59.811	...with risk of homelessness
		Z59.812	...homelessness in past 12 months
	Z59.82	Transportation insecurity	
	Z59.86	Financial insecurity	
Z63	**Other problems related to primary support group, including family circumstances**		
	Z63.0	Problems in relationship with spouse or partner	
	Z63.3	Absence of family member	
	Z63.4	Disappearance and death of family member	
	Z63.5	Disruption of family by separation and divorce	
	Z63.6	Dependent relative needing care at home	
	Z63.72	Alcoholism and drug addiction in family	
Z64	**Problems related to certain psychosocial circumstances**		
	Z64.0	Problems related to unwanted pregnancy	
	Z64.1	Problems related to multiparity	
Z65	**Problems related to other certain psychosocial circumstances**		
	Z65.0	Conviction in civil and criminal proceedings without imprisonment	
	Z65.1	Imprisonment and other incarceration	
	Z65.2	Problems related to release from prison	
	Z65.3	Problems related to other legal circumstances	
	Z65.4	Victim of crime and terrorism	
	Z65.5	Exposure to disaster, war and other hostilities	

PART II
Components of Correct Coding

Surgery Codes

CPT® CODE 10060

Incision and drainage of abscess (eg, carbuncle, suppurative hidradenitis, cutaneous or subcutaneous abscess, cyst, furuncle, or paronychia); simple or single

POLICY INDICATORS

Global Period
10 day post-op period

Assistants at Surgery
No assistant

Co-Surgeons Allowed
No co-surgeon

Reduction for Multiple Procedures
Subject to 50% reduction

Bilateral Surgery Payment
N/A

Applicable Medicare Policies

SURGERY

Relative Value Units (RVUs)

Work RVUs	1.22
Non-Facility Total	3.84
Facility Total	3.24

Coding Assistance

10060 includes:

- Positioning and prepping patient
- Examination of site after anesthesia
- Operative services, including inspections around site and closure
- Appropriate post-op E/M visit(s)

Abbreviated Case Note Example:

- A 22-year-old patient has a large vaginal cyst, posterior to the cervix.
- Procedure: The cyst is incised with a cruciate incision and the contents of the cyst are expelled; homeostasis is achieved; and wound closure with sutures is not required. An incision and drainage is performed.

Additional Notes

- Local anesthetic is applied.
- Hemostasis is achieved.

CPT® CODE 10061

Incision and drainage of abscess (eg, carbuncle, suppurative hidradenitis, cutaneous or subcutaneous abscess, cyst, furuncle, or paronychia); complicated or multiple

POLICY INDICATORS

Global Period
10 day post-op period

Assistants at Surgery
No assistant

Co-Surgeons Allowed
No co-surgeon

Reduction for Multiple Procedures
Subject to 50% reduction

Bilateral Surgery Payment
N/A

Applicable Medicare Policies

Relative Value Units (RVUs)

Work RVUs	2.45
Non-Facility Total	6.44
Facility Total	5.56

Coding Assistance

10061 includes:

- Positioning and prepping patient
- Examination of site after anesthesia
- Operative services, including inspections around site and closure
- Appropriate post-op E/M visit(s)

Abbreviated Case Note Example:

- A 54-year-old female patient presents with a diagnosis of short-bowel syndrome after multiple complex operations in the past. Examination reveals a vaginal cuff that is concerning for fistulization to a chronic pelvic abscess. She is brought to the operating room to examine the problem and drain the chronic pelvic abscess.
- Procedure: The abscess site is incised, purulent drainage expressed, and chronic sinus track in the lower abdomen cleaned out, thus debriding it in that fashion. The site is flushed out multiple times with dilute betadine and examined for additional purulence. A drain is placed and the wound is packed.

Additional Notes

- Local anesthetic is applied.
- Hemostasis is achieved.

SURGERY

CPT® CODE 10140

Incision and drainage of hematoma, seroma or fluid collection

POLICY INDICATORS

Global Period
10 day post-op period

Assistants at Surgery
No assistant

Co-Surgeons Allowed
No co-surgeon

Reduction for Multiple Procedures
Subject to 50% reduction

Bilateral Surgery Payment
N/A

Applicable Medicare Policies

Relative Value Units (RVUs)

Work RVUs	1.58
Non-Facility Total	5.09
Facility Total	3.60

Coding Assistance

10140 includes:

- Positioning and prepping patient
- Examination of site after anesthesia
- Operative services, including inspections around site and closure
- Appropriate post-op E/M visit(s)

Abbreviated Case Note Example:

- A 34-year-old woman presents to the office with a cesarean section wound. Operative drainage is performed.
- Procedure: An incision is made over the wound, and the wound is opened approximately 1 cm to the right lateral border. Large seroma fluid is drained. The wound is packed or closed with dressing.

Additional Notes

- Local anesthetic is applied.
- Hemostasis is achieved.

CPT® CODE 10180

Incision and drainage, complex, postoperative wound infection

POLICY INDICATORS

Global Period
10 day post-op period

Assistants at Surgery
No assistant

Co-Surgeons Allowed
No co-surgeon

Reduction for Multiple Procedures
Subject to 50% reduction

Bilateral Surgery Payment
N/A

Applicable Medicare Policies

Relative Value Units (RVUs)

Work RVUs	2.30
Non-Facility Total	7.91
Facility Total	5.44

Coding Assistance

10180 includes:

- Positioning and prepping patient
- Examination of site after anesthesia
- Operative services, including inspections around site and closure
- Appropriate post-op E/M visit(s)

CPT® CODE 11004

Debridement of skin, subcutaneous tissue, muscle and fascia for necrotizing soft tissue infection; external genitalia and perineum

POLICY INDICATORS

Global Period
0 day post-op period

Assistants at Surgery
No assistant

Co-Surgeons Allowed
No co-surgeon

Reduction for Multiple Procedures
Subject to 50% reduction

Bilateral Surgery Payment
N/A

Applicable Medicare Policies
Inpatient-only

Relative Value Units (RVUs)

Work RVUs	10.80
Non-Facility Total	Only valued for facility
Facility Total	16.91

Coding Assistance

11004 includes:

- Positioning and prepping patient
- Examination of site after anesthesia
- Operative services, including inspections around site and closure

Additional Notes

- Exam is performed under anesthesia

CPT® CODE 11005

Debridement of skin, subcutaneous tissue, muscle and fascia for necrotizing soft tissue infection; abdominal wall, with or without fascial closure

POLICY INDICATORS

Global Period
0 day post-op period

Assistants at Surgery
Submit reason for assistant

Co-Surgeons Allowed
No co-surgeon

Reduction for Multiple Procedures
Not subject to multiple surgery reduction

Bilateral Surgery Payment
N/A

Applicable Medicare Policies
Inpatient-only

Relative Value Units (RVUs)

Work RVUs	14.24
Non-Facility Total	Only valued for facility
Facility Total	23.02

Coding Assistance

11005 includes:

- Positioning and prepping patient
- Examination of site after anesthesia
- Operative services, including inspections around site and closure

CPT® CODE 11006

Debridement of skin, subcutaneous tissue, muscle and fascia for necrotizing soft tissue infection; external genitalia, perineum and abdominal wall, with or without fascial closure

POLICY INDICATORS

Global Period
0 day post-op period

Assistants at Surgery
No assistant

Co-Surgeons Allowed
No co-surgeon

Reduction for Multiple Procedures
Subject to 50% reduction

Bilateral Surgery Payment
N/A

Applicable Medicare Policies
Inpatient-only

Relative Value Units (RVUs)

Work RVUs	13.10
Non-Facility Total	Only valued for facility
Facility Total	20.90

Coding Assistance

11006 includes:

- Positioning and prepping patient
- Examination of site after anesthesia
- Operative services, including inspections around site and closure

Abbreviated Case Note Example:

- A 48-year-old female patient presents to the ER with full-thickness skin necrosis with surrounding erythema and crepitus involving large areas of the genitalia, perineum, and lower abdominal wall. Immediate debridement of all involved tissues is performed.
- Procedure: The patient is taken to the OR and placed in the supine position. Evaluation of the extent of the necrotic tissue is performed under anesthesia, and necrotic skin, subcutaneous tissue, fat, and muscle are resected and debrided back to healthy tissue. The genitalia and lower abdominal tissue are debrided as necessary. The Jackson-Pratt drains are placed, and the wounds are packed open with gauze.

SURGERY

CPT® CODE 11042

Debridement, subcutaneous tissue (includes epidermis and dermis, if performed); first 20 sq cm or less

POLICY INDICATORS

Global Period
0 day post-op period

Assistants at Surgery
No assistant

Co-Surgeons Allowed
No co-surgeon

Reduction for Multiple Procedures
Subject to 50% reduction

Bilateral Surgery Payment
N/A

Applicable Medicare Policies

Relative Value Units (RVUs)

Work RVUs	1.01
Non-Facility Total	3.87
Facility Total	1.82

Coding Assistance

11042 includes:

- Positioning and prepping patient
- Examination of site after anesthesia
- Operative services, including inspections around site and closure
- Active wound management (97597-97602)

Abbreviated Case Note Example:

- A 20-year-old woman with a history of foreign body/mesh/suture erosion presents with recurrence of necrosis and granulation tissue with associated pain and discharge.
- Procedure: The patient is taken to the OR and placed under general anesthesia. The left anterior side wall of the vagina area is readily identified. Moderate granulation and necrotic tissue are noted around a knotted-up permanent suture. The area is injected with 0.25% bupivacaine with epinephrine, and lateral incision is made above the area of granulation and necrotic tissue. The necrotic tissue is debrided, the incision edges are trimmed, and the area is irrigated. The skin was closed with running 3-0 vicryl.

Additional Notes

- Debridement is reported separately only when wound contamination requires either prolonged cleaning or removal of appreciable amounts of devitalized or contaminated tissue

CPT® CODE 11104

Punch biopsy of skin (including simple closure, when performed); single lesion

POLICY INDICATORS

Global Period
0 day post-op period

Assistants at Surgery
No assistant

Co-Surgeons Allowed
No co-surgeon

Reduction for Multiple Procedures
Subject to 50% reduction

Bilateral Surgery Payment
N/A

Applicable Medicare Policies

Relative Value Units (RVUs)

Work RVUs	0.83
Non-Facility Total	3.69
Facility Total	1.40

Coding Assistance

11104 includes:

- Positioning and prepping patient
- Examination of site after anesthesia
- Operative services, including inspections around site and closure

Abbreviated Case Note Example:

- A 48-year-old patient presents with a vulvar lesion. A punch biopsy is performed.
- Procedure: The affected area is treated with hurricane spray and injected with a 2% lidocaine solution. A 3-mm punch biopsy is performed on the affected area, and the specimen is prepared and sent to pathology. The biopsy site is treated with silver nitrate and pressure.

Additional Notes

- Exam is performed under anesthesia

CPT® CODE 11105

Punch biopsy of skin (including simple closure, when performed); each separate/additional lesion (List separately in addition to code for primary procedure)

POLICY INDICATORS

Global Period
Global for primary procedure applies

Assistants at Surgery
No assistant

Co-Surgeons Allowed
No co-surgeon

Reduction for Multiple Procedures
Not subject to multiple surgery reduction

Bilateral Surgery Payment
N/A

Applicable Medicare Policies

Relative Value Units (RVUs)

Work RVUs	0.45
Non-Facility Total	1.78
Facility Total	2.33

Coding Assistance

11105 includes:

- Positioning and prepping patient
- Examination of site after anesthesia
- Operative services, including inspections around site and closure
- Appropriate post-op E/M visit(s)

Abbreviated Case Note Example:

- A 48-year-old patient presents with a vulvar lesion. A punch biopsy is performed on each additional lesion. (Note: This is an add-on code for the additional physician work related to the biopsy of one additional lesion.)
- Procedure: The affected area is treated with hurricane spray and injected with a 2% lidocaine solution. A 3-mm punch biopsy was performed on the affected area, and the specimen is prepared and sent to pathology. The biopsy site is treated with silver nitrate and pressure.

SURGERY

CPT® CODE 11200

Removal of skin tags, multiple fibrocutaneous tags, any area; up to and including 15 lesions

POLICY INDICATORS

Global Period
10 day post-op period

Assistants at Surgery
No assistant

Co-Surgeons Allowed
No co-surgeon

Reduction for Multiple Procedures
Subject to 50% reduction

Bilateral Surgery Payment
N/A

Applicable Medicare Policies

Relative Value Units (RVUs)

Work RVUs	0.82
Non-Facility Total	2.79
Facility Total	2.33

Coding Assistance

11200 includes:

- Positioning and prepping patient
- Examination of site after anesthesia
- Operative services, including inspections around site and closure
- Appropriate post-op E/M visit(s)

Abbreviated Case Note Example:

- A 55-year-old female patient presents with complaints of growing skin lesions on her neck, which are irritated by her collar and sometimes catch in her necklace, causing bleeding. There is a total of 12 lesions from 3 to 6 mm in size on the anterior and sides of the neck, all typical for a diagnosis of skin tags. A removal is recommended.
- Procedure: The area is cleansed with alcohol and a 1% lidocaine is applied to each tag for anesthesia. The smaller neck lesions are excised with scissors and a topical aluminium chloride solution is applied for hemostasis. The larger neck lesions are then electrodessicated at their base to facilitate hemostasis prior to the scissors excision. Antibiotic ointment and dressing are applied.

Additional Notes

- If removing more than 25 total lesions, report 11201 for lesions 16-25 and 11201 again for lesions 26-35

SURGERY

CPT® CODE 11201

Removal of skin tags, multiple fibrocutaneous tags, any area; each additional 10 lesions, or part thereof (List separately in addition to code for primary procedure)

POLICY INDICATORS

Global Period
Global for primary procedure applies

Assistants at Surgery
No assistant

Co-Surgeons Allowed
No co-surgeon

Reduction for Multiple Procedures
Not subject to multiple surgery reduction

Bilateral Surgery Payment
N/A

Applicable Medicare Policies

Relative Value Units (RVUs)

Work RVUs	0.29
Non-Facility Total	0.55
Facility Total	0.48

Coding Assistance

11201 includes:

- Positioning and prepping patient
- Examination of site after anesthesia
- Operative services, including inspections around site and closure
- Appropriate post-op E/M visit(s)

Abbreviated Case Note Example:

- A 55-year-old female patient presents with complaints of growing skin lesions on her neck, which are irritated by her collar and sometimes catch in her necklace, causing bleeding. There is a total of 12 lesions ranging from 3 to 5 mm in size on the sides of the neck, and 11 lesions that are 2 to 6 mm in size in the axillary areas, all typical for a diagnosis of skin tags. A removal is recommended.
- Procedure: The area is cleansed with alcohol and a 1% lidocaine is applied to each tag for anesthesia. The smaller neck lesions are excised with scissors, and a topical aluminium chloride solution is applied for hemostasis. The larger neck lesions are then electrodessicated at their base to facilitate hemostasis prior to the scissors excision. Antibiotic ointment and dressing are applied.

CPT® CODE 11420

Excision, benign lesion including margins, except skin tag (unless listed elsewhere), scalp, neck, hands, feet, genitalia; excised diameter 0.5 cm or less

POLICY INDICATORS

Global Period
10 day post-op period

Assistants at Surgery
No assistant

Co-Surgeons Allowed
No co-surgeon

Reduction for Multiple Procedures
Subject to 50% reduction

Bilateral Surgery Payment
N/A

Applicable Medicare Policies

Relative Value Units (RVUs)

Work RVUs	1.03
Non-Facility Total	3.80
Facility Total	2.51

Coding Assistance

11420 includes:

- Positioning and prepping patient
- Examination of site after anesthesia
- Operative services, including inspections around site and closure
- Appropriate post-op E/M visit(s)

Abbreviated Case Note Example:

- A 35-year-old female patient presents for removal of a warty growth on the left labium majors.
- Procedure: The physician cleanses the area and delineates the extent of the excision, including appropriate margins, with a sterile surgical marker. The base of the lesion is injected with local 2% lidocaine, and the lesion is excised sharply at its base. The base is then cauterized with silver nitrate. EBL is minimal. Hemostasis is achieved with cautery or suture. Suture material is used to close the wound.

SURGERY

CPT® CODE 11421

Excision, benign lesion including margins, except skin tag (unless listed elsewhere), scalp, neck, hands, feet, genitalia; excised diameter 0.6 to 1.0 cm

POLICY INDICATORS

Global Period
10 day post-op period

Assistants at Surgery
No assistant

Co-Surgeons Allowed
No co-surgeon

Reduction for Multiple Procedures
Subject to 50% reduction

Bilateral Surgery Payment
N/A

Applicable Medicare Policies

Relative Value Units (RVUs)

Work RVUs	1.47
Non-Facility Total	4.78
Facility Total	3.31

Coding Assistance

11421 includes:

- Positioning and prepping patient
- Examination of site after anesthesia
- Operative services, including inspections around site and closure
- Appropriate post-op E/M visit(s)

Abbreviated Case Note Example:

- A 40-year-old female patient presents for an excision and revision of vaginal scar due to a persistent granulation following an obstetrical laceration.
- Procedure: The distal right implant at the distal posterior vagina is grasped with pickups, concurrent rectal exam elevated, and the area flattened. The extent of the area is confirmed, and the granulaton is trimmed and removed with tenotomy scissors. The excision site is circumferentially undermined, and the mucosa closed with interrupted sutures of 3-0 vicryl. Concurrent rectal exam is performed throughout the element of the procedure with no suture entry or injury. Mucosa edges are confirmed closed.
- Findings: Left sulcus granulation with interval resolution, distal posterior vagina, right of midline with 8 mm length at base.

CPT® CODE 11422

Excision, benign lesion including margins, except skin tag (unless listed elsewhere), scalp, neck, hands, feet, genitalia; excised diameter 1.1 to 2.0 cm

POLICY INDICATORS

Global Period
10 day post-op period

Assistants at Surgery
No assistant

Co-Surgeons Allowed
No co-surgeon

Reduction for Multiple Procedures
Subject to 50% reduction

Bilateral Surgery Payment
N/A

Applicable Medicare Policies

Relative Value Units (RVUs)

Work RVUs	1.68
Non-Facility Total	5.39
Facility Total	4.15

Coding Assistance

11422 includes:

- Positioning and prepping patient
- Examination of site after anesthesia
- Operative services, including inspections around site and closure
- Appropriate post-op E/M visit(s)

Abbreviated Case Note Example:

- A 55-year-old female patient presents for removal of a biopsy-proven vulvar lesion with an excised diameter of 1.5 cm.
- Procedure: The physician cleanses the area and delineates the extent of the excision, including appropriate margins, with a sterile surgical marker. After injecting local anesthetic, patient is reprepped, and draped, the lights are positioned, and a scapel is used to incise along the borders of the lesion. The excision of the vulvar lesion is carried out. Hemostasis is achieved with cautery or suture. The wound is closed with suture materials.

CPT® CODE 11423

Excision, benign lesion including margins, except skin tag (unless listed elsewhere), scalp, neck, hands, feet, genitalia; excised diameter 2.1 to 3.0 cm

POLICY INDICATORS

Global Period
10 day post-op period

Assistants at Surgery
No assistant

Co-Surgeons Allowed
No co-surgeon

Reduction for Multiple Procedures
Subject to 50% reduction

Bilateral Surgery Payment
N/A

Applicable Medicare Policies

Relative Value Units (RVUs)

Work RVUs	2.06
Non-Facility Total	6.21
Facility Total	4.81

Coding Assistance

11423 includes:

- Positioning and prepping patient
- Examination of site after anesthesia
- Operative services, including inspections around site and closure
- Appropriate post-op E/M visit(s)

Abbreviated Case Note Example:

- A 55-year-old female patient presents for an ongoing issue with a lesion in the left labia area, and multiple lesions consistent with genital warts. She presents today for removal of these lesions.
- Procedure: After general anesthesia is administered, the left labial lesion is grasped with 2 Allis clamps. An elliptical incision is made with the Bovie electrocautery utilizing pure cutting, the left labia lesion is removed first, and the defect is closed with 2-0 vicryl sutures placed about 5 mm apart. The perianal lesion is removed by dissection with Bovie electrocautery utilizing the pure cutting mode. Hemostasis is achieved. This area is not closed with sutures given its location.

SURGERY

CPT® CODE 11980

Subcutaneous hormone pellet implantation (implantation of estradiol and/or testosterone pellets beneath the skin)

POLICY INDICATORS

Global Period
0 day post-op period

Assistants at Surgery
No assistant

Co-Surgeons Allowed
No co-surgeon

Reduction for Multiple Procedures
Subject to 50% reduction

Bilateral Surgery Payment
N/A

Applicable Medicare Policies

Relative Value Units (RVUs)

Work RVUs	1.10
Non-Facility Total	2.83
Facility Total	1.65

Coding Assistance

11980 includes:

- Positioning and prepping patient
- Examination of site after anesthesia
- Operative services, including inspections around site and closure

CPT® CODE 11981

Insertion, drug-delivery implant (ie, bioresorbable, biodegradable, non-biodegradable)

POLICY INDICATORS

Global Period
0 day post-op period

Assistants at Surgery
Submit reason for assistant

Co-Surgeons Allowed
No co-surgeon

Reduction for Multiple Procedures
Subject to 50% reduction

Bilateral Surgery Payment
N/A

Applicable Medicare Policies

Relative Value Units (RVUs)

Work RVUs	1.14
Non-Facility Total	3.03
Facility Total	1.89

Coding Assistance

11981 includes:

- Positioning and prepping patient
- Examination of site after anesthesia
- Operative services, including inspections around site and closure

Abbreviated Case Note Example:

- A 34-year-old G2P2 woman presents with a desire for Nexplanon. The physician counsels her on the risks, benefits, and alternatives of the procedure.
- Procedure: After administering the general anesthesia without complication, an insertion point is identified at least 10 cm from the medial epicondyle in the intermuscular groove. The media arm is prepped with antiseptic, the insertion site and the length of the Nexplanon insertion are injected with 3 cc of 1% lidocaine plain. The Nexplanon device is opened in a sterile manner, and inserted in the left upper arm through the insertion site on the first attempt without difficulty. After placement, the implant is palpated by both the patient and the physician. Pressure is applied to the incision to help with hemostasis. Steri-strips are applied to the wound and a pressure dressing.

SURGERY

CPT® CODE 11982

Removal, non-biodegradable drug delivery implant

POLICY INDICATORS

Global Period
0 day post-op period

Assistants at Surgery
Submit reason for assistant

Co-Surgeons Allowed
No co-surgeon

Reduction for Multiple Procedures
Subject to 50% reduction

Bilateral Surgery Payment
N/A

Applicable Medicare Policies

Relative Value Units (RVUs)

Work RVUs	1.34
Non-Facility Total	3.31
Facility Total	2.18

Coding Assistance

11982 includes:

- Positioning and prepping patient
- Examination of site after anesthesia
- Operative services, including inspections around site and closure

Abbreviated Case Note Example:

- A 34-year-old female patient presents with a deep subdermal contraceptive implant that is embedded in the fascia/muscle. She is here for the removal of the contraceptive implant.
- Procedure: The patient consents and undergoes MAC without complication. The radiologist provides the ultrasound guidance, implant is located, and the skin is marked for localization. The patient's left arm is prepped and draped in sterile fashion. The skin is infused with 1 cc of 1% lidocaine epinephrine, and a 2-cm skin incision is made over the implant. The subcutaneous tissue is dissected with a hemostat to the level of the fascia, and the fascia is incised over the site of the implant. The implant is palpated within the triceps muscle tissue and grasped with vasectomy clamp. The implant is elevated, scar tissue and muscle dissected with a scapel, bluntly with gauze, and the implant is removed intact. The skin is closed using a 4-0 Biosyn and dressing applied.

CPT® CODE 11983

Removal with reinsertion, non-biodegradable drug delivery implant

POLICY INDICATORS

Global Period
0 day post-op period

Assistants at Surgery
Submit reason for assistant

Co-Surgeons Allowed
No co-surgeon

Reduction for Multiple Procedures
Subject to 50% reduction

Bilateral Surgery Payment
N/A

Applicable Medicare Policies

Relative Value Units (RVUs)

Work RVUs	1.91
Non-Facility Total	4.25
Facility Total	3.10

Coding Assistance

11983 includes:

- Positioning and prepping patient
- Examination of site after anesthesia
- Operative services, including inspections around site and closure

Abbreviated Case Note Example:

- A 28-year-old female patient presents for the removal and replacement of Nexplanon contraceptives.
- Procedure: The patient's left arm is prepped and draped in sterile fashion. The skin is infused with 1 cc of 1% lidocaine with epinephrine, and a small stab incision is made in the left arm. Visualization of the implant is obtained and the Nexplanon is inserted. The skin is closed with steri-strips and pressure bandage applied.

CPT® CODE 17250

Chemical cauterization of granulation tissue (ie, proud flesh)

POLICY INDICATORS

Global Period
0 day post-op period

Assistants at Surgery
No assistant

Co-Surgeons Allowed
No co-surgeon

Reduction for Multiple Procedures
Subject to 50% reduction

Bilateral Surgery Payment
N/A

Applicable Medicare Policies

Relative Value Units (RVUs)

Work RVUs	0.50
Non-Facility Total	2.54
Facility Total	1.13

Coding Assistance

17250 includes:

- Positioning and prepping patient
- Examination of site after anesthesia
- Operative services, including inspections around site and closure

CPT® CODE 19000

Puncture aspiration of cyst of breast

POLICY INDICATORS

Global Period
0 day post-op period

Assistants at Surgery
No assistant

Co-Surgeons Allowed
No co-surgeon

Reduction for Multiple Procedures
Subject to 50% reduction

Bilateral Surgery Payment
N/A

Applicable Medicare Policies

Relative Value Units (RVUs)

Work RVUs	0.84
Non-Facility Total	2.91
Facility Total	1.27

Coding Assistance

19000 includes:

- Positioning and prepping patient
- Examination of site after anesthesia
- Operative services, including inspections around site and closure

CPT® CODE 19001

Puncture aspiration of cyst of breast; each additional cyst (List separately in addition to code for primary procedure)

POLICY INDICATORS

Global Period
Global for primary procedure applies

Assistants at Surgery
No assistant

Co-Surgeons Allowed
No co-surgeon

Reduction for Multiple Procedures
Not subject to multiple surgery reduction

Bilateral Surgery Payment
N/A

Applicable Medicare Policies

Relative Value Units (RVUs)

Work RVUs	0.42
Non-Facility Total	0.78
Facility Total	0.61

Coding Assistance

19001 includes:

- Positioning and prepping patient
- Examination of site after anesthesia
- Operative services, including inspections around site and closure
- Appropriate post-op E/M visit(s)

CPT® CODE 20550

Injection(s); single tendon sheath, or ligament, aponeurosis (eg, plantar "fascia")

POLICY INDICATORS

Global Period
0 day post-op period

Assistants at Surgery
No assistant

Co-Surgeons Allowed
No co-surgeon

Reduction for Multiple Procedures
Subject to 50% reduction

Bilateral Surgery Payment
150% paid if bilateral

Applicable Medicare Policies

Relative Value Units (RVUs)

Work RVUs	0.75
Non-Facility Total	1.75
Facility Total	1.17

Coding Assistance

20550 includes:

- Positioning and prepping patient
- Examination of site after anesthesia
- Operative services, including inspections around site and closure

Abbreviated Case Note Example:

- A 50-year-old female patient is diagnosed with plantar fasciitis. She has failed to respond to nonsteroidal anti-inflammatory drugs (NSAIDs), modification in shoe gear, and stretching exercises. She consents to a steroid injection into the plantar fascia.
- Procedure: The injection site is prepared, and local anesthetic is infiltrated. The medial and lateral tubercles of the calcaneus are palpated, and the point of maximum tenderness is identified. The medial and central bands of the plantar fascia are localized. Using a medial approach, the injection is given superficial to the plantar fascia.

CPT® CODE 20552

Injection(s); single or multiple trigger point(s), 1 or 2 muscle(s)

POLICY INDICATORS

Global Period
0 day post-op period

Assistants at Surgery
No assistant

Co-Surgeons Allowed
No co-surgeon

Reduction for Multiple Procedures
Subject to 50% reduction

Bilateral Surgery Payment
N/A

Applicable Medicare Policies

Relative Value Units (RVUs)

Work RVUs	0.66
Non-Facility Total	1.57
Facility Total	1.09

Coding Assistance

20552 includes:

- Positioning and prepping patient
- Examination of site after anesthesia
- Operative services, including inspections around site and closure

Abbreviated Case Note Example:

- A 50-year-old female patient presents with 4-month history of pain in the left lower back, with radiation of pain into the left buttock. Muscle relaxants, NSAIDs, and physical therapy have not relieved her pain. She is diagnosed with iliopsosas myofascial dysfunction and consents for psoas muscle block.
- Procedure: Patient is placed on lateral position, and Iliac crest is identified. Curved transducer of ultrasound is placed and an anatomic survey is performed from medial to lateral. The muscle location is confirmed using hip flexion. A 22-gauge 5-inch spinal needle is placed through the skin and with in plain technique directed toward the anterior compartment of the psoas muscle. Three injection spots are chosen. 10 mL of 0.25% of Marcaine without epinephrine and 10 mg of Decadron are injected. Needle is removed and no complications are noted.

SURGERY

CPT® CODE 20553

Injection(s); single or multiple trigger point(s), 3 or more muscles

POLICY INDICATORS

Global Period
0 day post-op period

Assistants at Surgery
No assistant

Co-Surgeons Allowed
No co-surgeon

Reduction for Multiple Procedures
Subject to 50% reduction

Bilateral Surgery Payment
N/A

Applicable Medicare Policies

Relative Value Units (RVUs)

Work RVUs	0.75
Non-Facility Total	1.81
Facility Total	1.24

Coding Assistance

20553 includes:

- Positioning and prepping patient
- Examination of site after anesthesia
- Operative services, including inspections around site and closure

Abbreviated Case Note Example:

- A 40-year-old female patient presents with chronic bilateral lower back pain. She has completed a trial of physical therapy and NSAID therapy, but without relief of her pain. She is diagnosed with pelvic floor dysfunction and consents to pelvic floor Botox trigger point injections.
- Procedure: 100 units of Botox are reconstituted in 20 mL NS. Bilaretal pudendal block is performed with 5 mL 1% lidocaine plan per side. Using pudendal injection tray of 50 units, Botox in 10 mL NS is injected into each side levator ani, iliococcygeus, coccygeus, piriformis, and obturator internus muscle. Pressure is applied for hemostasis.

CPT® CODE 27040

Biopsy, soft tissue of pelvis and hip area; superficial

POLICY INDICATORS

Global Period
10 day post-op period

Assistants at Surgery
No assistant

Co-Surgeons Allowed
No co-surgeon

Reduction for Multiple Procedures
Subject to 50% reduction

Bilateral Surgery Payment
150% paid if bilateral

Applicable Medicare Policies

Relative Value Units (RVUs)

Work RVUs	2.92
Non-Facility Total	10.14
Facility Total	6.06

Coding Assistance

27040 includes:

- Positioning and prepping patient
- Examination of site after anesthesia
- Operative services, including inspections around site and closure
- Appropriate post-op E/M visit(s)

CPT® CODE 38500

Biopsy or excision of lymph node(s); open, superficial

POLICY INDICATORS

Global Period
10 day post-op period

Assistants at Surgery
No assistant

Co-Surgeons Allowed
No co-surgeon

Reduction for Multiple Procedures
Subject to 50% reduction

Bilateral Surgery Payment
150% paid if bilateral

Applicable Medicare Policies

Relative Value Units (RVUs)

Work RVUs	3.79
Non-Facility Total	10.12
Facility Total	7.73

Coding Assistance

38500 includes:

- Positioning and prepping patient
- Examination of site after anesthesia
- Operative services, including inspections around site and closure
- Appropriate post-op E/M visit(s)

Abbreviated Case Note Example:

- A 60-year-old female patient presents with a persistent enlarged superficial axillary nodes. She consents to a superficial axillary nodes biopsy.
- Procedure: After administering the anesthesia, a skin incision is made to carefully incise the subcutaneous tissues. The clavipectoral fascia overlying the pathological lymph node is carefully incised. Using a blunt, sharp, monopolar/bipolar electrocautery dissection, the pathological lymph node is dissected free circumferentially. The small lymphatics and bridging blood vessels are carefully dissected out and ligated with fine ties or cautery. The pathological lymph node is removed and bisected, and a portion is submitted for culture. The wound is inspected for hemostasis and irrigated. No drain is placed.

CPT® CODE 38530

Biopsy or excision of lymph node(s); open, internal mammary node(s)

POLICY INDICATORS

Global Period
90 day post-op period

Assistants at Surgery
Assistant allowed

Co-Surgeons Allowed
Submit reason for co-surgeon

Reduction for Multiple Procedures
Subject to 50% reduction

Bilateral Surgery Payment
150% paid if bilateral

Applicable Medicare Policies

Relative Value Units (RVUs)

Work RVUs	8.34
Non-Facility Total	Only valued for facility
Facility Total	17.31

Coding Assistance

38530 includes:

- Positioning and prepping patient
- Examination of site after anesthesia
- Operative services, including inspections around site and closure
- Appropriate post-op E/M visit(s)

CPT® CODE 38570

Laparoscopy, surgical; with retroperitoneal lymph node sampling (biopsy), single or multiple

POLICY INDICATORS

Global Period
10 day post-op period

Assistants at Surgery
Assistant allowed

Co-Surgeons Allowed
Co-surgeon allowed

Reduction for Multiple Procedures
Endoscopy payment rules apply

Bilateral Surgery Payment
N/A

Applicable Medicare Policies

Relative Value Units (RVUs)

Work RVUs	8.49
Non-Facility Total	Only valued for facility
Facility Total	15.59

Coding Assistance

38570 includes:

- Positioning and prepping patient
- Examination of site after anesthesia
- Operative services, including inspections around site and closure
- Appropriate post-op E/M visit(s)
- Photodocumentation
- Limited lymphadenectomy
- Exploration of retroperitoneum

Additional Notes

- A diagnostic laparoscopy is included in this procedure
- If a more extensive procedure is done, code for the more extensive procedure

CPT® CODE 38571

Laparoscopy, surgical; with bilateral total pelvic lymphadenectomy

POLICY INDICATORS

Global Period
10 day post-op period

Assistants at Surgery
Assistant allowed

Co-Surgeons Allowed
Co-surgeon allowed

Reduction for Multiple Procedures
Endoscopy payment rules apply

Bilateral Surgery Payment
Bilateral surgery

Applicable Medicare Policies

Relative Value Units (RVUs)

Work RVUs	12.00
Non-Facility Total	Only valued for facility
Facility Total	19.89

Coding Assistance

38571 includes:

- Positioning and prepping patient
- Examination of site after anesthesia
- Operative services, including inspections around site and closure
- Appropriate post-op E/M visit(s)
- Photodocumentation
- Pelvic lymphadenectomy
- Exploration of retroperitoneum
- Retroperitoneal lymph node sampling

Additional Notes

- A diagnostic laparoscopy is included in this procedure
- Postoperative counseling about chemotherapy and/or radiotherapy should be coded with the appropriate E/M code and modifier -24

CPT® CODE 38770

Pelvic lymphadenectomy, including external iliac, hypogastric, and obturator nodes (separate procedure)

POLICY INDICATORS

Global Period
90 day post-op period

Assistants at Surgery
Assistant allowed

Co-Surgeons Allowed
Submit reason for co-surgeon

Reduction for Multiple Procedures
Subject to 50% reduction

Bilateral Surgery Payment
150% paid if bilateral

Applicable Medicare Policies
Inpatient-only

Relative Value Units (RVUs)

Work RVUs	14.06
Non-Facility Total	Only valued for facility
Facility Total	24.25

Coding Assistance

38770 includes:

- Positioning and prepping patient
- Examination of site after anesthesia
- Operative services, including inspections around site and closure
- Appropriate post-op E/M visit(s)
- Photodocumentation
- Procedures on lymph nodes
- Exploration of retroperitoneum

Additional Notes

- If performed using a laparoscopy, see code 38571
- If performed with a hysterectomy, see codes 58200-58210, 58951, 58954
- Postoperative counseling about chemotherapy and/or radiotherapy should be coded with the appropriate E/M code and modifier -24

CPT® CODE 38900

Intraoperative identification (eg, mapping) of sentinel lymph node(s) includes injection of non-radioactive dye, when performed
(List separately in addition to code for primary procedure)

POLICY INDICATORS

Global Period
Global for primary procedure applies

Assistants at Surgery
Assistant allowed

Co-Surgeons Allowed
Submit reason for co-surgeon

Reduction for Multiple Procedures
Not subject to multiple surgery reduction

Bilateral Surgery Payment
150% paid if bilateral

Applicable Medicare Policies

Relative Value Units (RVUs)

Work RVUs	2.50
Non-Facility Total	4.11
Facility Total	4.11

Coding Assistance

38900 includes:

- Positioning and prepping patient
- Examination of site after anesthesia
- Operative services, including inspections around site and closure
- Appropriate post-op E/M visit(s)

Abbreviated Case Note Example:

- A 55-year-old female patient was recently diagnosed with vulvar squamous cell carcinoma. She undergoes vulvectomy with sentinel lymph node injection interoperative due to inability to tolerate injections.
- Procedure: After induction of general anesthesia without complication, the sentinel node injection with 1,100 microcuries of Tc-99m sulfur colloid in four divided doses is injected into the dermis of the lesion preoperatively. Sentinel node site is identified intraoperatively on the left using the gamma probe. Sentinel node site is not identified on the right. The vulvar lesion is injected with isosulfan blue. A 3-cm left groin node incision is made after injecting with 0.5% Marcaine. Using a gamma probe, a hot left inguinal sentinel is identified, and the sentinel node is excised. Ten-second count was 172. Minimal background residual is noted. The wound is irrigated and made hemostatic with electrocautery.

SURGERY

CPT® CODE 44955

Appendectomy; when done for indicated purpose at time of other major procedure (not as separate procedure)
(List separately in addition to code for primary procedure)

POLICY INDICATORS

Global Period
Global for primary procedure applies

Assistants at Surgery
Assistant allowed

Co-Surgeons Allowed
Submit reason for co-surgeon

Reduction for Multiple Procedures
Not subject to multiple surgery reduction

Bilateral Surgery Payment
N/A

Applicable Medicare Policies

Relative Value Units (RVUs)

Work RVUs	1.53
Non-Facility Total	Only valued for facility
Facility Total	2.49

Coding Assistance

44955 includes:

- Positioning and prepping patient
- Examination of site after anesthesia
- Operative services, including inspections around site and closure
- Appropriate post-op E/M visit(s)

CPT® CODE 44970

Laparoscopy, surgical, appendectomy

POLICY INDICATORS

Global Period
90 day post-op period

Assistants at Surgery
Assistant allowed

Co-Surgeons Allowed
Co-surgeon allowed

Reduction for Multiple Procedures
Subject to 50% reduction

Bilateral Surgery Payment
N/A

Applicable Medicare Policies

Relative Value Units (RVUs)

Work RVUs	9.45
Non-Facility Total	Only valued for facility
Facility Total	18.29

Coding Assistance

44970 includes:

- Positioning and prepping patient
- Examination of site after anesthesia
- Operative services, including inspections around site and closure
- Appropriate post-op E/M visit(s)
- Photodocumentation

Abbreviated Case Note Example:

- A 25-year-old female patient presents with right lower quadrant pain and elevated white blood cell (WBC) count, and she is diagnosed with acute appendicitis. She stays in observation for 4 hours, with an increasing WBC, symptoms, and frank rebound tenderness in the right lower quadrant. She is scheduled for laparoscopic appendectomy.
- Procedure: After proper positioning, the appendix is identified, mobilized with grasper instruments, and freed from surrounding adhesions by laparoscopic scissors. The blood supply is stapled or hemoclipped. The appendix is then sized for proper staple selection by means of a laparoscopic sizing instrument, and then resected by means of laparoscopic stapling instrument. The appendix is then placed in a laparoscopic specimen bag to avoid contamination of the abdomen and trocar insertions sites, and is then carefully extracted from the abdomen. The abdomen is then lavaged with saline and carefully inspected for hemostasis and presence of other abnormalities.

Additional Notes

- A diagnostic laparoscopy is included in this procedure
- Incidental appendectomy during a laparoscopic surgery does not usually warrant a separate code
- Postoperative counseling about chemotherapy and/or radiotherapy should be coded with the appropriate E/M code and modifier -24

CPT® CODE 49000

Exploratory laparotomy, exploratory celiotomy with or without biopsy(s) (separate procedure)

POLICY INDICATORS

Global Period
90 day post-op period

Assistants at Surgery
Assistant allowed

Co-Surgeons Allowed
Submit reason for co-surgeon

Reduction for Multiple Procedures
Subject to 50% reduction

Bilateral Surgery Payment
N/A

Applicable Medicare Policies
Inpatient-only

Relative Value Units (RVUs)

Work RVUs	12.54
Non-Facility Total	Only valued for facility
Facility Total	23.26

Coding Assistance

49000 includes:

- Positioning and prepping patient
- Examination of site after anesthesia
- Operative services, including inspections around site and closure
- Appropriate post-op E/M visit(s)
- Photodocumentation
- Peritoneal biopsy(ies)
- Pelvic examination under anesthesia

Abbreviated Case Note Example:

- A 30-year-old female patient was noted to be persistently hypotensive and tachycardic after her scheduled repeat cesarean section and bilateral tubal ligation. A normal postpartum lochia/vaginal bleeding is noted in the PACU. Patient becomes near syncopal and a decision is made to go to the OR for exploratory laparotomy for suspected intra-abdominal bleeding.
- Procedure: After patient undergoes general anesthesia, the abdomen is prepped and draped. Her Pfannenstiel incision is re-opened using scissors. A hemoperitoneum is immediately evident upon entry into the abdominal cavity. Blood transfusion is initiated. The hemoperitoneum is evacuated in an effort to identify the source of bleeding. Inspection of the hysterectomy repair and tubal sterilization sites appears hemostatic. A large 10 x 12-cm left broad ligament hematoma is identified, which is partially evacuated to help identify any active bleeding vessels. Two sites of bleeding are noted and figure-of-8 ligatures are placed to control the bleeding.

CPT® CODE 49002

Reopening of recent laparotomy

POLICY INDICATORS

Global Period
90 day post-op period

Assistants at Surgery
Assistant allowed

Co-Surgeons Allowed
Submit reason for co-surgeon

Reduction for Multiple Procedures
Subject to 50% reduction

Bilateral Surgery Payment
N/A

Applicable Medicare Policies
Inpatient-only

Relative Value Units (RVUs)

Work RVUs	17.63
Non-Facility Total	Only valued for facility
Facility Total	31.42

Coding Assistance

49002 includes:

- Positioning and prepping patient
- Examination of site after anesthesia
- Operative services, including inspections around site and closure
- Appropriate post-op E/M visit(s)
- Photodocumentation

Abbreviated Case Note Example:

- A 32-year-old female patient has just undergone an uncomplicated c-section. In the first postop hour, the patient has lower abdominal discomfort for which IV Dilaudid is given, to which her blood pressure dropping is attributed, and IV ephedrine is given. The patient then becomes tachycardic, and her blood pressure continues to drop, despite fluid bolus. We feel the need to take her urgently to the OR for surgical exploration to rule out intra-abdominal bleeding.
- Procedure: Patient is rushed to the OR and general anesthesia is performed without any difficulty. Staples from the previous Pfannenstiel incision are removed, subcutaneous and fascial stitch are cut and layers are opened up. There is no intra-abdominal or extrauterine bleeding. There is a large and tense right broad ligament hematoma, extending all the way to the pelvic side wall and possible retroperitoneal. Uterus itself is firm; no intrauterine bleeding or hematoma is noted.

CPT® CODE 49010

Exploration, retroperitoneal area with or without biopsy(s) (separate procedure)

POLICY INDICATORS

Global Period
90 day post-op period

Assistants at Surgery
Assistant allowed

Co-Surgeons Allowed
Submit reason for co-surgeon

Reduction for Multiple Procedures
Subject to 50% reduction

Bilateral Surgery Payment
N/A

Applicable Medicare Policies
Inpatient-only

Relative Value Units (RVUs)

Work RVUs	16.06
Non-Facility Total	Only valued for facility
Facility Total	27.86

Coding Assistance

49010 includes:

- Positioning and prepping patient
- Examination of site after anesthesia
- Operative services, including inspections around site and closure
- Appropriate post-op E/M visit(s)

CPT® CODE 49020

Drainage of peritoneal abscess or localized peritonitis, exclusive of appendiceal abscess, open

POLICY INDICATORS

Global Period
90 day post-op period

Assistants at Surgery
Assistant allowed

Co-Surgeons Allowed
No co-surgeon

Reduction for Multiple Procedures
Subject to 50% reduction

Bilateral Surgery Payment
N/A

Applicable Medicare Policies
Inpatient-only

Relative Value Units (RVUs)

Work RVUs	26.67
Non-Facility Total	Only valued for facility
Facility Total	48.01

Coding Assistance

49020 includes:

- Positioning and prepping patient
- Examination of site after anesthesia
- Operative services, including inspections around site and closure
- Appropriate post-op E/M visit(s)

CPT® CODE 49084

Peritoneal lavage, including imaging guidance, when performed

POLICY INDICATORS

Global Period
0 day post-op period

Assistants at Surgery
No assistant

Co-Surgeons Allowed
No co-surgeon

Reduction for Multiple Procedures
Subject to 50% reduction

Bilateral Surgery Payment
N/A

Applicable Medicare Policies

Relative Value Units (RVUs)

Work RVUs	2.00
Non-Facility Total	Only valued for facility
Facility Total	3.22

Coding Assistance

49084 includes:

- Positioning and prepping patient
- Examination of site after anesthesia
- Operative services, including inspections around site and closure

CPT® CODE 49186

Excision or destruction, open, intra-abdominal (ie, peritoneal, mesenteric, retroperitoneal), primary or secondary tumor(s) or cyst(s), sum of the maximum length of tumor(s) or cyst(s); 5 cm or less

POLICY INDICATORS

Global Period
90 day post-op period

Assistants at Surgery
Assistant allowed

Co-Surgeons Allowed
Submit reason for co-surgeon

Reduction for Multiple Procedures
Subject to 50% reduction

Bilateral Surgery Payment
N/A

Applicable Medicare Policies
Inpatient-only

Relative Value Units (RVUs)

Work RVUs	22.00
Non-Facility Total	Only valued for facility
Facility Total	39.50

Coding Assistance

49186 includes:

- Positioning and prepping patient
- Examination of site after anesthesia
- Operative services, including inspections around site and closure
- Appropriate post-op E/M visit(s)
- Cytoreduction
- Debulking

Additional Notes

- Report only the measured tumor(s) and cyst(s) in situ, not the tissue before excision or destruction.
- If open resection of recurrent ovarian, endometrial, tubal or primary peritoneal gynecologic malignancies without lymphadenectomy is performed, report 49186–49190.
- If another open resection of initial or recurrent ovarian, endometrial, tubal or primary peritoneal gynecologic malignancies are performed, report 58943, 58950–58960 instead.
- If an open excision or destruction of endometriomas is performed, report 58999.

SURGERY

CPT® CODE 49187

Excision or destruction, open, intra-abdominal (ie, peritoneal, mesenteric, retroperitoneal), primary or secondary tumor(s) or cyst(s), sum of the maximum length of tumor(s) or cyst(s); 5.1 to 10 cm

POLICY INDICATORS

Global Period
90 day post-op period

Assistants at Surgery
Assistant allowed

Co-Surgeons Allowed
Submit reason for co-surgeon

Reduction for Multiple Procedures
Subject to 50% reduction

Bilateral Surgery Payment
N/A

Applicable Medicare Policies
Inpatient-only

Relative Value Units (RVUs)

Work RVUs	28.65
Non-Facility Total	Only valued for facility
Facility Total	50.48

Coding Assistance

49187 includes:

- Positioning and prepping patient
- Examination of site after anesthesia
- Operative services, including inspections around site and closure
- Appropriate post-op E/M visit(s)
- Cytoreduction
- Debulking

Additional Notes

- Report only the measured tumor(s) and cyst(s) in situ, not the tissue before excision or destruction
- If open resection of recurrent ovarian, endometrial, tubal or primary peritoneal gynecologic malignancies without lymphadenectomy is performed, report 49186–49190
- If another open resection of initial or recurrent ovarian, endometrial, tubal or primary peritoneal gynecologic malignancies are performed, report 58943, 58950–58960 instead
- If an open excision or destruction of endometriomas is performed, report 58999

CPT® CODE 49188

Excision or destruction, open, intra-abdominal (ie, peritoneal, mesenteric, retroperitoneal), primary or secondary tumor(s) or cyst(s), sum of the maximum length of tumor(s) or cyst(s); 10.1 to 20 cm

POLICY INDICATORS

Global Period
90 day post-op period

Assistants at Surgery
Assistant allowed

Co-Surgeons Allowed
Submit reason for co-surgeon

Reduction for Multiple Procedures
Subject to 50% reduction

Bilateral Surgery Payment
N/A

Applicable Medicare Policies
Inpatient-only

Relative Value Units (RVUs)

Work RVUs	34.00
Non-Facility Total	Only valued for facility
Facility Total	60.32

Coding Assistance

49187 includes:

- Positioning and prepping patient
- Examination of site after anesthesia
- Operative services, including inspections around site and closure
- Appropriate post-op E/M visit(s)
- Cytoreduction
- Debulking

Additional Notes

- Report only the measured tumor(s) and cyst(s) in situ, not the tissue before excision or destruction
- If open resection of recurrent ovarian, endometrial, tubal or primary peritoneal gynecologic malignancies without lymphadenectomy is performed, report 49186–49190
- If another open resection of initial or recurrent ovarian, endometrial, tubal or primary peritoneal gynecologic malignancies are performed, report 58943, 58950–58960 instead
- If an open excision or destruction of endometriomas is performed, report 58999

CPT® CODE 49189

Excision or destruction, open, intra-abdominal (ie, peritoneal, mesenteric, retroperitoneal), primary or secondary tumor(s) or cyst(s), sum of the maximum length of tumor(s) or cyst(s); 20.1 to 30 cm

POLICY INDICATORS

Global Period
90 day post-op period

Assistants at Surgery
Assistant allowed

Co-Surgeons Allowed
Submit reason for co-surgeon

Reduction for Multiple Procedures
Subject to 50% reduction

Bilateral Surgery Payment
N/A

Applicable Medicare Policies
Inpatient-only

Relative Value Units (RVUs)

Work RVUs	40.00
Non-Facility Total	Only valued for facility
Facility Total	70.17

Coding Assistance

49189 includes:

- Positioning and prepping patient
- Examination of site after anesthesia
- Operative services, including inspections around site and closure
- Appropriate post-op E/M visit(s)
- Cytoreduction
- Debulking

Additional Notes

- Report only the measured tumor(s) and cyst(s) in situ, not the tissue before excision or destruction
- If open resection of recurrent ovarian, endometrial, tubal or primary peritoneal gynecologic malignancies without lymphadenectomy is performed, report 49186–49190
- If another open resection of initial or recurrent ovarian, endometrial, tubal or primary peritoneal gynecologic malignancies are performed, report 58943, 58950–58960 instead
- If an open excision or destruction of endometriomas is performed, report 58999

CPT® CODE 49190

Excision or destruction, open, intra-abdominal (ie, peritoneal, mesenteric, retroperitoneal), primary or secondary tumor(s) or cyst(s), sum of the maximum length of tumor(s) or cyst(s); greater than 30 cm

POLICY INDICATORS

Global Period
90 day post-op period

Assistants at Surgery
Assistant allowed

Co-Surgeons Allowed
Submit reason for co-surgeon

Reduction for Multiple Procedures
Subject to 50% reduction

Bilateral Surgery Payment
N/A

Applicable Medicare Policies
Inpatient-only

Relative Value Units (RVUs)

Work RVUs	50.00
Non-Facility Total	Only valued for facility
Facility Total	86.50

Coding Assistance

49189 includes:

- Positioning and prepping patient
- Examination of site after anesthesia
- Operative services, including inspections around site and closure
- Appropriate post-op E/M visit(s)
- Cytoreduction
- Debulking

Additional Notes

- Report only the measured tumor(s) and cyst(s) in situ, not the tissue before excision or destruction
- If open resection of recurrent ovarian, endometrial, tubal or primary peritoneal gynecologic malignancies without lymphadenectomy is performed, report 49186–49190.
- If another open resection of initial or recurrent ovarian, endometrial, tubal or primary peritoneal gynecologic malignancies are performed, report 58943, 58950–58960 instead.
- If an open excision or destruction of endometriomas is performed, report 58999

CPT® CODE 49203

Excision or destruction, open, intra-abdominal tumors, cysts or endometriomas, 1 or more peritoneal, mesenteric, or retroperitoneal primary or secondary tumors; largest tumor 5 cm diameter or less

POLICY INDICATORS

Global Period
90 day post-op period

Assistants at Surgery
Assistant allowed

Co-Surgeons Allowed
Submit reason for co-surgeon

Reduction for Multiple Procedures
Subject to 50% reduction

Bilateral Surgery Payment
N/A

Applicable Medicare Policies
Inpatient-only

Relative Value Units (RVUs)

Work RVUs	20.13
Non-Facility Total	Only valued for facility
Facility Total	35.85

Coding Assistance

49203 includes:

- Positioning and prepping patient
- Examination of site after anesthesia
- Operative services, including inspections around site and closure
- Appropriate post-op E/M visit(s)
- Photodocumentation
- Enterolysis
- Pelvic examination under anesthesia
- Exploration of retroperitoneum
- Omentectomy
- Excision of presacral or sacrococcygeal tumor

Abbreviated Case Note Example:

- A 27-year-old female patient presents with progressive pelvic pain and dysmenorrhea. She desires future fertility. A pelvic ultrasound shows a 3-cm right pelvic side-wall mass with morphology consistent with an endometrioma. The patient is scheduled for an open excision of intraperitoneal and extraperitoneal endometriomas.
- Procedure: The physician incises the skin using a sharp dissection, and achieves hemostasis using electrocautery and small ligatures as necessary. Grasp, elevate, and carefully incise the peritoneum to avoid injury to bowel. Enter the peritoneal cavity under direct vision. Clear adhesions by sharp dissection in order to expose all of the abdominal viscera. Perform a visual and manual complete exploration of the abdominal cavity and its contents. Carefully insert a self-retaining retractor while avoiding injury or entrapment of abdominal contents. Confirm the location and extent of the primary lesions. Pack away the abdominal contents, to the exclusion of the right colon, using laparotomy pads and place additional retractors for optimal exposure. Resect individually three 2- to 3-cm implanted masses using cautery. During this dissection, identify the right ureter and place a vessel loop for continual identification and protection of the ureter. Irrigate the abdominal cavity copiously with antibiotic solution and obtain hemostasis. Inspect the abdomen for injury and presence of any instruments. Return the abdominal organs to normal anatomical position. Close the fascia with running suture. Irrigate and close the skin.

Additional Notes

- Do not report with lymphadenectomy, renal or ovarian procedures

CPT® CODE 49204

Excision or destruction, open, intra-abdominal tumors, cysts or endometriomas, 1 or more peritoneal, mesenteric, or retroperitoneal primary or secondary tumors; largest tumor 5.1-10.0 cm diameter

POLICY INDICATORS

Global Period
90 day post-op period

Assistants at Surgery
Assistant allowed

Co-Surgeons Allowed
Submit reason for co-surgeon

Reduction for Multiple Procedures
Subject to 50% reduction

Bilateral Surgery Payment
N/A

Applicable Medicare Policies
Inpatient-only

Relative Value Units (RVUs)

Work RVUs	26.13
Non-Facility Total	Only valued for facility
Facility Total	45.67

Coding Assistance

49204 includes:

- Positioning and prepping patient
- Examination of site after anesthesia
- Operative services, including inspections around site and closure
- Appropriate post-op E/M visit(s)
- Photodocumentation
- Enterolysis
- Pelvic examination under anesthesia
- Exploration of retroperitoneum
- Omentectomy
- Excision of presacral or sacrococcygeal tumor

Abbreviated Case Note Example:

- A 34-year-old female patient with a history of endometriosis and previous total abdominal hysterectomy and bilateral salpingo-oophorectomy, now presents with progressive pelvic pain and tenesmus. She has been on unopposed estrogen therapy for 10 years. A pelvic ultrasound shows a 6-cm complex pelvic mass with moderately severe left hydronephrosis. A diagnostic laparoscopy shows pelvic endometriomas involving the left pelvic side wall, partially obstructing the left ureter, with obliteration of the pelvic cul-de-sac, and multiple implants over the pelvic and bladder peritoneum. The patient is scheduled for an open excision of intraperitoneal and extraperitoneal endometriomas.
- Procedure: The physician incises the skin using a sharp dissection; hemostasis is achieved using electrocautery and small ligatures as necessary. Grasp, elevate, and carefully incise the peritoneum to avoid injury to bowel. Enter the peritoneal cavity under direct vision. Clear adhesions by sharp dissection in order to expose all of the abdominal viscera. Perform a visual and manual complete exploration of the abdominal cavity and its contents. Carefully insert a self-retaining retractor while avoiding injury or entrapment of abdominal contents. Confirm the location and extent of the primary lesions. Pack away the abdominal contents, to the exclusion of the right colon, using laparotomy pads and place additional retractors for optimal exposure. A 7-cm mass is identified in the mesentery adjacent to above-mentioned small bowel lesions. Carefully dissect it from the retroperitoneal tissues. Identify the right ureter and place a vessel loop for continual identification and protection of the ureter. Dissect the mass completely away from the duodenum and mesenteric vessels as well as the ureter. Resect the two small bowel lesions en bloc from the mesentery of the small bowel. Irrigate the abdominal cavity copiously with antibiotic solution, and obtain hemostasis. Inspect the abdomen for injury and presence of any instruments. Return the abdominal organs to normal anatomical position. Close the fascia with running suture. Irrigate and close the skin.

Additional Notes

- Do not report with lymphadenectomy, renal or ovarian procedures

CPT® CODE 49205

Excision or destruction, open, intra-abdominal tumors, cysts or endometriomas, 1 or more peritoneal, mesenteric, or retroperitoneal primary or secondary tumors; largest tumor greater than 10.0 cm diameter

POLICY INDICATORS

Global Period
90 day post-op period

Assistants at Surgery
Assistant allowed

Co-Surgeons Allowed
Submit reason for co-surgeon

Reduction for Multiple Procedures
Subject to 50% reduction

Bilateral Surgery Payment
N/A

Applicable Medicare Policies
Inpatient-only

Relative Value Units (RVUs)

Work RVUs	30.13
Non-Facility Total	Only valued for facility
Facility Total	52.39

Coding Assistance

49205 includes:

- Positioning and prepping patient
- Examination of site after anesthesia
- Operative services, including inspections around site and closure
- Appropriate post-op E/M visit(s)
- Photodocumentation
- Enterolysis
- Laparotomy
- Omentectomy
- Pelvic examination under anesthesia
- Ureterolysis

Additional Notes

- Do not report with lymphadenectomy, renal or ovarian procedures

CPT® CODE 49320

Laparoscopy, abdomen, peritoneum, and omentum, diagnostic, with or without collection of specimen(s) by brushing or washing (separate procedure)

POLICY INDICATORS

Global Period
10 day post-op period

Assistants at Surgery
Assistant allowed

Co-Surgeons Allowed
No co-surgeon

Reduction for Multiple Procedures
Subject to 50% reduction

Bilateral Surgery Payment
N/A

Applicable Medicare Policies

Relative Value Units (RVUs)

Work RVUs	5.14
Non-Facility Total	Only valued for facility
Facility Total	10.03

Coding Assistance

49320 includes:

- Positioning and prepping patient
- Examination of site after anesthesia
- Operative services, including inspections around site and closure
- Appropriate post-op E/M visit(s)
- Photodocumentation
- Cervical dilation

Abbreviated Case Note Example:

- A 25-year-old female patient with a history of endometriosis presents with right lower quadrant pain with direct rebound tenderness and an elevated white blood cell count. The following day, her white blood cell count returns to normal, but she still has direct and rebound tenderness. She consents to undergo laparoscopy.
- Procedure: The physician performs a bimanual pelvic examination to assess uterine size, position, and nobility before a uterine cannula is inserted. Exposure of the cervix, and grasping the anterior lip of the cervix with a tenaculum attached to an intrauterine cannula is obtained; achieving pneumoperitoneum by inserting a Veress or Touhy needle at the inferior rim of the umbilicus through a 2-mm incision. The peritoneal space is insufflated with carbon dioxide gas to a pressure of 10 mm Hg, and extending the 2-mm incision to 1 cm once satisfactory displacement of organs is achieved. Then insert the laparoscope trocar and sleeve through the rectus fascia, removing the trocar from the sleeve, and documenting the proper placement as the operating laparoscope is advanced down the trocar sleeve into the pelvis. The entire abdomen and pelvis are viewed systematically, noting and/or photodocumenting the pathology. The trocars are removed under direct vision, the site is observed for bleeding, the abdomen is deflated, the fascia separately, and the skin wounds are closed.

Additional Notes

- If additional procedures are performed through the laparoscope, do not report this procedure

SURGERY

CPT® CODE 49321

Laparoscopy, surgical; with biopsy (single or multiple)

POLICY INDICATORS

Global Period
10 day post-op period

Assistants at Surgery
Assistant allowed

Co-Surgeons Allowed
Co-surgeon allowed

Reduction for Multiple Procedures
Endoscopy payment rules apply

Bilateral Surgery Payment
N/A

Applicable Medicare Policies

Relative Value Units (RVUs)

Work RVUs	5.44
Non-Facility Total	Only valued for facility
Facility Total	10.45

Coding Assistance

49321 includes:

- Positioning and prepping patient
- Examination of site after anesthesia
- Operative services, including inspections around site and closure
- Appropriate post-op E/M visit(s)
- Photodocumentation

Abbreviated Case Note Example:

- A 30-year-old female patient is evaluated for increasing dysmenorrhea unresponsive to nonsteroidal anti-inflammatory drugs (NSAIDs). She is intolerant to oral contraceptives. Diagnostic laparoscopy demonstrates probable endometriosis with power burn and re-berrry lesions identified in the cul-de-sac and broad ligaments. She is scheduled for laparoscopy with a biopsy of these areas.
- Procedure: A bimanual pelvic examination is performed to assess uterine size, position, and mobility before insertion of a uterine cannula. Expose the cervix to achieve pneumoperitoneum by inserting a Veress or Tuohy needle at the inferior rim of the umbilicus through a 2-mm incision. After satisfactory displacement of organs is achieved, extend the 2-mm incision to 1 cm, and insert the laparoscope trocar and sleeve through the rectus fascia. Remove the trocar from the sleeve and document proper placement as the operating laparoscope is advanced down the trocar sleeve into the pelvis. After the laparoscope has been inserted, view the entire abdomen and pelvis systematically and note any pathology, which may be photodocumented. Upon completion of the exploration, select areas of abnormal pathology for biopsy specimens, and achieve hemostasis as needed. Remove trocars under direct vision and observe sites for bleeding. Deflate abdomen, and close the fascia separately and the skin wounds.

Additional Notes

- A diagnostic laparoscopy is included in this procedure
- If a more extensive procedure is done, code for the more extensive procedure
- This code is used to report a biopsy of the ovary or fallopian tube

CPT® CODE 49322

Laparoscopy, surgical; with aspiration of cavity or cyst (eg, ovarian cyst) (single or multiple)

POLICY INDICATORS

Global Period
10 day post-op period

Assistants at Surgery
Assistant allowed

Co-Surgeons Allowed
Co-surgeon allowed

Reduction for Multiple Procedures
Endoscopy payment rules apply

Bilateral Surgery Payment
N/A

Applicable Medicare Policies

Relative Value Units (RVUs)

Work RVUs	6.01
Non-Facility Total	Only valued for facility
Facility Total	11.35

Coding Assistance

49322 includes:

- Positioning and prepping patient
- Examination of site after anesthesia
- Operative services, including inspections around site and closure
- Appropriate post-op E/M visit(s)
- Photodocumentation

Abbreviated Case Note Example:

- A 35-year-old female patient presented 2 months ago with complaints of left lower quadrant pain for the past week. Examination and ultrasound demonstrated a large left adnexal mass that appeared to be a simple ovarian cyst without signs of malignancy. Patient is evaluated 2 months later. A repeat ultrasound performed 2 months after the initial presentation and after a normal menses demonstrates persistent cysts that have not changed in size. The patient is now taken to the OR.
- Procedure: After induction of general anesthesia, a pelvic examination is performed, and a uterine manipulator is placed on the cervix. Laparoscopy is performed, which shows a simple-appearing 5-cm cyst of the left ovary. The fallopian tubes appear normal, and chromotubation is performed, demonstrating bilateral tubal patency. There are no findings to suggest that the cyst is malignant. A needle is passed through the second port, and the cyst is aspirated of clear yellow fluid.

Additional Notes

- A diagnostic laparoscopy is included in this procedure
- If a more extensive procedure is done, code for the more extensive procedure

SURGERY

CPT® CODE 49323

Laparoscopy, surgical; with drainage of lymphocele to peritoneal cavity

POLICY INDICATORS

Global Period
90 day post-op period

Assistants at Surgery
Assistant allowed

Co-Surgeons Allowed
Co-surgeon allowed

Reduction for Multiple Procedures
Endoscopy payment rules apply

Bilateral Surgery Payment
N/A

Applicable Medicare Policies

Relative Value Units (RVUs)

Work RVUs	10.23
Non-Facility Total	Only valued for facility
Facility Total	19.40

Coding Assistance

49323 includes:

- Positioning and prepping patient
- Examination of site after anesthesia
- Operative services, including inspections around site and closure
- Appropriate post-op E/M visit(s)

CPT® CODE 49324

Laparoscopy, surgical; with insertion of tunneled intraperitoneal catheter

POLICY INDICATORS

Global Period
10 day post-op period

Assistants at Surgery
Assistant allowed

Co-Surgeons Allowed
Co-surgeon allowed

Reduction for Multiple Procedures
Endoscopy payment rules apply

Bilateral Surgery Payment
N/A

Applicable Medicare Policies

Relative Value Units (RVUs)

Work RVUs	6.32
Non-Facility Total	Only valued for facility
Facility Total	11.66

Coding Assistance

49324 includes:

- Positioning and prepping patient
- Examination of site after anesthesia
- Operative services, including inspections around site and closure
- Appropriate post-op E/M visit(s)

Abbreviated Case Note Example:

- A 45-year-old female patient with end-stage renal disease caused by diabetic nephropathy needs to initiate dialysis therapy. The patient has a surgical history of cesarean section and open cholecystectomy. She is referred for placement of a peritoneal dialysis catheter.
- Procedure: A skin incision is made and carried through the subcutaneous tissues, and hemostasis is obtained. The midline fascia is exposed to either side of the midline and incised vertically. The peritoneum is opened under direct vision, and a 10-mm trocar is placed. The abdomen is insufflated with carbon dioxide, and the appropriate camera is inserted. A thorough exploration of the abdominal cavity is performed, local anesthesia is injected, and a trocar is placed in the right upper quadrant immediately adjacent to the midline with two additional 5-mm ports. Laparoscopic exploration is performed to identify a space to which the peritoneal dialysis catheter will be directed. The intraperitoneal catheter is inserted, the extraperitoneal portion is tunneled subcutaneously from the abdominal insertion location to a skin exit site and tested. The skin incisions are closed in a subcuticular fashion.

CPT® CODE 50715

Ureterolysis, with or without repositioning of ureter for retroperitoneal fibrosis

POLICY INDICATORS

Global Period
90 day post-op period

Assistants at Surgery
Assistant allowed

Co-Surgeons Allowed
Submit reason for co-surgeon

Reduction for Multiple Procedures
Subject to 50% reduction

Bilateral Surgery Payment
150% paid if bilateral

Applicable Medicare Policies
Inpatient-only list

Relative Value Units (RVUs)

Work RVUs	20.64
Non-Facility Total	Only valued for facility
Facility Total	36.38

Coding Assistance

50715 includes:

- Positioning and prepping patient
- Examination of site after anesthesia
- Operative services, including inspections around site and closure
- Appropriate post-op E/M visit(s)

CPT® CODE 50722

Ureterolysis for ovarian vein syndrome

POLICY INDICATORS

Global Period
90 day post-op period

Assistants at Surgery
Assistant allowed

Co-Surgeons Allowed
Submit reason for co-surgeon

Reduction for Multiple Procedures
Subject to 50% reduction

Bilateral Surgery Payment
N/A

Applicable Medicare Policies
Inpatient-only list

Relative Value Units (RVUs)

Work RVUs	17.95
Non-Facility Total	Only valued for facility
Facility Total	30.64

Coding Assistance

50722 includes:

- Positioning and prepping patient
- Examination of site after anesthesia
- Operative services, including inspections around site and closure
- Appropriate post-op E/M visit(s)

CPT® CODE 50727

Revision of urinary-cutaneous anastomosis (any type urostomy)

POLICY INDICATORS

Global Period
90 day post-op period

Assistants at Surgery
Assistant allowed

Co-Surgeons Allowed
Co-surgeon allowed

Reduction for Multiple Procedures
Subject to 50% reduction

Bilateral Surgery Payment
N/A

Applicable Medicare Policies

Relative Value Units (RVUs)

Work RVUs	8.28
Non-Facility Total	Only valued for facility
Facility Total	15.43

Coding Assistance

50727 includes:

- Positioning and prepping patient
- Examination of site after anesthesia
- Operative services, including inspections around site and closure
- Appropriate post-op E/M visit(s)

CPT® CODE 50760

Ureteroureterostomy

POLICY INDICATORS

Global Period
90 day post-op period

Assistants at Surgery
Assistant allowed

Co-Surgeons Allowed
Submit reason for co-surgeon

Reduction for Multiple Procedures
Subject to 50% reduction

Bilateral Surgery Payment
150% paid if bilateral

Applicable Medicare Policies
Inpatient-only list

Relative Value Units (RVUs)

Work RVUs	20.07
Non-Facility Total	Only valued for facility
Facility Total	33.84

Coding Assistance

50760 includes:

- Positioning and prepping patient
- Examination of site after anesthesia
- Operative services, including inspections around site and closure
- Appropriate post-op E/M visit(s)

SURGERY

CPT® CODE 50770

Transureteroureterostomy, anastomosis of ureter to contralateral ureter

POLICY INDICATORS

Global Period
90 day post-op period

Assistants at Surgery
Assistant allowed

Co-Surgeons Allowed
Submit reason for co-surgeon

Reduction for Multiple Procedures
Subject to 50% reduction

Bilateral Surgery Payment
N/A

Applicable Medicare Policies
Inpatient-only list

Relative Value Units (RVUs)

Work RVUs	21.22
Non-Facility Total	Only valued for facility
Facility Total	34.49

Coding Assistance

50770 includes:

- Positioning and prepping patient
- Examination of site after anesthesia
- Operative services, including inspections around site and closure
- Appropriate post-op E/M visit(s)

CPT® CODE 50780

Ureteroneocystostomy; anastomosis of single ureter to bladder

POLICY INDICATORS

Global Period
90 day post-op period

Assistants at Surgery
Assistant allowed

Co-Surgeons Allowed
Submit reason for co-surgeon

Reduction for Multiple Procedures
Subject to 50% reduction

Bilateral Surgery Payment
150% paid if bilateral

Applicable Medicare Policies
Inpatient-only list

Relative Value Units (RVUs)

Work RVUs	19.95
Non-Facility Total	Only valued for facility
Facility Total	33.39

Coding Assistance

50780 includes:

- Positioning and prepping patient
- Examination of site after anesthesia
- Operative services, including inspections around site and closure
- Appropriate post-op E/M visit(s)

CPT® CODE 50785

Ureteroneocystostomy; with vesico-psoas hitch or bladder flap

POLICY INDICATORS

Global Period
90 day post-op period

Assistants at Surgery
Assistant allowed

Co-Surgeons Allowed
Submit reason for co-surgeon

Reduction for Multiple Procedures
Subject to 50% reduction

Bilateral Surgery Payment
150% paid if bilateral

Applicable Medicare Policies
Inpatient-only list

Relative Value Units (RVUs)

Work RVUs	22.23
Non-Facility Total	Only valued for facility
Facility Total	36.39

Coding Assistance

50785 includes:

- Positioning and prepping patient
- Examination of site after anesthesia
- Operative services, including inspections around site and closure
- Appropriate post-op E/M visit(s)

CPT® CODE 50800

Ureteroenterostomy, direct anastomosis of ureter to intestine

POLICY INDICATORS

Global Period
90 day post-op period

Assistants at Surgery
Assistant allowed

Co-Surgeons Allowed
Submit reason for co-surgeon

Reduction for Multiple Procedures
Subject to 50% reduction

Bilateral Surgery Payment
150% paid if bilateral

Applicable Medicare Policies
Inpatient-only list

Relative Value Units (RVUs)

Work RVUs	16.41
Non-Facility Total	Only valued for facility
Facility Total	27.69

Coding Assistance

50800 includes:

- Positioning and prepping patient
- Examination of site after anesthesia
- Operative services, including inspections around site and closure
- Appropriate post-op E/M visit(s)

CPT® CODE 50810

Ureterosigmoidostomy, with creation of sigmoid bladder and establishment of abdominal or perineal colostomy, including intestine anastomosis

POLICY INDICATORS

Global Period
90 day post-op period

Assistants at Surgery
Assistant allowed

Co-Surgeons Allowed
Submit reason for co-surgeon

Reduction for Multiple Procedures
Subject to 50% reduction

Bilateral Surgery Payment
N/A

Applicable Medicare Policies
Inpatient-only list

Relative Value Units (RVUs)

Work RVUs	22.61
Non-Facility Total	Only valued for facility
Facility Total	42.52

Coding Assistance

50810 includes:

- Positioning and prepping patient
- Examination of site after anesthesia
- Operative services, including inspections around site and closure
- Appropriate post-op E/M visit(s)

CPT® CODE 50815

Ureterocolon conduit, including intestine anastomosis

POLICY INDICATORS

Global Period
90 day post-op period

Assistants at Surgery
Assistant allowed

Co-Surgeons Allowed
Submit reason for co-surgeon

Reduction for Multiple Procedures
Subject to 50% reduction

Bilateral Surgery Payment
150% paid if bilateral

Applicable Medicare Policies
Inpatient-only list

Relative Value Units (RVUs)

Work RVUs	22.26
Non-Facility Total	Only valued for facility
Facility Total	36.67

Coding Assistance

50815 includes:

- Positioning and prepping patient
- Examination of site after anesthesia
- Operative services, including inspections around site and closure
- Appropriate post-op E/M visit(s)

CPT® CODE 50820

Ureteroileal conduit (ileal bladder), including intestine anastomosis (Bricker operation)

POLICY INDICATORS

Global Period
90 day post-op period

Assistants at Surgery
Assistant allowed

Co-Surgeons Allowed
Submit reason for co-surgeon

Reduction for Multiple Procedures
Subject to 50% reduction

Bilateral Surgery Payment
150% paid if bilateral

Applicable Medicare Policies
Inpatient-only list

Relative Value Units (RVUs)

Work RVUs	24.07
Non-Facility Total	Only valued for facility
Facility Total	39.29

Coding Assistance

50820 includes:

- Positioning and prepping patient
- Examination of site after anesthesia
- Operative services, including inspections around site and closure
- Appropriate post-op E/M visit(s)

CPT® CODE 50825

Continent diversion, including intestine anastomosis using any segment of small and/or large intestine (Kock pouch or Camey enterocystoplasty)

POLICY INDICATORS

Global Period
90 day post-op period

Assistants at Surgery
Assistant allowed

Co-Surgeons Allowed
Submit reason for co-surgeon

Reduction for Multiple Procedures
Subject to 50% reduction

Bilateral Surgery Payment
N/A

Applicable Medicare Policies
Inpatient-only list

Relative Value Units (RVUs)

Work RVUs	30.68
Non-Facility Total	Only valued for facility
Facility Total	49.16

Coding Assistance

50825 includes:

- Positioning and prepping patient
- Examination of site after anesthesia
- Operative services, including inspections around site and closure
- Appropriate post-op E/M visit(s)

CPT® CODE 50830

Urinary undiversion (eg, taking down of ureteroileal conduit, ureterosigmoidostomy or ureteroenterostomy with ureteroureterostomy or ureteroneocystostomy)

POLICY INDICATORS

Global Period
90 day post-op period

Assistants at Surgery
Assistant allowed

Co-Surgeons Allowed
Submit reason for co-surgeon

Reduction for Multiple Procedures
Subject to 50% reduction

Bilateral Surgery Payment
N/A

Applicable Medicare Policies
Inpatient-only list

Relative Value Units (RVUs)

Work RVUs	33.77
Non-Facility Total	Only valued for facility
Facility Total	53.73

Coding Assistance

50830 includes:

- Positioning and prepping patient
- Examination of site after anesthesia
- Operative services, including inspections around site and closure
- Appropriate post-op E/M visit(s)

CPT® CODE 50900

Ureterorrhaphy, suture of ureter (separate procedure)

POLICY INDICATORS

Global Period
90 day post-op period

Assistants at Surgery
Assistant allowed

Co-Surgeons Allowed
Submit reason for co-surgeon

Reduction for Multiple Procedures
Subject to 50% reduction

Bilateral Surgery Payment
150% paid if bilateral

Applicable Medicare Policies
Inpatient-only list

Relative Value Units (RVUs)

Work RVUs	15.04
Non-Facility Total	Only valued for facility
Facility Total	25.32

Coding Assistance

50900 includes:

- Positioning and prepping patient
- Examination of site after anesthesia
- Operative services, including inspections around site and closure
- Appropriate post-op E/M visit(s)

CPT® CODE 50947

Laparoscopy, surgical; ureteroneocystostomy with cystoscopy and ureteral stent placement

POLICY INDICATORS

Global Period
90 day post-op period

Assistants at Surgery
Assistant allowed

Co-Surgeons Allowed
Submit reason for co-surgeon

Reduction for Multiple Procedures
Subject to 50% reduction

Bilateral Surgery Payment
150% paid if bilateral

Applicable Medicare Policies

Relative Value Units (RVUs)

Work RVUs	25.78
Non-Facility Total	Only valued for facility
Facility Total	41.28

Coding Assistance

50947 includes:

- Positioning and prepping patient
- Examination of site after anesthesia
- Operative services, including inspections around site and closure
- Appropriate post-op E/M visit(s)

Abbreviated Case Note Example:

- A 15-year-old female patient with recurrent UTIs is found to have grade III left-sided vesicoureteral reflux. Due to breakthrough UTIs and recurrent left pyelonephritis, ureteral implant is recommended. The parents have elected for a laparoscopic left ureteral reimplant rather than an open procedure.
- Procedure: A periumbilical incision is made in a circumferential direction inferior to the umbilicus. Introduce a disposable trocar and laparoscope and insufflate the abdomen. Three 5-mm instruments are introduced. After these ports are placed, dissect to mobilize the ureter just proximal to the broad ligament and down to the ureterovesical junction. Incise along the left lateral aspect of the bladder in a direction such that the ureter can lie in a nonkinking position into the trough. Insert a cystoscope into the bladder and advance a French ureteral stent up the left ureter to the kidney. Under laparoscopic vision, the stent is seen to slide up the ureter with ease. The urethral catheter is placed, all scopes are removed, and the abdominal wound is closed.

CPT® CODE 51040

Cystostomy, cystotomy with drainage

POLICY INDICATORS

Global Period
90 day post-op period

Assistants at Surgery
Assistant allowed

Co-Surgeons Allowed
Submit reason for co-surgeon

Reduction for Multiple Procedures
Subject to 50% reduction

Bilateral Surgery Payment
N/A

Applicable Medicare Policies

Relative Value Units (RVUs)

Work RVUs	4.49
Non-Facility Total	Only valued for facility
Facility Total	8.86

Coding Assistance

51040 includes:

- Positioning and prepping patient
- Examination of site after anesthesia
- Operative services, including inspections around site and closure
- Appropriate post-op E/M visit(s)

CPT® CODE 51045

Cystotomy, with insertion of ureteral catheter or stent (separate procedure)

POLICY INDICATORS

Global Period
90 day post-op period

Assistants at Surgery
Assistant allowed

Co-Surgeons Allowed
No co-surgeon

Reduction for Multiple Procedures
Subject to 50% reduction

Bilateral Surgery Payment
N/A

Applicable Medicare Policies

Relative Value Units (RVUs)

Work RVUs	7.81
Non-Facility Total	Only valued for facility
Facility Total	14.86

Coding Assistance

51045 includes:

- Positioning and prepping patient
- Examination of site after anesthesia
- Operative services, including inspections around site and closure
- Appropriate post-op E/M visit(s)

CPT® CODE 51050

Cystolithotomy, cystotomy with removal of calculus, without vesical neck resection

POLICY INDICATORS

Global Period
90 day post-op period

Assistants at Surgery
Assistant allowed

Co-Surgeons Allowed
Submit reason for co-surgeon

Reduction for Multiple Procedures
Subject to 50% reduction

Bilateral Surgery Payment
N/A

Applicable Medicare Policies

Relative Value Units (RVUs)

Work RVUs	7.97
Non-Facility Total	Only valued for facility
Facility Total	14.30

Coding Assistance

51050 includes:

- Positioning and prepping patient
- Examination of site after anesthesia
- Operative services, including inspections around site and closure
- Appropriate post-op E/M visit(s)

CPT® CODE 51600

Injection procedure for cystography or voiding urethrocystography

POLICY INDICATORS

Global Period
0 day post-op period

Assistants at Surgery
No assistant

Co-Surgeons Allowed
No co-surgeon

Reduction for Multiple Procedures
Subject to 50% reduction

Bilateral Surgery Payment
N/A

Applicable Medicare Policies

Relative Value Units (RVUs)

Work RVUs	0.88
Non-Facility Total	6.12
Facility Total	1.28

Coding Assistance

51600 includes:

- Positioning and prepping patient
- Examination of site after anesthesia
- Operative services, including inspections around site and closure

Abbreviated Case Note Example:

- A 45-year-old female patient has had chronic urinary tract infections and stress urinary incontinence with a history of two previous operations for urinary incontinence.
- Procedure: A #16 Foley catheter is placed. The bladder is filled with contrast under fluoroscopy. The catheter is removed, and the patient voids in the upright position. A video recording is made.

CPT® CODE 51700

Bladder irrigation, simple, lavage and/or instillation

POLICY INDICATORS

Global Period
0 day post-op period

Assistants at Surgery
No assistant

Co-Surgeons Allowed
No co-surgeon

Reduction for Multiple Procedures
Subject to 50% reduction

Bilateral Surgery Payment
N/A

Applicable Medicare Policies

Relative Value Units (RVUs)

Work RVUs	0.60
Non-Facility Total	2.27
Facility Total	0.89

Coding Assistance

51700 includes:

- Positioning and prepping patient
- Examination of site after anesthesia
- Operative services, including inspections around site and closure

Abbreviated Case Note Example:

- A 57-year-old female patient with a long history of a female urethral syndrome and interstitial cystitis is treated with dimethyl sulfoxide (DMSO).
- Procedure: A urinary catheter is placed, and the bladder is drained. Then 50 cc of DMSO or other medication is placed in the bladder, and the catheter is clamped. The bladder is drained, and the catheter is removed.

CPT® CODE 51701

Insertion of non-indwelling bladder catheter (eg, straight catheterization for residual urine)

POLICY INDICATORS

Global Period
0 day post-op period

Assistants at Surgery
No assistant

Co-Surgeons Allowed
No co-surgeon

Reduction for Multiple Procedures
Subject to 50% reduction

Bilateral Surgery Payment
N/A

Applicable Medicare Policies

Relative Value Units (RVUs)

Work RVUs	0.50
Non-Facility Total	1.32
Facility Total	0.75

Coding Assistance

51701 includes:

- Positioning and prepping patient
- Examination of site after anesthesia
- Operative services, including inspections around site and closure

Abbreviated Case Note Example:

- A 72-year-old patient presents with incomplete bladder emptying. A postvoid residual urine with straight catherization is performed to determine the amount of urine left in the bladder.
- Procedure: Insert the catheter via urethra into the bladder. Drain urine from the bladder into a graduated cylinder. Measure the residual urine in milliliters. Remove the temporary catheter from the patient's bladder/urethra and discard. Remove the scrub solution from the patient's genitalia.

CPT® CODE 51702

Insertion of temporary indwelling bladder catheter; simple (eg, Foley)

POLICY INDICATORS

Global Period
0 day post-op period

Assistants at Surgery
No assistant

Co-Surgeons Allowed
No co-surgeon

Reduction for Multiple Procedures
Subject to 50% reduction

Bilateral Surgery Payment
N/A

Applicable Medicare Policies

Relative Value Units (RVUs)

Work RVUs	0.50
Non-Facility Total	1.85
Facility Total	0.74

Coding Assistance

51702 includes:

- Positioning and prepping patient
- Examination of site after anesthesia
- Operative services, including inspections around site and closure

Abbreviated Case Note Example:

- A 60-year-old patient presents with retention of urine. An in-dwelling catheter with bag is placed to allow bladder drainage.
- Procedure: Insert the catheter via urethra into the bladder. Inflate the balloon of the catheter to ensure it does not fall out. Drain urine from the bladder into the collection bag and measure residual urine in milliliters. Secure the catheter to the patient's suprapubic region or inner thigh with a catheter-secure device. Discard the remaining catheter supplies. Remove the scrub solution from the patient's genitalia.

CPT® CODE 51703

Insertion of temporary indwelling bladder catheter; complicated (eg, altered anatomy, fractured catheter/balloon)

POLICY INDICATORS

Global Period
0 day post-op period

Assistants at Surgery
No assistant

Co-Surgeons Allowed
No co-surgeon

Reduction for Multiple Procedures
Subject to 50% reduction

Bilateral Surgery Payment
N/A

Applicable Medicare Policies

Relative Value Units (RVUs)

Work RVUs	1.47
Non-Facility Total	4.43
Facility Total	2.27

Coding Assistance

51703 includes:

- Positioning and prepping patient
- Examination of site after anesthesia
- Operative services, including inspections around site and closure

CPT® CODE 51705

Change of cystostomy tube; simple

POLICY INDICATORS

Global Period
0 day post-op period

Assistants at Surgery
No assistant

Co-Surgeons Allowed
No co-surgeon

Reduction for Multiple Procedures
Subject to 50% reduction

Bilateral Surgery Payment
N/A

Applicable Medicare Policies

Relative Value Units (RVUs)

Work RVUs	0.90
Non-Facility Total	2.93
Facility Total	1.57

Coding Assistance

51705 includes:

- Positioning and prepping patient
- Examination of site after anesthesia
- Operative services, including inspections around site and closure

CPT® CODE 51710

Change of cystostomy tube; complicated

POLICY INDICATORS

Global Period
0 day post-op period

Assistants at Surgery
No assistant

Co-Surgeons Allowed
No co-surgeon

Reduction for Multiple Procedures
Subject to 50% reduction

Bilateral Surgery Payment
N/A

Applicable Medicare Policies

Relative Value Units (RVUs)

Work RVUs	1.35
Non-Facility Total	4.06
Facility Total	2.40

Coding Assistance

51710 includes:

- Positioning and prepping patient for catheter change
- Examination of tube site after anesthesia
- Operative services, including inspections around tube site and closure

CPT® CODE 51715

Endoscopic injection of implant material into the submucosal tissues of the urethra and/or bladder neck

POLICY INDICATORS

Global Period
0 day post-op period

Assistants at Surgery
Submit reason for assistant

Co-Surgeons Allowed
No co-surgeon

Reduction for Multiple Procedures
Subject to 50% reduction

Bilateral Surgery Payment
N/A

Applicable Medicare Policies

Relative Value Units (RVUs)

Work RVUs	3.73
Non-Facility Total	10.52
Facility Total	5.95

Coding Assistance

51715 includes:

- Positioning and prepping patient
- Examination of site after anesthesia
- Operative services, including inspections around site and closure

CPT® CODE 51720

Bladder instillation of anticarcinogenic agent (including retention time)

POLICY INDICATORS

Global Period
0 day post-op period

Assistants at Surgery
No assistant

Co-Surgeons Allowed
No co-surgeon

Reduction for Multiple Procedures
Subject to 50% reduction

Bilateral Surgery Payment
N/A

Applicable Medicare Policies

Relative Value Units (RVUs)

Work RVUs	0.87
Non-Facility Total	2.67
Facility Total	1.31

Coding Assistance

51720 includes:

- Positioning and prepping patient
- Examination of site after anesthesia
- Operative services, including inspections around site and closure

CPT® CODE 51800

Cystoplasty or cystourethroplasty, plastic operation on bladder and/or vesical neck (anterior Y-plasty, vesical fundus resection), any procedure, with or without wedge resection of posterior vesical neck

POLICY INDICATORS

Global Period
90 day post-op period

Assistants at Surgery
Assistant allowed

Co-Surgeons Allowed
Submit reason for co-surgeon

Reduction for Multiple Procedures
Subject to 50% reduction

Bilateral Surgery Payment
N/A

Applicable Medicare Policies
Inpatient-only list

Relative Value Units (RVUs)

Work RVUs	18.89
Non-Facility Total	Only valued for facility
Facility Total	31.10

Coding Assistance

51800 includes:

- Positioning and prepping patient
- Examination of site after anesthesia
- Operative services, including inspections around site and closure
- Appropriate post-op E/M visit(s)

CPT® CODE 51820

Cystourethroplasty with unilateral or bilateral ureteroneocystostomy

POLICY INDICATORS

Global Period
90 day post-op period

Assistants at Surgery
Assistant allowed

Co-Surgeons Allowed
Submit reason for co-surgeon

Reduction for Multiple Procedures
Subject to 50% reduction

Bilateral Surgery Payment
Bilateral surgery

Applicable Medicare Policies
Inpatient-only list

Relative Value Units (RVUs)

Work RVUs	19.59
Non-Facility Total	Only valued for facility
Facility Total	32.53

Coding Assistance

51820 includes:

- Positioning and prepping patient
- Examination of site after anesthesia
- Operative services, including inspections around site and closure
- Appropriate post-op E/M visit(s)

Additional Notes

- If a paravaginal defect repair is performed, report 58284 instead

CPT® CODE 51840

Anterior vesicourethropexy, or urethropexy (eg, Marshall-Marchetti-Krantz, Burch); simple

POLICY INDICATORS

Global Period
90 day post-op period

Assistants at Surgery
Assistant allowed

Co-Surgeons Allowed
Submit reason for co-surgeon

Reduction for Multiple Procedures
Subject to 50% reduction

Bilateral Surgery Payment
N/A

Applicable Medicare Policies
Inpatient-only list

Relative Value Units (RVUs)

Work RVUs	11.36
Non-Facility Total	Only valued for facility
Facility Total	20.90

Coding Assistance

51840 includes:

- Positioning and prepping patient
- Examination of site after anesthesia
- Operative services, including inspections around site and closure
- Appropriate post-op E/M visit(s)

Additional Notes

- If a paravaginal defect repair is performed, report 58284 instead

CPT® CODE 51841

Anterior vesicourethropexy, or urethropexy (eg, Marshall-Marchetti-Krantz, Burch); complicated (eg, secondary repair)

POLICY INDICATORS

Global Period
90 day post-op period

Assistants at Surgery
Assistant allowed

Co-Surgeons Allowed
Submit reason for co-surgeon

Reduction for Multiple Procedures
Subject to 50% reduction

Bilateral Surgery Payment
N/A

Applicable Medicare Policies
Inpatient-only list

Relative Value Units (RVUs)

Work RVUs	13.68
Non-Facility Total	Only valued for facility
Facility Total	24.15

Coding Assistance

51841 includes:

- Positioning and prepping patient
- Examination of site after anesthesia
- Operative services, including inspections around site and closure
- Appropriate post-op E/M visit(s)
- Cystoscopy to ensure bladder integrity

CPT® CODE 51845

Abdomino-vaginal vesical neck suspension, with or without endoscopic control (eg, Stamey, Raz, modified Pereyra)

POLICY INDICATORS

Global Period
90 day post-op period

Assistants at Surgery
Assistant allowed

Co-Surgeons Allowed
Submit reason for co-surgeon

Reduction for Multiple Procedures
Subject to 50% reduction

Bilateral Surgery Payment
N/A

Applicable Medicare Policies

Relative Value Units (RVUs)

Work RVUs	10.15
Non-Facility Total	Only valued for facility
Facility Total	17.58

Coding Assistance

51845 includes:

- Positioning and prepping patient
- Examination of site after anesthesia
- Operative services, including inspections around site and closure
- Appropriate post-op E/M visit(s)
- Photodocumentation
- Cystoscopy to ensure bladder integrity

CPT® CODE 51860

Cystorrhaphy, suture of bladder wound, injury or rupture; simple

POLICY INDICATORS

Global Period
90 day post-op period

Assistants at Surgery
Assistant allowed

Co-Surgeons Allowed
Submit reason for co-surgeon

Reduction for Multiple Procedures
Subject to 50% reduction

Bilateral Surgery Payment
N/A

Applicable Medicare Policies

Relative Value Units (RVUs)

Work RVUs	12.60
Non-Facility Total	Only valued for facility
Facility Total	22.39

Coding Assistance

51860 includes:

- Positioning and prepping patient
- Examination of site after anesthesia
- Operative services, including inspections around site and closure
- Appropriate post-op E/M visit(s)

CPT® CODE 51865

Cystorrhaphy, suture of bladder wound, injury or rupture; complicated

POLICY INDICATORS

Global Period
90 day post-op period

Assistants at Surgery
Assistant allowed

Co-Surgeons Allowed
Submit reason for co-surgeon

Reduction for Multiple Procedures
Subject to 50% reduction

Bilateral Surgery Payment
N/A

Applicable Medicare Policies
Inpatient-only list

Relative Value Units (RVUs)

Work RVUs	15.80
Non-Facility Total	Only valued for facility
Facility Total	26.85

Coding Assistance

51865 includes:

- Positioning and prepping patient
- Examination of site after anesthesia
- Operative services, including inspections around site and closure
- Appropriate post-op E/M visit(s)

CPT® CODE 51880

Closure of cystostomy (separate procedure)

POLICY INDICATORS

Global Period
90 day post-op period

Assistants at Surgery
Assistant allowed

Co-Surgeons Allowed
Submit reason for co-surgeon

Reduction for Multiple Procedures
Subject to 50% reduction

Bilateral Surgery Payment
N/A

Applicable Medicare Policies

Relative Value Units (RVUs)

Work RVUs	7.87
Non-Facility Total	Only valued for facility
Facility Total	14.03

Coding Assistance

51880 includes:

- Positioning and prepping patient
- Examination of site after anesthesia
- Operative services, including inspections around site and closure
- Appropriate post-op E/M visit(s)

CPT® CODE 51900

Closure of vesicovaginal fistula, abdominal approach

POLICY INDICATORS

Global Period
90 day post-op period

Assistants at Surgery
Assistant allowed

Co-Surgeons Allowed
Submit reason for co-surgeon

Reduction for Multiple Procedures
Subject to 50% reduction

Bilateral Surgery Payment
N/A

Applicable Medicare Policies
Inpatient-only list

Relative Value Units (RVUs)

Work RVUs	14.63
Non-Facility Total	Only valued for facility
Facility Total	24.80

Coding Assistance

51900 includes:

- Positioning and prepping patient
- Examination of site after anesthesia
- Operative services, including inspections around site and closure
- Appropriate post-op E/M visit(s)

CPT® CODE 51925

Closure of vesicouterine fistula; with hysterectomy

POLICY INDICATORS

Global Period
90 day post-op period

Assistants at Surgery
Assistant allowed

Co-Surgeons Allowed
Submit reason for co-surgeon

Reduction for Multiple Procedures
Subject to 50% reduction

Bilateral Surgery Payment
N/A

Applicable Medicare Policies
Inpatient-only list

Relative Value Units (RVUs)

Work RVUs	17.53
Non-Facility Total	Only valued for facility
Facility Total	32.31

Coding Assistance

51925 includes:

- Positioning and prepping patient
- Examination of site after anesthesia
- Operative services, including inspections around site and closure
- Appropriate post-op E/M visit(s)

CPT® CODE 51980

Cutaneous vesicostomy

POLICY INDICATORS

Global Period
90 day post-op period

Assistants at Surgery
Assistant allowed

Co-Surgeons Allowed
Submit reason for co-surgeon

Reduction for Multiple Procedures
Subject to 50% reduction

Bilateral Surgery Payment
N/A

Applicable Medicare Policies
Inpatient-only list

Relative Value Units (RVUs)

Work RVUs	12.57
Non-Facility Total	Only valued for facility
Facility Total	21.48

Coding Assistance

51980 includes:

- Positioning and prepping patient
- Examination of site after anesthesia
- Operative services, including inspections around site and closure
- Appropriate post-op E/M visit(s)

CPT® CODE 51990

Laparoscopy, surgical; urethral suspension for stress incontinence

POLICY INDICATORS

Global Period
90 day post-op period

Assistants at Surgery
Assistant allowed

Co-Surgeons Allowed
Submit reason for co-surgeon

Reduction for Multiple Procedures
Subject to 50% reduction

Bilateral Surgery Payment
N/A

Applicable Medicare Policies

Relative Value Units (RVUs)

Work RVUs	13.36
Non-Facility Total	Only valued for facility
Facility Total	22.37

Coding Assistance

51990 includes:

- Positioning and prepping patient
- Examination of site after anesthesia
- Operative services, including inspections around site and closure
- Appropriate post-op E/M visit(s)

Abbreviated Case Note Example:

- A 45-year-old female patient who presents with a genuine stress urinary incontinence has failed medical therapy and wears four to five pads a day. Urodynamic testing reveals a compliant bladder without uninhibited contractions and good detrusor activity. She has tried Kegel exercises without success. Open surgery and laparoscopic repair are offered, but the patient consents to the laparoscopic urethral suspension.
- Procedure: An extraperitoneal or transperitoneal approach using four trocar-sheath units is placed in a diamond configuration to access the pelvic organs; place two stitches of 2-0 nonabsorbable suture laparoscopically into the endopelvic fascia at the bladder neck region on each side and secure them to the ipsilateral Cooper's ligament. Tie the sutures with extracorporeal or intracorporeal knots so as to create a hammock-type suspension of the bladder neck, and remove the ports. Close the sites in the usual fashion.

Additional Notes

- A diagnostic laparoscopy is included in this procedure
- This code is used to report a laparoscopic Burch procedure

CPT® CODE 51992

Laparoscopy, surgical; sling operation for stress incontinence (eg, fascia or synthetic)

POLICY INDICATORS

Global Period
90 day post-op period

Assistants at Surgery
Assistant allowed

Co-Surgeons Allowed
Submit reason for co-surgeon

Reduction for Multiple Procedures
Subject to 50% reduction

Bilateral Surgery Payment
N/A

Applicable Medicare Policies

Relative Value Units (RVUs)

Work RVUs	14.87
Non-Facility Total	Only valued for facility
Facility Total	25.09

Coding Assistance

51992 includes:

- Positioning and prepping patient
- Examination of site after anesthesia
- Operative services, including inspections around site and closure
- Appropriate post-op E/M visit(s)
- Photodocumentation

Abbreviated Case Note Example:

- A 55-year-old female patient presents with genuine stress urinary incontinence that has failed medical therapy and wears four to five pads a day. Urodynamic testing reveals a compliant bladder without uninhibited contractions and good detrusor activity. She has tried Kegel exercises without success. She consents and is scheduled for a laparoscopic sling operation.
- Procedure: Using an extraperitoneal or transperitoneal approach with five trocar sheaths, expose the bladder neck and Cooper's ligament. Open the endopelvic fascia and dissect a tunnel between the urethra and vagina mucosa. Then pass sling material (cadaver or synthetic) and secure to Cooper's ligament bilaterally. Remove the ports and close the sites in the usual fashion.

Additional Notes

- A diagnostic laparoscopy is included in this procedure

CPT® CODE 52000

Cystourethroscopy (separate procedure)

POLICY INDICATORS

Global Period
0 day post-op period

Assistants at Surgery
No assistant

Co-Surgeons Allowed
No co-surgeon

Reduction for Multiple Procedures
Subject to 50% reduction

Bilateral Surgery Payment
N/A

Applicable Medicare Policies

Relative Value Units (RVUs)

Work RVUs	1.53
Non-Facility Total	6.59
Facility Total	2.39

Coding Assistance

52000 includes:

- Positioning and prepping patient
- Examination of site after anesthesia
- Operative services, including inspections around site and closure
- Photodocumentation

Abbreviated Case Note Example:

- A 55-year-old patient presents with gross hematuria. A diagnostic cystourethroscopy is performed to evaluate the bladder.
- Procedure: Insert the endoscope into the urethra, and inspect the relevant urethral anatomy, including the external urinary sphincter. Assess the bladder neck, inspect the trigone, and identify the ureteral orifices. A check for efflux of urine from each ureteral orifice is made. The bladder mucosa is inspected, and the bladder capacity, compliance, and sensation is made. A retroflex scope, if flexible, is used to inspect the bladder's dome. The bladder is drained, and the endoscope is removed.

SURGERY

CPT® CODE 52001

Cystourethroscopy with irrigation and evacuation of multiple obstructing clots

POLICY INDICATORS

Global Period
0 day post-op period

Assistants at Surgery
No assistant

Co-Surgeons Allowed
No co-surgeon

Reduction for Multiple Procedures
Endoscopy payment rules apply

Bilateral Surgery Payment
N/A

Applicable Medicare Policies

Relative Value Units (RVUs)

Work RVUs	5.44
Non-Facility Total	12.59
Facility Total	8.51

Coding Assistance

52001 includes:

- Positioning and prepping patient
- Examination of site after anesthesia
- Operative services, including inspections around site and closure

Abbreviated Case Note Example:

- A 55-year-old patient presents with lower abdominal pain and copious amounts of feculent material. On physical examination, her bladder is tender and distended. Several urethra catheters are placed, but they rapidly obstruct secondary to clots.
- Procedure: General anesthesia is given and found to be adequate. Copious amounts of feculent material is evacuated from the patient's vagina. A 70-degree cystoscope is placed in the patient's bladder and significant feculent material is visualized. The bladder is irrigated with approximately 2 L of sterile water until visualization improves. An extremely thorough survey of the bladder reveals no evidence of discrete fistula. Scattered small to medium diverticula are notable. There is some evidence of brisk left ureteral jets, which appear somewhat discolored, but no clear feculent material is emanating from this area. All instruments are removed from the bladder.

CPT® CODE 52005

Cystourethroscopy, with ureteral catheterization, with or without irrigation, instillation, or ureteropyelography, exclusive of radiologic service

POLICY INDICATORS

Global Period
0 day post-op period

Assistants at Surgery
No assistant

Co-Surgeons Allowed
No co-surgeon

Reduction for Multiple Procedures
Endoscopy payment rules apply

Bilateral Surgery Payment
N/A

Applicable Medicare Policies

Relative Value Units (RVUs)

Work RVUs	2.37
Non-Facility Total	8.51
Facility Total	3.98

Coding Assistance

52005 includes:

- Positioning and prepping patient
- Examination of site after anesthesia
- Operative services, including inspections around site and closure

Abbreviated Case Note Example:

- A 55-year-old patient presents with lower abdominal pain and copious amounts of feculent material. On physical examination, her bladder is tender and distended. Several urethra catheters are placed, but they rapidly obstruct secondary to clots.
- Procedure: General anesthesia is given and found to be adequate. Copious amounts of feculent material is evacuated from the patient's vagina. A 70-degree cystoscope is placed in the patient's bladder and significant feculent material is visualized. The bladder is irrigated with approximately 2 L of sterile water until visualization improves. An extremely thorough survey of the bladder reveals no evidence of discrete fistula. Scattered small to medium diverticula are notable. There is some evidence of brisk left ureteral jets, which appear somewhat discolored, but no clear feculent material is emanating from this area. All instruments are removed from the bladder.

CPT® CODE 52007

Cystourethroscopy, with ureteral catheterization, with or without irrigation, instillation, or ureteropyelography, exclusive of radiologic service; with brush biopsy of ureter and/or renal pelvis

POLICY INDICATORS

Global Period
0 day post-op period

Assistants at Surgery
No assistant

Co-Surgeons Allowed
No co-surgeon

Reduction for Multiple Procedures
Endoscopy payment rules apply

Bilateral Surgery Payment
150% paid if bilateral

Applicable Medicare Policies

Relative Value Units (RVUs)

Work RVUs	3.02
Non-Facility Total	12.73
Facility Total	4.96

Coding Assistance

52007 includes:

- Positioning and prepping patient
- Examination of site after anesthesia
- Operative services, including inspections around site and closure

CPT® CODE 52010

Cystourethroscopy, with ejaculatory duct catheterization, with or without irrigation, instillation, or duct radiography, exclusive of radiologic service

POLICY INDICATORS

Global Period
0 day post-op period

Assistants at Surgery
No assistant

Co-Surgeons Allowed
No co-surgeon

Reduction for Multiple Procedures
Endoscopy payment rules apply

Bilateral Surgery Payment
N/A

Applicable Medicare Policies

Relative Value Units (RVUs)

Work RVUs	3.02
Non-Facility Total	10.82
Facility Total	4.94

Coding Assistance

52010 includes:

- Positioning and prepping patient
- Examination of site after anesthesia
- Operative services, including inspections around site and closure

CPT® CODE 52204

Cystourethroscopy, with biopsy(s)

POLICY INDICATORS

Global Period
0 day post-op period

Assistants at Surgery
No assistant

Co-Surgeons Allowed
No co-surgeon

Reduction for Multiple Procedures
Endoscopy payment rules apply

Bilateral Surgery Payment
N/A

Applicable Medicare Policies

Relative Value Units (RVUs)

Work RVUs	2.59
Non-Facility Total	10.61
Facility Total	4.21

Coding Assistance

52204 includes:

- Positioning and prepping patient
- Examination of site after anesthesia
- Operative services, including inspections around site and closure

CPT® CODE 52214

Cystourethroscopy, with fulguration (including cryosurgery or laser surgery) of trigone, bladder neck, prostatic fossa, urethra, or periurethral glands

POLICY INDICATORS

Global Period
0 day post-op period

Assistants at Surgery
No assistant

Co-Surgeons Allowed
No co-surgeon

Reduction for Multiple Procedures
Endoscopy payment rules apply

Bilateral Surgery Payment
N/A

Applicable Medicare Policies

Relative Value Units (RVUs)

Work RVUs	3.50
Non-Facility Total	21.21
Facility Total	5.20

Coding Assistance

52214 includes:

- Positioning and prepping patient
- Examination of site after anesthesia
- Operative services, including inspections around site and closure

CPT® CODE 52224

Cystourethroscopy, with fulguration (including cryosurgery or laser surgery) or treatment of MINOR (less than 0.5 cm) lesion(s) with or without biopsy

POLICY INDICATORS

Global Period
0 day post-op period

Assistants at Surgery
No assistant

Co-Surgeons Allowed
No co-surgeon

Reduction for Multiple Procedures
Endoscopy payment rules apply

Bilateral Surgery Payment
N/A

Applicable Medicare Policies

Relative Value Units (RVUs)

Work RVUs	4.05
Non-Facility Total	22.20
Facility Total	6.01

Coding Assistance

52224 includes:

- Positioning and prepping patient
- Examination of site after anesthesia
- Operative services, including inspections around site and closure

CPT® CODE 52234

Cystourethroscopy, with fulguration (including cryosurgery or laser surgery) and/or resection of; SMALL bladder tumor(s) (0.5 up to 2.0 cm)

POLICY INDICATORS

Global Period
0 day post-op period

Assistants at Surgery
No assistant

Co-Surgeons Allowed
No co-surgeon

Reduction for Multiple Procedures
Endoscopy payment rules apply

Bilateral Surgery Payment
N/A

Applicable Medicare Policies

Relative Value Units (RVUs)

Work RVUs	4.62
Non-Facility Total	Only valued for facility
Facility Total	7.30

Coding Assistance

52234 includes:

- Positioning and prepping patient
- Examination of site after anesthesia
- Operative services, including inspections around site and closure

Abbreviated Case Note Example:

- A 52-year-old female patient presents with painless hematuria. Previous cystoscopy demonstrated a 1-cm bladder tumor. Transurethral resection and fulguration of the bladder tumor is performed.
- Procedure: Under general anesthesia, a cystoscope is inserted and the bladder is completely visualized to assess the tumor burden. The ureteral orifices are identified in relation to the location of the tumor(s). The cystoscope is removed and a resectoscope is inserted. The tumor(s) is resected, the base of the tumor(s) is fulgurated, and the specimen(s) is retrieved. A Foley catheter may be placed. If cryosurgery, laser ablation, or fulguration is planned, the appropriate energy source will be passed through the cystoscope and the tumor(s) treated.

CPT® CODE 52235

Cystourethroscopy, with fulguration (including cryosurgery or laser surgery) and/or resection of; MEDIUM bladder tumor(s) (2.0 to 5.0 cm)

POLICY INDICATORS

Global Period
0 day post-op period

Assistants at Surgery
No assistant

Co-Surgeons Allowed
No co-surgeon

Reduction for Multiple Procedures
Endoscopy payment rules apply

Bilateral Surgery Payment
N/A

Applicable Medicare Policies

Relative Value Units (RVUs)

Work RVUs	5.44
Non-Facility Total	Only valued for facility
Facility Total	8.55

Coding Assistance

52235 includes:

- Positioning and prepping patient
- Examination of site after anesthesia
- Operative services, including inspections around site and closure

CPT® CODE 52240

Cystourethroscopy, with fulguration (including cryosurgery or laser surgery) and/or resection of; LARGE bladder tumor(s)

POLICY INDICATORS

Global Period
0 day post-op period

Assistants at Surgery
No assistant

Co-Surgeons Allowed
No co-surgeon

Reduction for Multiple Procedures
Endoscopy payment rules apply

Bilateral Surgery Payment
N/A

Applicable Medicare Policies

Relative Value Units (RVUs)

Work RVUs	7.50
Non-Facility Total	Only valued for facility
Facility Total	11.60

Coding Assistance

52240 includes:

- Positioning and prepping patient
- Examination of site after anesthesia
- Operative services, including inspections around site and closure

SURGERY

CPT® CODE 52260

Cystourethroscopy, with dilation of bladder for interstitial cystitis; general or conduction (spinal) anesthesia

POLICY INDICATORS

Global Period
0 day post-op period

Assistants at Surgery
No assistant

Co-Surgeons Allowed
No co-surgeon

Reduction for Multiple Procedures
Endoscopy payment rules apply

Bilateral Surgery Payment
N/A

Applicable Medicare Policies

Relative Value Units (RVUs)

Work RVUs	3.91
Non-Facility Total	Only valued for facility
Facility Total	6.26

Coding Assistance

52260 includes:

- Positioning and prepping patient
- Examination of site after anesthesia
- Operative services, including inspections around site and closure

CPT® CODE 52265

Cystourethroscopy, with dilation of bladder for interstitial cystitis; local anesthesia

POLICY INDICATORS

Global Period
0 day post-op period

Assistants at Surgery
No assistant

Co-Surgeons Allowed
No co-surgeon

Reduction for Multiple Procedures
Endoscopy payment rules apply

Bilateral Surgery Payment
N/A

Applicable Medicare Policies

Relative Value Units (RVUs)

Work RVUs	2.94
Non-Facility Total	10.46
Facility Total	4.84

Coding Assistance

52265 includes:

- Positioning and prepping patient
- Examination of site after anesthesia
- Operative services, including inspections around site and closure

CPT® CODE 52270

Cystourethroscopy, with internal urethrotomy; female

POLICY INDICATORS

Global Period
0 day post-op period

Assistants at Surgery
No assistant

Co-Surgeons Allowed
No co-surgeon

Reduction for Multiple Procedures
Endoscopy payment rules apply

Bilateral Surgery Payment
N/A

Applicable Medicare Policies

Relative Value Units (RVUs)

Work RVUs	3.36
Non-Facility Total	11.92
Facility Total	5.42

Coding Assistance

52270 includes:

- Positioning and prepping patient
- Examination of site after anesthesia
- Operative services, including inspections around site and closure

CPT® CODE 52276

Cystourethroscopy with direct vision internal urethrotomy

POLICY INDICATORS

Global Period
0 day post-op period

Assistants at Surgery
No assistant

Co-Surgeons Allowed
No co-surgeon

Reduction for Multiple Procedures
Endoscopy payment rules apply

Bilateral Surgery Payment
N/A

Applicable Medicare Policies

Relative Value Units (RVUs)

Work RVUs	4.99
Non-Facility Total	Only valued for facility
Facility Total	7.85

Coding Assistance

52276 includes:

- Positioning and prepping patient
- Examination of site after anesthesia
- Operative services, including inspections around site and closure

CPT® CODE 52281

Cystourethroscopy, with calibration and/or dilation of urethral stricture or stenosis, with or without meatotomy, with or without injection procedure for cystography, male or female

POLICY INDICATORS

Global Period
0 day post-op period

Assistants at Surgery
No assistant

Co-Surgeons Allowed
No co-surgeon

Reduction for Multiple Procedures
Endoscopy payment rules apply

Bilateral Surgery Payment
N/A

Applicable Medicare Policies

Relative Value Units (RVUs)

Work RVUs	2.75
Non-Facility Total	9.18
Facility Total	4.54

Coding Assistance

52281 includes:

- Positioning and prepping patient
- Examination of site after anesthesia
- Operative services, including inspections around site and closure

CPT® CODE 52283

Cystourethroscopy, with steroid injection into stricture

POLICY INDICATORS

Global Period
0 day post-op period

Assistants at Surgery
No assistant

Co-Surgeons Allowed
No co-surgeon

Reduction for Multiple Procedures
Endoscopy payment rules apply

Bilateral Surgery Payment
N/A

Applicable Medicare Policies

Relative Value Units (RVUs)

Work RVUs	3.73
Non-Facility Total	10.08
Facility Total	6.02

Coding Assistance

52283 includes:

- Positioning and prepping patient
- Examination of site after anesthesia
- Operative services, including inspections around site and closure

CPT® CODE 52285

Cystourethroscopy for treatment of the female urethral syndrome with any or all of the following: urethral meatotomy, urethral dilation, internal urethrotomy, lysis of urethrovaginal septal fibrosis, lateral incisions of the bladder neck, and fulguration

POLICY INDICATORS

Global Period
0 day post-op period

Assistants at Surgery
No assistant

Co-Surgeons Allowed
No co-surgeon

Reduction for Multiple Procedures
Endoscopy payment rules apply

Bilateral Surgery Payment
N/A

Applicable Medicare Policies

Relative Value Units (RVUs)

Work RVUs	3.60
Non-Facility Total	9.96
Facility Total	5.87

Coding Assistance

52285 includes:

- Positioning and prepping patient
- Examination of site after anesthesia
- Operative services, including inspections around site and closure

CPT® CODE 52287

Cystourethroscopy, with injection(s) for chemodenervation of the bladder

POLICY INDICATORS

Global Period
0 day post-op period

Assistants at Surgery
No assistant

Co-Surgeons Allowed
No co-surgeon

Reduction for Multiple Procedures
Endoscopy payment rules apply

Bilateral Surgery Payment
N/A

Applicable Medicare Policies

Relative Value Units (RVUs)

Work RVUs	3.20
Non-Facility Total	10.97
Facility Total	5.04

Coding Assistance

52287 includes:

- Positioning and prepping patient
- Examination of site after anesthesia
- Operative services, including inspections around site and closure
- Photodocumentation

Abbreviated Case Note Example:

- A 36-year-old female patient has failed conservative (drug therapy) for urinary urgency and urge urinary incontinence secondary to neurogenic detrusor overactivity. After it is explained to her, she consents to cystourethroscopy, with chemodenervation of the bladder by multiple intravesical injections of bladder muscle.
- Procedure: Prior to the injection, attach the syringe containing the reconstituted drug to the cystoscopic injection needle, which is then primed with approximately 1-mL of diluted drug to remove any air. Insert the cystoscope through the patient's urethra into the bladder under direct visualization. Distend the urinary bladder to near capacity with approximately 300 cc of cystoscopic irrigant using sterile normal saline. Under direct vision, place the cystoscopic needle at 2 to 4 mm of depth into the bladder detrussor muscle ensuring the needle depth has not perforated the bladder. At the end of the injection procedure, drain the bladder and reinsert the cystoscope to refill the bladder and observe for any bleeding and ensure there is no perforation or injuries. Redrain the bladder at the end of the procedure.

CPT® CODE 52310

Cystourethroscopy, with removal of foreign body, calculus, or ureteral stent from urethra or bladder (separate procedure); simple

POLICY INDICATORS

Global Period
0 day post-op period

Assistants at Surgery
No assistant

Co-Surgeons Allowed
No co-surgeon

Reduction for Multiple Procedures
Endoscopy payment rules apply

Bilateral Surgery Payment
N/A

Applicable Medicare Policies

Relative Value Units (RVUs)

Work RVUs	2.81
Non-Facility Total	9.04
Facility Total	4.52

Coding Assistance

52310 includes:

- Positioning and prepping patient
- Examination of site after anesthesia
- Operative services, including inspections around site and closure

CPT® CODE 52315

Cystourethroscopy, with removal of foreign body, calculus, or ureteral stent from urethra or bladder (separate procedure); complicated

POLICY INDICATORS

Global Period
0 day post-op period

Assistants at Surgery
No assistant

Co-Surgeons Allowed
No co-surgeon

Reduction for Multiple Procedures
Endoscopy payment rules apply

Bilateral Surgery Payment
N/A

Applicable Medicare Policies

Relative Value Units (RVUs)

Work RVUs	5.20
Non-Facility Total	13.51
Facility Total	8.14

Coding Assistance

52315 includes:

- Positioning and prepping patient
- Examination of site after anesthesia
- Operative services, including inspections around site and closure

CPT® CODE 52317

Litholapaxy: crushing or fragmentation of calculus by any means in bladder and removal of fragments; simple or small (less than 2.5 cm)

POLICY INDICATORS

Global Period
0 day post-op period

Assistants at Surgery
No assistant

Co-Surgeons Allowed
No co-surgeon

Reduction for Multiple Procedures
Endoscopy payment rules apply

Bilateral Surgery Payment
N/A

Applicable Medicare Policies

Relative Value Units (RVUs)

Work RVUs	6.71
Non-Facility Total	25.39
Facility Total	10.28

Coding Assistance

52317 includes:

- Positioning and prepping patient
- Examination of site after anesthesia
- Operative services, including inspections around site and closure

CPT® CODE 52318

Litholapaxy: crushing or fragmentation of calculus by any means in bladder and removal of fragments; complicated or large (over 2.5 cm)

POLICY INDICATORS

Global Period
0 day post-op period

Assistants at Surgery
No assistant

Co-Surgeons Allowed
No co-surgeon

Reduction for Multiple Procedures
Endoscopy payment rules apply

Bilateral Surgery Payment
N/A

Applicable Medicare Policies

Relative Value Units (RVUs)

Work RVUs	9.18
Non-Facility Total	Only valued for facility
Facility Total	14.02

Coding Assistance

52318 includes:

- Positioning and prepping patient
- Examination of site after anesthesia
- Operative services, including inspections around site and closure

CPT® CODE 52320

Cystourethroscopy (including ureteral catheterization); with removal of ureteral calculus

POLICY INDICATORS

Global Period
0 day post-op period

Assistants at Surgery
No assistant

Co-Surgeons Allowed
No co-surgeon

Reduction for Multiple Procedures
Endoscopy payment rules apply

Bilateral Surgery Payment
150% paid if bilateral

Applicable Medicare Policies

Relative Value Units (RVUs)

Work RVUs	4.69
Non-Facility Total	Only valued for facility
Facility Total	7.32

Coding Assistance

52320 includes:

- Positioning and prepping patient
- Examination of site after anesthesia
- Operative services, including inspections around site and closure

CPT® CODE 52327

Cystourethroscopy (including ureteral catheterization); with subureteric injection of implant material

POLICY INDICATORS

Global Period
0 day post-op period

Assistants at Surgery
No assistant

Co-Surgeons Allowed
No co-surgeon

Reduction for Multiple Procedures
Endoscopy payment rules apply

Bilateral Surgery Payment
150% paid if bilateral

Applicable Medicare Policies

Relative Value Units (RVUs)

Work RVUs	5.18
Non-Facility Total	Only valued for facility
Facility Total	7.67

Coding Assistance

52327 includes:

- Positioning and prepping patient
- Examination of site after anesthesia
- Operative services, including inspections around site and closure

CPT® CODE 52330

Cystourethroscopy (including ureteral catheterization); with manipulation, without removal of ureteral calculus

POLICY INDICATORS

Global Period
0 day post-op period

Assistants at Surgery
No assistant

Co-Surgeons Allowed
No co-surgeon

Reduction for Multiple Procedures
Endoscopy payment rules apply

Bilateral Surgery Payment
150% paid if bilateral

Applicable Medicare Policies

Relative Value Units (RVUs)

Work RVUs	5.03
Non-Facility Total	17.27
Facility Total	7.81

Coding Assistance

52330 includes:

- Positioning and prepping patient
- Examination of site after anesthesia
- Operative services, including inspections around site and closure

CPT® CODE 52332

Cystourethroscopy, with insertion of indwelling ureteral stent (eg, Gibbons or double-J type)

POLICY INDICATORS

Global Period
0 day post-op period

Assistants at Surgery
No assistant

Co-Surgeons Allowed
No co-surgeon

Reduction for Multiple Procedures
Endoscopy payment rules apply

Bilateral Surgery Payment
150% paid if bilateral

Applicable Medicare Policies

Relative Value Units (RVUs)

Work RVUs	2.82
Non-Facility Total	11.21
Facility Total	4.64

Coding Assistance

52332 includes:

- Positioning and prepping patient
- Examination of site after anesthesia
- Operative services, including inspections around site and closure
- Appropriate post-op E/M visit(s)

Abbreviated Case Note Example:

- A 45-year-old female patient presents with severe right flank pain for 24 hours. Urinalysis shows blood. A non-contrast CT shows an 8-mm stone at the right ureteropelvic junction with severe hydronephrosis. It is elected to place an in-dwelling J-stent to relieve the hydronephrosis and pain.
- Procedure: Place a 21 Fr cystoscope at the meatus and pass into the bladder. Inspect the bladder with the 30- and 70-degree lenses, which shows a normal trigone and bladder wall with no stone debris in the bladder lumen. Place an angle-tipped catheter in the right orifice and pass a 0.35 guidewire through the catheter and up the ureter to the level of the stone. Once the guidewire's position beyond the stone is confirmed, remove the angle-tipped catheter leaving the guidewire in place. Under fluoroscopy, a 6-Fr by 26-cm open-ended J-stent is then passed over the guidewire through the cystoscope and up the right ureter. At the level of the stone, manipulate the J-stent into the right renal pelvis, being careful not to perforate the ureter. Once it is is confirmed that the distal end of the J-stent is in the renal pelvis and the proximized end is in the bladder, remove the guidewire. If the J-stent is not perfectly positioned, utilize grasping forceps to manipulate the distal end of the J-stent and achieve the correct positioning. Then, empty the bladder, remove the cystoscope, and place the Foley catheter.

CPT® CODE 53060

Drainage of Skene's gland abscess or cyst

POLICY INDICATORS

Global Period
10 day post-op period

Assistants at Surgery
No assistant

Co-Surgeons Allowed
No co-surgeon

Reduction for Multiple Procedures
Subject to 50% reduction

Bilateral Surgery Payment
N/A

Applicable Medicare Policies

Relative Value Units (RVUs)

Work RVUs	2.68
Non-Facility Total	5.74
Facility Total	5.04

Coding Assistance

53060 includes:

- Positioning and prepping patient
- Examination of site after anesthesia
- Operative services, including inspections around site and closure
- Appropriate post-op E/M visit(s)

CPT® CODE 53200

Biopsy of urethra

POLICY INDICATORS

Global Period
0 day post-op period

Assistants at Surgery
No assistant

Co-Surgeons Allowed
No co-surgeon

Reduction for Multiple Procedures
Subject to 50% reduction

Bilateral Surgery Payment
N/A

Applicable Medicare Policies

Relative Value Units (RVUs)

Work RVUs	2.59
Non-Facility Total	4.82
Facility Total	4.26

Coding Assistance

53200 includes:

- Positioning and prepping patient
- Examination of site after anesthesia
- Operative services, including inspections around site and closure

CPT® CODE 53210

Urethrectomy, total, including cystostomy; female

POLICY INDICATORS

Global Period
90 day post-op period

Assistants at Surgery
Assistant allowed

Co-Surgeons Allowed
Submit reason for co-surgeon

Reduction for Multiple Procedures
Subject to 50% reduction

Bilateral Surgery Payment
N/A

Applicable Medicare Policies

Relative Value Units (RVUs)

Work RVUs	13.72
Non-Facility Total	Only valued for facility
Facility Total	23.53

Coding Assistance

53210 includes:

- Positioning and prepping patient
- Examination of site after anesthesia
- Operative services, including inspections around site and closure
- Appropriate post-op E/M visit(s)

CPT® CODE 53220

Excision or fulguration of carcinoma of urethra

POLICY INDICATORS

Global Period
90 day post-op period

Assistants at Surgery
Submit reason for assistant

Co-Surgeons Allowed
No co-surgeon

Reduction for Multiple Procedures
Subject to 50% reduction

Bilateral Surgery Payment
N/A

Applicable Medicare Policies

Relative Value Units (RVUs)

Work RVUs	7.63
Non-Facility Total	Only valued for facility
Facility Total	13.66

Coding Assistance

53220 includes:

- Positioning and prepping patient
- Examination of site after anesthesia
- Operative services, including inspections around site and closure
- Appropriate post-op E/M visit(s)

SURGERY

CPT® CODE 53230

Excision of urethral diverticulum (separate procedure); female

POLICY INDICATORS

Global Period
90 day post-op period

Assistants at Surgery
Assistant allowed

Co-Surgeons Allowed
Submit reason for co-surgeon

Reduction for Multiple Procedures
Subject to 50% reduction

Bilateral Surgery Payment
N/A

Applicable Medicare Policies

Relative Value Units (RVUs)

Work RVUs	10.44
Non-Facility Total	Only valued for facility
Facility Total	18.40

Coding Assistance

53230 includes:

- Positioning and prepping patient
- Examination of site after anesthesia
- Operative services, including inspections around site and closure
- Appropriate post-op E/M visit(s)

CPT® CODE 53250

Excision of bulbourethral gland (Cowper's gland)

POLICY INDICATORS

Global Period
90 day post-op period

Assistants at Surgery
No assistant

Co-Surgeons Allowed
No co-surgeon

Reduction for Multiple Procedures
Subject to 50% reduction

Bilateral Surgery Payment
N/A

Applicable Medicare Policies

Relative Value Units (RVUs)

Work RVUs	6.52
Non-Facility Total	Only valued for facility
Facility Total	12.03

Coding Assistance

53250 includes:

- Positioning and prepping patient
- Examination of site after anesthesia
- Operative services, including inspections around site and closure
- Appropriate post-op E/M visit(s)

CPT® CODE 53260

Excision or fulguration; urethral polyp(s), distal urethra

POLICY INDICATORS

Global Period
10 day post-op period

Assistants at Surgery
No assistant

Co-Surgeons Allowed
No co-surgeon

Reduction for Multiple Procedures
Subject to 50% reduction

Bilateral Surgery Payment
N/A

Applicable Medicare Policies

Relative Value Units (RVUs)

Work RVUs	3.03
Non-Facility Total	6.29
Facility Total	5.49

Coding Assistance

53260 includes:

- Positioning and prepping patient
- Examination of site after anesthesia
- Operative services, including inspections around site and closure
- Appropriate post-op E/M visit(s)

CPT® CODE 53270

Excision or fulguration; Skene's glands

POLICY INDICATORS

Global Period
10 day post-op period

Assistants at Surgery
No assistant

Co-Surgeons Allowed
No co-surgeon

Reduction for Multiple Procedures
Subject to 50% reduction

Bilateral Surgery Payment
N/A

Applicable Medicare Policies

Relative Value Units (RVUs)

Work RVUs	3.14
Non-Facility Total	6.44
Facility Total	5.61

Coding Assistance

53270 includes:

- Positioning and prepping patient
- Examination of site after anesthesia
- Operative services, including inspections around site and closure
- Appropriate post-op E/M visit(s)

CPT® CODE 53275

Excision or fulguration; urethral prolapse

POLICY INDICATORS

Global Period
10 day post-op period

Assistants at Surgery
No assistant

Co-Surgeons Allowed
No co-surgeon

Reduction for Multiple Procedures
Subject to 50% reduction

Bilateral Surgery Payment
N/A

Applicable Medicare Policies

Relative Value Units (RVUs)

Work RVUs	4.57
Non-Facility Total	Only valued for facility
Facility Total	7.90

Coding Assistance

53275 includes:

- Positioning and prepping patient
- Examination of site after anesthesia
- Operative services, including inspections around site and closure
- Appropriate post-op E/M visit(s)

CPT® CODE 53400

Urethroplasty; first stage, for fistula, diverticulum, or stricture (eg, Johannsen type)

POLICY INDICATORS

Global Period
90 day post-op period

Assistants at Surgery
Assistant allowed

Co-Surgeons Allowed
Submit reason for co-surgeon

Reduction for Multiple Procedures
Subject to 50% reduction

Bilateral Surgery Payment
N/A

Applicable Medicare Policies

Relative Value Units (RVUs)

Work RVUs	14.13
Non-Facility Total	Only valued for facility
Facility Total	24.11

Coding Assistance

53400 includes:

- Positioning and prepping patient
- Examination of site after anesthesia
- Operative services, including inspections around site and closure
- Appropriate post-op E/M visit(s)

CPT® CODE 53430

Urethroplasty, reconstruction of female urethra

POLICY INDICATORS

Global Period
90 day post-op period

Assistants at Surgery
Assistant allowed

Co-Surgeons Allowed
Submit reason for co-surgeon

Reduction for Multiple Procedures
Subject to 50% reduction

Bilateral Surgery Payment
N/A

Applicable Medicare Policies

Relative Value Units (RVUs)

Work RVUs	17.43
Non-Facility Total	Only valued for facility
Facility Total	29.21

Coding Assistance

53430 includes:

- Positioning and prepping patient
- Examination of site after anesthesia
- Operative services, including inspections around site and closure
- Appropriate post-op E/M visit(s)

CPT® CODE 53460

Urethromeatoplasty, with partial excision of distal urethral segment (Richardson type procedure)

POLICY INDICATORS

Global Period
90 day post-op period

Assistants at Surgery
Submit reason for assistant

Co-Surgeons Allowed
No co-surgeon

Reduction for Multiple Procedures
Subject to 50% reduction

Bilateral Surgery Payment
N/A

Applicable Medicare Policies

Relative Value Units (RVUs)

Work RVUs	7.75
Non-Facility Total	Only valued for facility
Facility Total	13.83

Coding Assistance

53460 includes:

- Positioning and prepping patient
- Examination of site after anesthesia
- Operative services, including inspections around site and closure
- Appropriate post-op E/M visit(s)

CPT® CODE 53500

Urethrolysis, transvaginal, secondary, open, including cystourethroscopy (eg, postsurgical obstruction, scarring)

POLICY INDICATORS

Global Period
90 day post-op period

Assistants at Surgery
Assistant allowed

Co-Surgeons Allowed
Submit reason for co-surgeon

Reduction for Multiple Procedures
Subject to 50% reduction

Bilateral Surgery Payment
N/A

Applicable Medicare Policies

Relative Value Units (RVUs)

Work RVUs	13.00
Non-Facility Total	Only valued for facility
Facility Total	22.50

Coding Assistance

53500 includes:

- Positioning and prepping patient
- Examination of site after anesthesia
- Operative services, including inspections around site and closure
- Appropriate post-op E/M visit(s)

Abbreviated Case Note Example:

- A 52-year-old female patient presents with history of bladder neck suspension. She developed progressive urinary obstructive symptoms, including decreased force of stream, straining to void, and double voiding. Workup demonstrates significant bladder outlet obstruction secondary to urethral scarring and fibrosis. After counseling, the patient elects for an open transvaginal ureterolysis to be performed.
- Procedure: Insert a 16-Fr Foley catheter in the bladder. Make a vaginal incision and dissect the periurethral and vesicovaginal space with special care being taken to avoid injury to the urethra and bladder neck. Perform dissection, lysis, or removal of the associated fibrosis. Perform meticulous hemostasis to prevent refibrosis of the urethra. Close the incision in multiple layers. Gently position a vaginal pack, leave the Foley catheter in place, and place drains as necessary.

CPT® CODE 53502

Urethrorrhaphy, suture of urethral wound or injury, female

POLICY INDICATORS

Global Period
90 day post-op period

Assistants at Surgery
No assistant

Co-Surgeons Allowed
No co-surgeon

Reduction for Multiple Procedures
Subject to 50% reduction

Bilateral Surgery Payment
N/A

Applicable Medicare Policies

Relative Value Units (RVUs)

Work RVUs	8.26
Non-Facility Total	Only valued for facility
Facility Total	14.71

Coding Assistance

53502 includes:

- Positioning and prepping patient
- Examination of site after anesthesia
- Operative services, including inspections around site and closure
- Appropriate post-op E/M visit(s)

CPT® CODE 53660

Dilation of female urethra including suppository and/or instillation; initial

POLICY INDICATORS

Global Period
0 day post-op period

Assistants at Surgery
No assistant

Co-Surgeons Allowed
No co-surgeon

Reduction for Multiple Procedures
Subject to 50% reduction

Bilateral Surgery Payment
N/A

Applicable Medicare Policies

Relative Value Units (RVUs)

Work RVUs	0.71
Non-Facility Total	2.27
Facility Total	1.24

Coding Assistance

53660 includes:

- Positioning and prepping patient
- Examination of site after anesthesia
- Operative services, including inspections around site and closure

CPT® CODE 53661

Dilation of female urethra including suppository and/or instillation; subsequent

POLICY INDICATORS

Global Period
0 day post-op period

Assistants at Surgery
No assistant

Co-Surgeons Allowed
No co-surgeon

Reduction for Multiple Procedures
Subject to 50% reduction

Bilateral Surgery Payment
N/A

Applicable Medicare Policies

Relative Value Units (RVUs)

Work RVUs	0.72
Non-Facility Total	2.24
Facility Total	1.20

Coding Assistance

53661 includes:

- Positioning and prepping patient
- Examination of site after anesthesia
- Operative services, including inspections around site and closure

CPT® CODE 53665

Dilation of female urethra, general or conduction (spinal) anesthesia

POLICY INDICATORS

Global Period
0 day post-op period

Assistants at Surgery
No assistant

Co-Surgeons Allowed
No co-surgeon

Reduction for Multiple Procedures
Subject to 50% reduction

Bilateral Surgery Payment
N/A

Applicable Medicare Policies

Relative Value Units (RVUs)

Work RVUs	0.76
Non-Facility Total	Only valued for facility
Facility Total	1.11

Coding Assistance

53665 includes:

- Positioning and prepping patient
- Examination of site after anesthesia
- Operative services, including inspections around site and closure

CPT® CODE 56405

Incision and drainage of vulva or perineal abscess

POLICY INDICATORS

Global Period
10 day post-op period

Assistants at Surgery
No assistant

Co-Surgeons Allowed
Co-surgeon allowed

Reduction for Multiple Procedures
Subject to 50% reduction

Bilateral Surgery Payment
N/A

Applicable Medicare Policies

Relative Value Units (RVUs)

Work RVUs	1.49
Non-Facility Total	4.38
Facility Total	3.85

Coding Assistance

56405 includes:

- Positioning and prepping patient
- Examination of site after anesthesia
- Operative services, including inspections around site and closure
- Appropriate post-op E/M visit(s)

Abbreviated Case Note Example:

- A 23-year-old female patient presents with fever, leukocytosis, and pelvic pain, and is diagnosed with clitoral hood abscess.
- Procedure: General anesthesia is performed without difficulty. Purulent material is noted to be spontaneously draining from a 1- to 2-mm well-epithelialized opening on the dorsal surface of the clitoris. This is further manually expressed. A gonorrhea/chlamydia and genital swab are collected and sent to pathology. Vaginal retractors are used to perform a thorough exam of the patient's vaginal walls and cervix, which appear normal. Attention is turned to the clitoral hood, where a laminar duct probe is inserted into the epithelialized opening and tracked to the right to the pubic bone for 4 cm. After injection of 5 cc of 2% lidocaine with 1:100,000 epinephrine bilaterally along the clitoral hood, a scapel is used to extend the pinpoint epithelialized opening superficially along the skin superiorly for 2 cm in an attempt to locate the source of the abscess without success. A spinal needle is then inserted retropubically along the patient's right lateral pubic mons with no return of pus. The Foley is removed, and no fluctuant collection palpated internally along her anterior vaginal mucosa. A cystoscopy is performed, and no sign of bladder mucosa injury. The Foley is replaced.

Additional Notes

- Whenever an abscess is present in the vulvar or perianal area, the service should be reported with CPT code 56405. If the abscess is located anywhere else on the body, it should be reported with 10060.

CPT® CODE 56420

Incision and drainage of Bartholin's gland abscess

POLICY INDICATORS

Global Period
10 day post-op period

Assistants at Surgery
No assistant

Co-Surgeons Allowed
No co-surgeon

Reduction for Multiple Procedures
Subject to 50% reduction

Bilateral Surgery Payment
N/A

Applicable Medicare Policies

Relative Value Units (RVUs)

Work RVUs	1.44
Non-Facility Total	5.53
Facility Total	3.32

Coding Assistance

56420 includes:

- Positioning and prepping patient
- Examination of site after anesthesia
- Operative services, including inspections around site and closure
- Appropriate post-op E/M visit(s)

Abbreviated Case Note Example:

- A 25-year-old patient presents with pain starting 4 days ago, getting worse with time, and is diagnosed with vulvar abscess. She consents to incision and drainage of vulvar abscess.
- Procedure: General anesthesia is performed without difficulty. Vulva and surrounding areas are draped in sterile manner. Bladder is drained. Right Bartholin gland abscess is incised with 15 blade. Cultures are obtained. Left labial abscess is incised with 15-blade. Purulent fluid is expressed. Both abscess cavities are packed with 1/4-inch iodoform gauze. Hemostasis is confirmed. Edema is present on right side and no significant cellulitis is encountered.

Additional Notes

- If Skene's gland is also affected, report code 53060 and 56420-51
- Most third-party payers, including Medicare, do not reimburse separately for supplies or equipment that are typically required to perform the service. Generally, it is inappropriate to report supplies when this service is performed in an emergency room. For physician offices, it may be appropriate to report supplies using the appropriate HCPCS Level II code. Be sure to check with the specific payer(s) to determine coverage.

CPT® CODE 56440

Marsupialization of Bartholin's gland cyst

POLICY INDICATORS

Global Period
10 day post-op period

Assistants at Surgery
No assistant

Co-Surgeons Allowed
No co-surgeon

Reduction for Multiple Procedures
Subject to 50% reduction

Bilateral Surgery Payment
N/A

Applicable Medicare Policies

Relative Value Units (RVUs)

Work RVUs	2.89
Non-Facility Total	Only valued for facility
Facility Total	5.50

Coding Assistance

56440 includes:

- Positioning and prepping patient
- Examination of site after anesthesia
- Operative services, including inspections around site and closure
- Appropriate post-op E/M visit(s)
- Incision and drainage of Bartholin's abscess if done on the same side

CPT® CODE 56441

Lysis of labial adhesions

POLICY INDICATORS

Global Period
10 day post-op period

Assistants at Surgery
Submit reason for assistant

Co-Surgeons Allowed
No co-surgeon

Reduction for Multiple Procedures
Subject to 50% reduction

Bilateral Surgery Payment
N/A

Applicable Medicare Policies

Relative Value Units (RVUs)

Work RVUs	2.02
Non-Facility Total	5.47
Facility Total	4.68

Coding Assistance

56441 includes:

- Positioning and prepping patient
- Examination of site after anesthesia
- Operative services, including inspections around site and closure
- Appropriate post-op E/M visit(s)
- Application of topical medication

Abbreviated Case Note Example:

- A 20-year-old female patient presents with labia fusion. She consents to a correction of labia fusion.
- Procedure: Labia are prepped with betadine; the area of labial fusion is ~2 cm in length and 3 mm in thickness; 2-cm region is infiltrated with ~3 cc of 1% lidocaine with epi; #15 scalpel is used to separate the labia at the midline. 4-0 vicryl is placed subcuticularly to reapproximate the raw edges at each labia.

CPT® CODE 56442

Hymenotomy, simple incision

POLICY INDICATORS

Global Period
0 day post-op period

Assistants at Surgery
Submit reason for assistant

Co-Surgeons Allowed
No co-surgeon

Reduction for Multiple Procedures
Subject to 50% reduction

Bilateral Surgery Payment
N/A

Applicable Medicare Policies

Relative Value Units (RVUs)

Work RVUs	0.68
Non-Facility Total	Only valued for facility
Facility Total	1.45

Coding Assistance

56442 includes:

- Positioning and prepping patient
- Examination of site after anesthesia
- Operative services, including inspections around site and closure
- Preoperative needle aspiration of intact membrane

CPT® CODE 56501

Destruction of lesion(s), vulva; simple (eg, laser surgery, electrosurgery, cryosurgery, chemosurgery)

POLICY INDICATORS

Global Period
10 day post-op period

Assistants at Surgery
No assistant

Co-Surgeons Allowed
No co-surgeon

Reduction for Multiple Procedures
Subject to 50% reduction

Bilateral Surgery Payment
N/A

Applicable Medicare Policies

Relative Value Units (RVUs)

Work RVUs	1.58
Non-Facility Total	5.73
Facility Total	4.04

Coding Assistance

56501 includes:

- Positioning and prepping patient
- Examination of site after anesthesia
- Operative services, including inspections around site and closure
- Appropriate post-op E/M visit(s)
- Application of topical medication

Abbreviated Case Note Example:

- A 35-year-old patient presents with an ongoing issue with a lesion in the left labial area. She also has multiple lesions consistent with genital warts. She consented to the removal of these lesions.
- Procedure: General anesthesia is administered without difficulty. The left labial lesion is removed and this is grasped with 2 Allis clamps. An elliptical incision is made with the Bovie electrocautery utilizing pure cutting. This is removed. The defect is closed with multiple interrupted 2-0 Vicryl sutures placed about 5 mm apart. This completes the removal of the left labial lesion. Silvadene cream is applied liberally to all sites.

Additional Notes

- Appropriate to use for the destruction of simple lesions on the vulva with an ultrasonic aspirator.

CPT® CODE 56515

Destruction of lesion(s), vulva; extensive (eg, laser surgery, electrosurgery, cryosurgery, chemosurgery)

POLICY INDICATORS

Global Period
10 day post-op period

Assistants at Surgery
No assistant

Co-Surgeons Allowed
No co-surgeon

Reduction for Multiple Procedures
Subject to 50% reduction

Bilateral Surgery Payment
N/A

Applicable Medicare Policies

Relative Value Units (RVUs)

Work RVUs	3.08
Non-Facility Total	8.30
Facility Total	6.42

Coding Assistance

56515 includes:

- Positioning and prepping patient
- Examination of site after anesthesia
- Operative services, including inspections around site and closure
- Appropriate post-op E/M visit(s)

Abbreviated Case Note Example:

- A 45-year-old female patient presents with biopsy-proven carcinoma in situ of the vulva with multifocal nature of the changes on the vulva. She consents to undergoing laser destruction procedure.
- Procedure: Local anesthesia is administered without difficulty. Destruction of multiple or extensive vulvar lesions, any method, is carried out.

CPT® CODE 56605

Biopsy of vulva or perineum (separate procedure); 1 lesion

POLICY INDICATORS

Global Period
0 day post-op period

Assistants at Surgery
No assistant

Co-Surgeons Allowed
Co-surgeon allowed

Reduction for Multiple Procedures
Subject to 50% reduction

Bilateral Surgery Payment
N/A

Applicable Medicare Policies

Relative Value Units (RVUs)

Work RVUs	1.10
Non-Facility Total	2.87
Facility Total	1.77

Coding Assistance

56605 includes:

- Positioning and prepping patient
- Examination of site after anesthesia
- Operative services, including inspections around site and closure

Abbreviated Case Note Example:

- A 50-year-old female patient presents with vulvar lesion. An examination of the vulva and perineum reveal a 0.5-cm dysplastic-appearing lesion. She consents to a vulvar biopsy.
- Procedure: Using local anesthesia, prepare the vulva with an antiseptic solution. Using a scalpel or punch biopsy instrument, incise or completely excise the lesion. Simple suturing may be required.

Additional Notes

- If a colposcopy is also performed, report 56821 instead

CPT® CODE 56606

Biopsy of vulva or perineum (separate procedure); each separate additional lesion
(List separately in addition to code for primary procedure)

POLICY INDICATORS

Global Period
Global for primary procedure applies

Assistants at Surgery
No assistant

Co-Surgeons Allowed
Co-surgeon allowed

Reduction for Multiple Procedures
Not subject to multiple surgery reduction

Bilateral Surgery Payment
N/A

Applicable Medicare Policies

Relative Value Units (RVUs)

Work RVUs	0.55
Non-Facility Total	1.13
Facility Total	0.86

Coding Assistance

56606 includes:

- Positioning and prepping patient
- Examination of site after anesthesia
- Operative services, including inspections around site and closure
- Appropriate post-op E/M visit(s)

Add-On Code:

- Follow Primary Code Policies

CPT® CODE 56620

Vulvectomy simple; partial

POLICY INDICATORS

Global Period
90 day post-op period

Assistants at Surgery
Assistant allowed

Co-Surgeons Allowed
Submit reason for co-surgeon

Reduction for Multiple Procedures
Subject to 50% reduction

Bilateral Surgery Payment
N/A

Applicable Medicare Policies

Relative Value Units (RVUs)

Work RVUs	7.53
Non-Facility Total	Only valued for facility
Facility Total	17.74

Coding Assistance

56620 includes:

- Positioning and prepping patient
- Examination of site after anesthesia
- Operative services, including inspections around site and closure
- Appropriate post-op E/M visit(s)
- Photodocumentation

Abbreviated Case Note Example:

- A 35-year-old female patient presents with biopsy-proven vulvar intraepithelial neoplasia III, raised erythematous left vulvar lesion involving the labia majora and minora, extending to the posterior forchette. She consents to partial vulvectomy to excise the lesion.
- Procedure: Identify the vulvar lesion, and incise the skin around the lesion including a 1-cm margin if a preinvasive lesion is indicated. Excision includes epidermis, dermis, and superficial subcutaneous tissue. Then close the defect in layers.

Additional Notes

- If a complete vulvectomy is performed, report 56625 instead
- For a postoperative counseling visit about sexual function, use the appropriate E/M with modifier 24

CPT® CODE 56625

Vulvectomy simple; complete

POLICY INDICATORS

Global Period
90 day post-op period

Assistants at Surgery
Assistant allowed

Co-Surgeons Allowed
Submit reason for co-surgeon

Reduction for Multiple Procedures
Subject to 50% reduction

Bilateral Surgery Payment
N/A

Applicable Medicare Policies

Relative Value Units (RVUs)

Work RVUs	9.68
Non-Facility Total	Only valued for facility
Facility Total	20.20

Coding Assistance

56625 includes:

- Positioning and prepping patient
- Examination of site after anesthesia
- Operative services, including inspections around site and closure
- Appropriate post-op E/M visit(s)
- Photodocumentation

Additional Notes

- If a complete vulvectomy is performed, report 56625 instead
- For a postoperative counseling visit about sexual function, use the appropriate E/M with modifier 24

CPT® CODE 56630

Vulvectomy, radical, partial

POLICY INDICATORS

Global Period
90 day post-op period

Assistants at Surgery
Assistant allowed

Co-Surgeons Allowed
Submit reason for co-surgeon

Reduction for Multiple Procedures
Subject to 50% reduction

Bilateral Surgery Payment
N/A

Applicable Medicare Policies
Inpatient-only list

Relative Value Units (RVUs)

Work RVUs	14.80
Non-Facility Total	Only valued for facility
Facility Total	29.00

Coding Assistance

56630 includes:

- Positioning and prepping patient
- Examination of site after anesthesia
- Operative services, including inspections around site and closure
- Appropriate post-op E/M visit(s)
- Photodocumentation
- Primary wound closure

Abbreviated Case Note Example:

- A 55-year-old female patient presents with notable lesion of the right vulva on the external genitalia. A radical partial vulvectomy is recommended.
- Procedure: General endotracheal anesthesia is obtained without difficulty. Incise the skin with a scapel and ligate the vulvar vascular pedicles down to the deep investing fascia. The right vulvar lesion is excised with a 5-mm margin with the scapel. The incision is closed in a subcuticular fashion.

Additional Notes

- If a unilateral or bilateral lymphadenectomy is performed, report 56631 or 56632
- For a postoperative counseling visit about sexual function, use the appropriate E/M with modifier 24
- Report 38531 when an inguinofemoral lymph node biopsy is performed without a complete inguinofemoral lymphadenectomy

CPT® CODE 56631

Vulvectomy, radical, partial; with unilateral inguinofemoral lymphadenectomy

POLICY INDICATORS

Global Period
90 day post-op period

Assistants at Surgery
Assistant allowed

Co-Surgeons Allowed
Co-surgeon allowed

Reduction for Multiple Procedures
Subject to 50% reduction

Bilateral Surgery Payment
N/A

Applicable Medicare Policies
Inpatient-only list

Relative Value Units (RVUs)

Work RVUs	18.99
Non-Facility Total	Only valued for facility
Facility Total	35.90

Coding Assistance

56631 includes:

- Positioning and prepping patient
- Examination of site after anesthesia
- Operative services, including inspections around site and closure
- Appropriate post-op E/M visit(s)
- Photodocumentation
- Primary wound closure
- Inginofemoral lymphadenectomy
- Vulvectomy

Abbreviated Case Note Example:

- A 45-year-old female patient presents with biopsy-proven vulvar squamous cell carcinoma. She consents to radical partial vulvectomy, with unilateral inguinofemoral lymphadenectomy.
- Procedure: Inject the sentinel node and identify the site using the gamma probe. The vulvar lesion is injected with isosulfan blue, and the sentinel node is excised. Vulvar lesion is identified on the left labia majora. Skin is injected with 1% lidocaine with epinephrine, and the lesion is excised with scalpel using a Bovie electrosurgical device and Harmonic.

Additional Notes

- If a bilateral lymphadenectomy is performed, use 56632 instead
- For a postoperative counseling visit about sexual function, use the appropriate E/M with modifier 24
- Report 38531 when an inguinofemoral lymph node biopsy is performed without a complete inguinofemoral lymphadenectomy
- This is a radical procedure, which includes the removal of skin and deep subcutaneous tissue, a partial procedure (less than 80% of the vulvar area), and lymph node removal.

CPT® CODE 56632

Vulvectomy, radical, partial; with bilateral inguinofemoral lymphadenectomy

POLICY INDICATORS

Global Period
90 day post-op period

Assistants at Surgery
Assistant allowed

Co-Surgeons Allowed
Co-surgeon allowed

Reduction for Multiple Procedures
Subject to 50% reduction

Bilateral Surgery Payment
Bilateral surgery

Applicable Medicare Policies
Inpatient-only list

Relative Value Units (RVUs)

Work RVUs	21.86
Non-Facility Total	Only valued for facility
Facility Total	43.35

Coding Assistance

56632 includes:

- Positioning and prepping patient
- Examination of site after anesthesia
- Operative services, including inspections around site and closure
- Appropriate post-op E/M visit(s)
- Primary wound closure
- Inginofemoral lymphadenectomy
- Vulvectomy

Abbreviated Case Note Example:

- A 34-year-old patient with biopsy-proven invasive cancer confined to the vulva of up to 2 cm in greatest diameter, involving midline structures of the perineum and clitoris.
- Procedure: A bilateral lymphadenectomy and nodes dissected away from the femoral artery, nerve, and femoral vein. The procedure is repeated on the other side. A partial radical vulvectomy is performed to remove the primary tumor (removal of less than 80% of the vulvar area). The excised areas may include the labial fold(s), clitoris, and/or perianal skin.

Additional Notes

- If a complete vulvectomy is performed, report 56634 instead
- For a postoperative counseling visit about sexual function, use the appropriate E/M with modifier 24
- Report 38531 when an inguinofemoral lymph node biopsy is performed without a complete inguinofemoral lymphadenectomy

CPT® CODE 56633

Vulvectomy, radical, complete

POLICY INDICATORS

Global Period
90 day post-op period

Assistants at Surgery
Assistant allowed

Co-Surgeons Allowed
Co-surgeon allowed

Reduction for Multiple Procedures
Subject to 50% reduction

Bilateral Surgery Payment
N/A

Applicable Medicare Policies
Inpatient-only list

Relative Value Units (RVUs)

Work RVUs	19.62
Non-Facility Total	Only valued for facility
Facility Total	34.92

Coding Assistance

56633 includes:

- Positioning and prepping patient
- Examination of site after anesthesia
- Operative services, including inspections around site and closure
- Appropriate post-op E/M visit(s)
- Photodocumentation

Abbreviated Case Note Example:

- A 75-year-old female patient presents with biopsy-proven differentiated verrucous carcinoma. Complete radical vulvectomy is indicated due to the extent of disease.
- Procedure: A radical vulvectomy using a scalpel or cautery is performed. The specimen includes the labia majora, labia minora, and clitoris to the level of fascia. Identify specimens and send to pathologist. Primary closure and drains may be placed.

Additional Notes

- If a unilateral or bilateral lymphadenectomy is performed, report 56634 or 56637
- For a postoperative counseling visit about sexual function, use the appropriate E/M with modifier 24
- Report 38531 when an inguinofemoral lymph node biopsy is performed without a complete inguinofemoral lymphadenectomy

CPT® CODE 56634

Vulvectomy, radical, complete; with unilateral inguinofemoral lymphadenectomy

POLICY INDICATORS

Global Period
90 day post-op period

Assistants at Surgery
Assistant allowed

Co-Surgeons Allowed
Co-surgeon allowed

Reduction for Multiple Procedures
Subject to 50% reduction

Bilateral Surgery Payment
N/A

Applicable Medicare Policies
Inpatient-only list

Relative Value Units (RVUs)

Work RVUs	20.66
Non-Facility Total	Only valued for facility
Facility Total	39.22

Coding Assistance

56634 includes:

- Positioning and prepping patient
- Examination of site after anesthesia
- Operative services, including inspections around site and closure
- Appropriate post-op E/M visit(s)
- Photodocumentation
- Primary wound closure
- Inginofemoral lymphadenectomy
- Vulvectomy

Additional Notes

- If a bilateral lymphadenectomy is performed, use 56637 instead
- For a postoperative counseling visit about sexual function, use the appropriate E/M with modifier 24
- Report 38531 when an inguinofemoral lymph node biopsy is performed without a complete inguinofemoral lymphadenectomy

CPT® CODE 56637

Vulvectomy, radical, complete; with bilateral inguinofemoral lymphadenectomy

POLICY INDICATORS

Global Period
90 day post-op period

Assistants at Surgery
Assistant allowed

Co-Surgeons Allowed
Co-surgeon allowed

Reduction for Multiple Procedures
Subject to 50% reduction

Bilateral Surgery Payment
N/A

Applicable Medicare Policies
Inpatient-only list

Relative Value Units (RVUs)

Work RVUs	24.75
Non-Facility Total	Only valued for facility
Facility Total	45.94

Coding Assistance

56637 includes:

- Positioning and prepping patient
- Examination of site after anesthesia
- Operative services, including inspections around site and closure
- Appropriate post-op E/M visit(s)
- Photodocumentation
- Inguinofemoral lymphadenectomy (38760)
- Vulvectomy

Additional Notes

- If iliac and pelvic lymphadenectomy is performed, report 56640 instead
- For a postoperative counseling visit about sexual function, use the appropriate E/M with modifier 24
- Report 38531 when an inguinofemoral lymph node biopsy is performed without a complete inguinofemoral lymphadenectomy

SURGERY

CPT® CODE 56640

Vulvectomy, radical, complete, with inguinofemoral, iliac, and pelvic lymphadenectomy

POLICY INDICATORS

Global Period
90 day post-op period

Assistants at Surgery
Assistant allowed

Co-Surgeons Allowed
Submit reason for co-surgeon

Reduction for Multiple Procedures
Subject to 50% reduction

Bilateral Surgery Payment
150% paid if bilateral

Applicable Medicare Policies
Inpatient-only list

Relative Value Units (RVUs)

Work RVUs	24.78
Non-Facility Total	Only valued for facility
Facility Total	46.13

Coding Assistance

56640 includes:

- Positioning and prepping patient
- Examination of site after anesthesia
- Operative services, including inspections around site and closure
- Appropriate post-op E/M visit(s)
- Photodocumentation
- Lymphadenectomy
- Exploration of retroperitoneum
- Vulvectomy

Additional Notes

- For a postoperative counseling visit about sexual function, use the appropriate E/M with modifier 24

CPT® CODE 56700

Partial hymenectomy or revision of hymenal ring

POLICY INDICATORS

Global Period
10 day post-op period

Assistants at Surgery
Assistant allowed

Co-Surgeons Allowed
Submit reason for co-surgeon

Reduction for Multiple Procedures
Subject to 50% reduction

Bilateral Surgery Payment
N/A

Applicable Medicare Policies

Relative Value Units (RVUs)

Work RVUs	2.84
Non-Facility Total	Only valued for facility
Facility Total	6.14

Coding Assistance

56700 includes:

- Positioning and prepping patient
- Examination of site after anesthesia
- Operative services, including inspections around site and closure
- Appropriate post-op E/M visit(s)
- Vaginal dilation

Abbreviated Case Note Example:

- A 28-year-old female patient presents with complaint of hymenal tissue getting caught with tampon insertion or removal. She consents to excision of hymen remnant.
- Procedure: Inject with lidocaine 2% with epi at 11 and 7 o'clock. Attach 4 cm x 1 cm from the 11-o'clock area of the hymen to the 7-o'clock area. Excise with knife at the 11- and 7-o'clock areas, and amputate the excess tissue.

CPT® CODE 56740

Excision of Bartholin's gland or cyst

POLICY INDICATORS

Global Period
10 day post-op period

Assistants at Surgery
No assistant

Co-Surgeons Allowed
No co-surgeon

Reduction for Multiple Procedures
Subject to 50% reduction

Bilateral Surgery Payment
150% paid if bilateral

Applicable Medicare Policies

Relative Value Units (RVUs)

Work RVUs	4.88
Non-Facility Total	Only valued for facility
Facility Total	9.47

Coding Assistance

56740 includes:

- Positioning and prepping patient
- Examination of site after anesthesia
- Operative services, including inspections around site and closure
- Appropriate post-op E/M visit(s)
- Incision and drainage of Bartholin's abscess if done on same side

Abbreviated Case Note Example:

- A 35-year-old female patient presents with a cyst/abscess of the Bartholin's gland and duct, previously treated with incision and drainage, marsupialization, and word catheter epithelialization. She consents to an excision of a Bartholin's gland and duct cyst, or abscess.
- Procedure: Under anesthesia, the skin is incised, and Bartholin's gland or cyst is excised.

CPT® CODE 56800

Plastic repair of introitus

POLICY INDICATORS

Global Period
10 day post-op period

Assistants at Surgery
Assistant allowed

Co-Surgeons Allowed
Submit reason for co-surgeon

Reduction for Multiple Procedures
Subject to 50% reduction

Bilateral Surgery Payment
N/A

Applicable Medicare Policies

Relative Value Units (RVUs)

Work RVUs	3.93
Non-Facility Total	Only valued for facility
Facility Total	7.66

Coding Assistance

56800 includes:

- Positioning and prepping patient
- Examination of site after anesthesia
- Operative services, including inspections around site and closure
- Appropriate post-op E/M visit(s)
- Perineoplasty

Additional Notes

- If posterior colporrhaphy is performed, report 57250 instead

CPT® CODE 56805

Clitoroplasty for intersex state

POLICY INDICATORS

Global Period
90 day post-op period

Assistants at Surgery
Assistant allowed

Co-Surgeons Allowed
Submit reason for co-surgeon

Reduction for Multiple Procedures
Subject to 50% reduction

Bilateral Surgery Payment
N/A

Applicable Medicare Policies

Relative Value Units (RVUs)

Work RVUs	19.88
Non-Facility Total	Only valued for facility
Facility Total	35.00

Coding Assistance

56805 includes:

- Positioning and prepping patient
- Examination of site after anesthesia
- Operative services, including inspections around site and closure
- Appropriate post-op E/M visit(s)

CPT® CODE 56810

Perineoplasty, repair of perineum, nonobstetrical (separate procedure)

POLICY INDICATORS

Global Period
10 day post-op period

Assistants at Surgery
Assistant allowed

Co-Surgeons Allowed
Co-surgeon allowed

Reduction for Multiple Procedures
Subject to 50% reduction

Bilateral Surgery Payment
N/A

Applicable Medicare Policies

Relative Value Units (RVUs)

Work RVUs	4.29
Non-Facility Total	Only valued for facility
Facility Total	8.19

Coding Assistance

56810 includes:

- Positioning and prepping patient
- Examination of site after anesthesia
- Operative services, including inspections around site and closure
- Appropriate post-op E/M visit(s)
- Photodocumentation
- Repair of introitus

Abbreviated Case Note Example:

- A 34-year-old female patient presents for surgical repair of a nonhealing perineal scar from vaginal birth trauma. She consents to perineoplasty.
- Procedure: Attention is turned to posterior fourchette. Midline vertical incision is made to release the skin bridge, the granulation tissue is removed, and the underlying scar is released. A vaginal advancement flap is created to help the tissue heal without excessive tension to the skin edges., and the skin is released from the underlying muscle with curved Mayo scissors. Incision is closed, and the perineum is cleansed and dried.

Additional Notes

- If posterior colporrhaphy is performed, report 57250 instead
- For repair of wounds to genitalia, use 12000-12007, 12041-12047, or 13131-13133
- For repair of recent injury to vagina and perineum, non-obstetrical, use 57210 instead of this code

SURGERY

CPT® CODE 56820

Colposcopy of the vulva

POLICY INDICATORS

Global Period
0 day post-op period

Assistants at Surgery
No assistant

Co-Surgeons Allowed
No co-surgeon

Reduction for Multiple Procedures
Subject to 50% reduction

Bilateral Surgery Payment
N/A

Applicable Medicare Policies

Relative Value Units (RVUs)

Work RVUs	1.50
Non-Facility Total	3.77
Facility Total	2.53

Coding Assistance

56820 includes:

- Positioning and prepping patient
- Examination of site after anesthesia
- Operative services, including inspections around site and closure

Abbreviated Case Note Example:

- A 45-year-old female patient presents with history of vulvar irritation and itching. She has a past history of HPV changes to Pap smear, and cyrotherapy of the cervix. Evaluation of the vulva to exclude vulvar intraepithelial neoplasia is performed.
- Procedure: Colposcope is directed at the vulva under appropriate magnification. The entire vulva is visualized with the colposcope at several magnifications. No suspicious lesions are found, and biopsies are not performed.

Additional Notes

- If colposcopy and biopsy of vulva is performed, report 56821 instead

CPT® CODE 56821

Colposcopy of the vulva; with biopsy(s)

POLICY INDICATORS

Global Period
0 day post-op period

Assistants at Surgery
No assistant

Co-Surgeons Allowed
No co-surgeon

Reduction for Multiple Procedures
Subject to 50% reduction

Bilateral Surgery Payment
N/A

Applicable Medicare Policies

Relative Value Units (RVUs)

Work RVUs	2.05
Non-Facility Total	5.04
Facility Total	3.41

Coding Assistance

56821 includes:

- Positioning and prepping patient
- Examination of site after anesthesia
- Operative services, including inspections around site and closure

Abbreviated Case Note Example:

- A 43-year-old female patient with history of vulvar intraepithelial neoplasia complains of vulvar itching. Physical examination does not reveal an obvious lesion.
- Procedure: Acetic acid is applied to the vulva and a colposcopic examination of the entire vulva is performed. Abnormal area suspicious for cancer is identified. An area of acetowhite epithelium is identified. The area is infiltrated with 1% lidocaine and 4-mm punch biopsy is obtained. Hemostasis is obtained with silver nitrate.

CPT® CODE 57000

Colpotomy; with exploration

POLICY INDICATORS

Global Period
10 day post-op period

Assistants at Surgery
Submit reason for assistant

Co-Surgeons Allowed
No co-surgeon

Reduction for Multiple Procedures
Subject to 50% reduction

Bilateral Surgery Payment
N/A

Applicable Medicare Policies

Relative Value Units (RVUs)

Work RVUs	3.02
Non-Facility Total	Only valued for facility
Facility Total	6.09

Coding Assistance

57000 includes:

- Positioning and prepping patient
- Examination of site after anesthesia
- Operative services, including inspections around site and closure
- Appropriate post-op E/M visit(s)
- Photodocumentation
- Irrigation of vagina

Additional Notes

- If transvaginal tubal ligation is performed, report 58600 instead
- If transvaginal drainage of ovarian cyst(s) is performed, report 58800 instead

CPT® CODE 57010

Colpotomy; with drainage of pelvic abscess

POLICY INDICATORS

Global Period
90 day post-op period

Assistants at Surgery
Submit reason for assistant

Co-Surgeons Allowed
No co-surgeon

Reduction for Multiple Procedures
Subject to 50% reduction

Bilateral Surgery Payment
N/A

Applicable Medicare Policies

Relative Value Units (RVUs)

Work RVUs	6.84
Non-Facility Total	Only valued for facility
Facility Total	13.81

Coding Assistance

57010 includes:

- Positioning and prepping patient
- Examination of site after anesthesia
- Operative services, including inspections around site and closure
- Appropriate post-op E/M visit(s)
- Photodocumentation
- Irrigation of vagina

Additional Notes

- If drainage of ovarian abscess is performed, report 58820 instead
- Requires incision and the drainage and exploration of the pelvic/peritoneal cavity.

CPT® CODE 57020

Colpocentesis (separate procedure)

POLICY INDICATORS

Global Period
0 day post-op period

Assistants at Surgery
Submit reason for assistant

Co-Surgeons Allowed
No co-surgeon

Reduction for Multiple Procedures
Subject to 50% reduction

Bilateral Surgery Payment
N/A

Applicable Medicare Policies

Relative Value Units (RVUs)

Work RVUs	1.50
Non-Facility Total	3.71
Facility Total	2.37

Coding Assistance

57020 includes:

- Positioning and prepping patient
- Examination of site after anesthesia
- Operative services, including inspections around site and closure

CPT® CODE 57022

Incision and drainage of vaginal hematoma; obstetrical/postpartum

POLICY INDICATORS

Global Period
10 day post-op period

Assistants at Surgery
Submit reason for assistant

Co-Surgeons Allowed
No co-surgeon

Reduction for Multiple Procedures
Subject to 50% reduction

Bilateral Surgery Payment
N/A

Applicable Medicare Policies

Relative Value Units (RVUs)

Work RVUs	2.73
Non-Facility Total	Only valued for facility
Facility Total	5.48

Coding Assistance

57022 includes:

- Positioning and prepping patient
- Examination of site after anesthesia
- Operative services, including inspections around site and closure
- Appropriate post-op E/M visit(s)
- Repair of vaginal lacerations
- Revision of episiotomy repair

Abbreviated Case Note Example:

- A 45-year-old female patient with recent vaginal delivery presents with complaint of vaginal pain. Examination reveals large hematoma in the vaginal canal.
- Procedure: Vaginal wall is incised and the hematoma evacuated under anesthesia. Bleeding vessels are ligated with suture and cavity irrigated.

Additional Notes

- If hematoma is not obstetrical or postpartal, report 57023 instead

CPT® CODE 57023

Incision and drainage of vaginal hematoma; non-obstetrical (eg, post-trauma, spontaneous bleeding)

POLICY INDICATORS

Global Period
10 day post-op period

Assistants at Surgery
Submit reason for assistant

Co-Surgeons Allowed
No co-surgeon

Reduction for Multiple Procedures
Subject to 50% reduction

Bilateral Surgery Payment
N/A

Applicable Medicare Policies

Relative Value Units (RVUs)

Work RVUs	5.18
Non-Facility Total	Only valued for facility
Facility Total	9.64

Coding Assistance

57023 includes:

- Positioning and prepping patient
- Examination of site after anesthesia
- Operative services, including inspections around site and closure
- Appropriate post-op E/M visit(s)
- Repair of vaginal lacerations

Abbreviated Case Note Example:

- A premenstrual female patient had a straddle injury with contusions and ecchymosis of the vulva, with vaginal bleeding. Examination reveals a large, lateral vaginal wall hematoma actively bleeding.
- Procedure: Vaginal wall is incised and the hematoma evacuated under anesthesia. Active bleeding vessels are identified and hemostasis obtained. Drain is placed in the defect and the vaginal mucosa is repaired.

Additional Notes

- If hematoma is not obstetrical or postpartal, report 57022 instead

CPT® CODE 57061

Destruction of vaginal lesion(s); simple (eg, laser surgery, electrosurgery, cryosurgery, chemosurgery)

POLICY INDICATORS

Global Period
10 day post-op period

Assistants at Surgery
No assistant

Co-Surgeons Allowed
No co-surgeon

Reduction for Multiple Procedures
Subject to 50% reduction

Bilateral Surgery Payment
N/A

Applicable Medicare Policies

Relative Value Units (RVUs)

Work RVUs	1.30
Non-Facility Total	4.99
Facility Total	3.49

Coding Assistance

57061 includes:

- Positioning and prepping patient
- Examination of site after anesthesia
- Operative services, including inspections around site and closure
- Appropriate post-op E/M visit(s)
- Photodocumentation
- Irrigation of vagina

Additional Notes

- If the lesion destruction is extensive, report 57065 instead

CPT® CODE 57065

Destruction of vaginal lesion(s); extensive (eg, laser surgery, electrosurgery, cryosurgery, chemosurgery)

POLICY INDICATORS

Global Period
10 day post-op period

Assistants at Surgery
No assistant

Co-Surgeons Allowed
No co-surgeon

Reduction for Multiple Procedures
Subject to 50% reduction

Bilateral Surgery Payment
N/A

Applicable Medicare Policies

Relative Value Units (RVUs)

Work RVUs	2.66
Non-Facility Total	7.37
Facility Total	5.61

Coding Assistance

57065 includes:

- Positioning and prepping patient
- Examination of site after anesthesia
- Operative services, including inspections around site and closure
- Appropriate post-op E/M visit(s)
- Irrigation of vagina
- Introduction of hemostatic agent or pack
- Catheter insertion
- Extensive destruction of lesions by any method
- Wound closure
- Injection of local anesthesia

Abbreviated Case Note Example:

- A 46-year-old female patient presents with a biopsy-proven verrucoid lesion compatible with vulvar condylomas. She consents to CO_2 laser ablation of the vaginal vault.
- Procedure: General anesthesia is performed without difficulty. A CO_2 laser is used to vaporize the condylomas around the urethra opening and a speculum is placed inside the vagina, which reveals a complete involvement of the vaginal cuff, left and right vaginal side walls, and the posterior vaginal mucosal tissue. A CO_2 laser is used to vaporize all these tissues, and hemostasis is achieved.

Additional Notes

- Do not report 57061 with this code

SURGERY

CPT® CODE 57100

Biopsy of vaginal mucosa; simple (separate procedure)

POLICY INDICATORS

Global Period
0 day post-op period

Assistants at Surgery
No assistant

Co-Surgeons Allowed
No co-surgeon

Reduction for Multiple Procedures
Subject to 50% reduction

Bilateral Surgery Payment
N/A

Applicable Medicare Policies

Relative Value Units (RVUs)

Work RVUs	1.20
Non-Facility Total	3.10
Facility Total	1.97

Coding Assistance

57100 includes:

- Positioning and prepping patient
- Examination of site after anesthesia
- Operative services, including inspections around site and closure
- Catheter insertion
- Biopsy of vaginal mucosa
- Hemostasis
- Wound closure
- Injection of local anesthesia

Abbreviated Case Note Example:

- A 40-year-old female patient with history of hysterectomy and carcinoma in situ presents with an abnormal Pap smear. Visible lesions at the apex of the vagina are observed. They turn white with an acetic acid swab.
- Procedure: Under local anesthesia, biopsies of the vaginal mucosa are taken and hemostasis is achieved.

CPT® CODE 57105

Biopsy of vaginal mucosa; extensive, requiring suture (including cysts)

POLICY INDICATORS

Global Period
10 day post-op period

Assistants at Surgery
No assistant

Co-Surgeons Allowed
No co-surgeon

Reduction for Multiple Procedures
Subject to 50% reduction

Bilateral Surgery Payment
N/A

Applicable Medicare Policies

Relative Value Units (RVUs)

Work RVUs	1.74
Non-Facility Total	5.29
Facility Total	4.42

Coding Assistance

57105 includes:

- Positioning and prepping patient
- Examination of site after anesthesia
- Operative services, including inspections around site and closure
- Appropriate post-op E/M visit(s)
- Catheter insertion
- Biopsy of vaginal mucosa
- Removal of vaginal cysts
- Hemostasis
- Wound closure
- Injection of local anesthesia

CPT® CODE 57106

Vaginectomy, partial removal of vaginal wall

POLICY INDICATORS

Global Period
90 day post-op period

Assistants at Surgery
Assistant allowed

Co-Surgeons Allowed
Submit reason for co-surgeon

Reduction for Multiple Procedures
Subject to 50% reduction

Bilateral Surgery Payment
N/A

Applicable Medicare Policies

Relative Value Units (RVUs)

Work RVUs	7.50
Non-Facility Total	Only valued for facility
Facility Total	16.23

Coding Assistance

57106 includes:

- Positioning and prepping patient
- Examination of site after anesthesia
- Operative services, including inspections around site and closure
- Appropriate post-op E/M visit(s)
- Photodocumentation
- Irrigation of vagina
- Introduction of hemostatic agent or pack
- Ureterolysis
- Catheter insertion
- Biopsy of vaginal mucosa
- Excision of vaginal septum
- Hemostasis
- Wound closure
- Removal of portion of vagina

Additional Notes

- If a complete colpectomy is performed, report 57110 instead
- If a vaginal tumor is excised, 57135 may be more appropriate
- For a postoperative counseling visit about sexual function, use the appropriate E/M with modifier 24

CPT® CODE 57107

Vaginectomy, partial removal of vaginal wall; with removal of paravaginal tissue (radical vaginectomy)

POLICY INDICATORS

Global Period
90 day post-op period

Assistants at Surgery
Assistant allowed

Co-Surgeons Allowed
Submit reason for co-surgeon

Reduction for Multiple Procedures
Subject to 50% reduction

Bilateral Surgery Payment
N/A

Applicable Medicare Policies

Relative Value Units (RVUs)

Work RVUs	24.56
Non-Facility Total	Only valued for facility
Facility Total	43.91

Coding Assistance

57107 includes:

- Positioning and prepping patient
- Examination of site after anesthesia
- Operative services, including inspections around site and closure
- Appropriate post-op E/M visit(s)
- Photodocumentation
- Ureterolysis
- Vaginal procedures
- Catheter insertion
- Dissection of rectum or bladder from vaginal wall
- Abdominal wall incision
- Removal of a portion of the vagina
- Hemostasis
- Development of paravaginal and pararectal spaces

Abbreviated Case Note Example:

- A 55-year-old female patient presents with a history of hysterectomy for severe menorrhagia and superficially invasive cancer in the vaginal apex. She consents to radical partial vaginectomy without lymphadenectomy.
- Procedure: Patient is examined under anesthesia. Upper half of the vagina is removed by dissecting the bladder off the anterior vaginal wall and the rectum off the posterior vaginal wall, followed by dissection of the ureters from the parametria. The ligamentous supports for the vagina is performed by cutting, clamping, and suturing the vascular structures surrounding them. The peritoneal cavity is irrigated, and hemostasis is secured.

Additional Notes

- If a total radical vaginectomy is performed, report 57111 instead
- If a lymphadenectomy is performed, report 57109 instead
- For a postoperative counseling visit about sexual function, use the appropriate E/M with modifier 24

SURGERY

CPT® CODE 57109

Vaginectomy, partial removal of vaginal wall; with removal of paravaginal tissue (radical vaginectomy) with bilateral total pelvic lymphadenectomy and para-aortic lymph node sampling (biopsy)

POLICY INDICATORS

Global Period
90 day post-op period

Assistants at Surgery
Assistant allowed

Co-Surgeons Allowed
Submit reason for co-surgeon

Reduction for Multiple Procedures
Subject to 50% reduction

Bilateral Surgery Payment
Bilateral surgery

Applicable Medicare Policies

Relative Value Units (RVUs)

Work RVUs	28.40
Non-Facility Total	Only valued for facility
Facility Total	52.30

Coding Assistance

57109 includes:

- Positioning and prepping patient
- Examination of site after anesthesia
- Operative services, including inspections around site and closure
- Appropriate post-op E/M visit(s)
- Photodocumentation
- Ureterolysis
- Vaginal procedures
- Catheter insertion
- Abdominal wall incision
- Dissection of bladder and rectum from vaginal wall
- Development of paravaginal and perirectal spaces
- Removal of pelvic lymph nodes bilaterally
- Sampling of lover para-aortic lymph nodes
- Removal of a portion of vagina
- Hemostasis
- Wound closure

Abbreviated Case Note Example:

- A 55-year-old female patient with history of vaginal hysterectomy for carcinoma, is found to have invasive squamous cell carcinoma in the vaginal apex.
- Procedure: Patient is examined under anesthesia. Upper half of the vagina is removed by dissecting the bladder off the anterior vaginal wall and the rectum off the posterior vaginal wall followed by dissection of the ureters from the parametria. The ligamentous supports for the vagina are incised lateral and posterior. A radical bilateral pelvic lymphadenectomy skeletonizes the common iliac, external iliac, hypogastric, and obturator vessels in order to remove all of the lymph nodes that drain the upper vagina. Hemostasis is secured.

Additional Notes

- If a partial radical vaginectomy without lymphadenectomy is performed, report 57017 instead
- For a postoperative counseling visit about sexual function, use the appropriate E/M with modifier 24

SURGERY

CPT® CODE 57110

Vaginectomy, complete removal of vaginal wall

POLICY INDICATORS

Global Period
90 day post-op period

Assistants at Surgery
Assistant allowed

Co-Surgeons Allowed
Submit reason for co-surgeon

Reduction for Multiple Procedures
Subject to 50% reduction

Bilateral Surgery Payment
N/A

Applicable Medicare Policies
Inpatient-only list

Relative Value Units (RVUs)

Work RVUs	15.48
Non-Facility Total	Only valued for facility
Facility Total	27.16

Coding Assistance

57110 includes:

- Positioning and prepping patient
- Examination of site after anesthesia
- Operative services, including inspections around site and closure
- Appropriate post-op E/M visit(s)
- Photodocumentation
- Ureterolysis
- Vaginal procedures
- Catheter insertion
- Incision into vaginal mucosa or submucosa
- Hemostasis
- Wound closure

Abbreviated Case Note Example:

- A 60-year-old female patient with history of total abdominal hysterectomy, is found to have an extensive vaginal carcinoma in situ involving the upper three-quarters of the entire vagina. She is sexually inactive with underlying invasive cancer not to be ruled out. She consents to a complete vaginectomy.
- Procedure: Using a scalpel or cautery, complete vaginectomy is performed. Specimen includes the entire length of the vagina, with dissection of the urethra, bladder, and rectum, and primary closure of the defect.

Additional Notes

- If a vaginal tumor is excised, 57135 may be more appropriate
- For a postoperative counseling visit about sexual function, use the appropriate E/M with modifier 24
- If a partial vaginectomy is performed, report 57106 instead of this code.

CPT® CODE 57111

Vaginectomy, complete removal of vaginal wall; with removal of paravaginal tissue (radical vaginectomy)

POLICY INDICATORS

Global Period
90 day post-op period

Assistants at Surgery
Assistant allowed

Co-Surgeons Allowed
Submit reason for co-surgeon

Reduction for Multiple Procedures
Subject to 50% reduction

Bilateral Surgery Payment
Bilateral surgery

Applicable Medicare Policies
Inpatient-only list

Relative Value Units (RVUs)

Work RVUs	28.40
Non-Facility Total	Only valued for facility
Facility Total	52.30

Coding Assistance

57111 includes:

- Positioning and prepping patient
- Examination of site after anesthesia
- Operative services, including inspections around site and closure
- Appropriate post-op E/M visit(s)
- Photodocumentation
- Ureterolysis
- Vaginal procedures
- Abdominal wall incision
- Catheter insertion
- Dissection of rectum or catheter from vaginal wall
- Development of paravaginal or pararectal space
- Removal of vagina
- Hemostasis
- Wound closure

Abbreviated Case Note Example:

- A 65-year-old female patient with history of hysterectomy, a verrucous vaginal cancer involving the middle and lower one-third of the vagina. Recommend total radical vaginectomy without a lymphadenectomy.
- Procedure: Patient is examined under anesthesia. Exploration of the abdomen, pelvis, and retroperitoneal areas; bladder, rectum, and ureters are dissected. Ligamentous support is cut and vascular pedicles must be clamped and sutured. A separate incision at the vaginal introits and a tissue plane lateral to the vaginal wall is developed, with great care being taken to avoid injury to the bladder and rectum. Vagina and paravaginal tissues are excised. The peritoneal cavity is then irrigated, and hemostasis is secured.

Additional Notes

- If a partial radical vaginectomy without lymphadenectomy is performed, report 57017 instead
- For a postoperative counseling visit about sexual function, use the appropriate E/M with modifier 24

SURGERY

CPT® CODE 57120

Colpocleisis (Le Fort type)

POLICY INDICATORS

Global Period
90 day post-op period

Assistants at Surgery
Assistant allowed

Co-Surgeons Allowed
Submit reason for co-surgeon

Reduction for Multiple Procedures
Subject to 50% reduction

Bilateral Surgery Payment
N/A

Applicable Medicare Policies

Relative Value Units (RVUs)

Work RVUs	8.28
Non-Facility Total	Only valued for facility
Facility Total	16.01

Coding Assistance

57120 includes:

- Positioning and prepping patient
- Examination of site after anesthesia
- Operative services, including inspections around site and closure
- Appropriate post-op E/M visit(s)
- Photodocumentation
- Biopsy of vaginal mucosa
- Excision of vaginal septum
- Irrigation of vagina
- Hemostatic agent or pack
- Wound closure
- Catheter insertion
- Incision of vaginal mucosa or submucosa
- Removal of rectangular tissue section in anterior and posterior vaginal wall

Abbreviated Case Note Example:

- A 55-year-old female patient was found to have a stage III pelvic organ prolapse and diagnosed with vaginal vault prolapse.
- Procedure: The anterior and posterior sections of the vagina are marked using electrocautery to make small dots on the mucosa, and a thin layer of the vaginal mucosa is dissected off.

CPT® CODE 57130

Excision of vaginal septum

POLICY INDICATORS

Global Period
10 day post-op period

Assistants at Surgery
Assistant allowed

Co-Surgeons Allowed
Submit reason for co-surgeon

Reduction for Multiple Procedures
Subject to 50% reduction

Bilateral Surgery Payment
N/A

Applicable Medicare Policies

Relative Value Units (RVUs)

Work RVUs	2.46
Non-Facility Total	6.88
Facility Total	5.23

Coding Assistance

57130 includes:

- Positioning and prepping patient
- Examination of site after anesthesia
- Operative services, including inspections around site and closure
- Appropriate post-op E/M visit(s)
- Photodocumentation
- Biopsy of vaginal mucosa
- Excision of vaginal wall septum
- Irrigation of vagina
- Hemostasis
- Wound closure
- Catheter insertion

Additional Notes

- For a postoperative counseling visit about sexual function, use the appropriate E/M with modifier 24

CPT® CODE 57135

Excision of vaginal cyst or tumor

POLICY INDICATORS

Global Period
10 day post-op period

Assistants at Surgery
No assistant

Co-Surgeons Allowed
No co-surgeon

Reduction for Multiple Procedures
Subject to 50% reduction

Bilateral Surgery Payment
N/A

Applicable Medicare Policies

Relative Value Units (RVUs)

Work RVUs	2.70
Non-Facility Total	7.42
Facility Total	5.69

Coding Assistance

57135 includes:

- Positioning and prepping patient
- Examination of site after anesthesia
- Operative services, including inspections around site and closure
- Appropriate post-op E/M visit(s)
- Photodocumentation
- Excision of vaginal cyst or tumor
- Hemostasis
- Wound closure
- Catheter insertion
- Injection of local anesthesia

Abbreviated Case Note Example:

- A 35-year-old female patient is diagnosed with vaginal cyst, malignancy. Recommended incision and drainage of the vaginal cyst.
- Procedure: General anesthesia is initiated without difficulty. Large vaginal cyst, approximately 10 cm, is adherent to surrounding vaginal mucosa. Using the scalpel to incise and drain the cyst, approximately 500 cc of purulent fluid is drained from the vaginal mucosa. Cyst wall is excised and sent to pathology.

CPT® CODE 57150

Irrigation of vagina and/or application of medicament for treatment of bacterial, parasitic, or fungoid disease

POLICY INDICATORS

Global Period
0 day post-op period

Assistants at Surgery
No assistant

Co-Surgeons Allowed
No co-surgeon

Reduction for Multiple Procedures
Subject to 50% reduction

Bilateral Surgery Payment
N/A

Applicable Medicare Policies

Relative Value Units (RVUs)

Work RVUs	0.50
Non-Facility Total	1.69
Facility Total	0.76

Coding Assistance

57150 includes:

- Positioning and prepping patient
- Examination of site after anesthesia
- Operative services, including inspections around site and closure
- Injection of local anesthesia

Abbreviated Case Note Example:

- A 36-year-old female patient presents for treatment of resistant monilial vaginitis.
- Procedure: Using an irrigating syringe and appropriate fluid, irrigate the vaginal canal until clear of discharge and visualize the vaginal mucosa adequately. Apply appropriate medication to the vaginal mucosa of the apex, sulci, and angles and length of the vaginal walls bilaterally.

CPT® CODE 57155

Insertion of uterine tandem and/or vaginal ovoids for clinical brachytherapy

POLICY INDICATORS

Global Period
0 day post-op period

Assistants at Surgery
No assistant

Co-Surgeons Allowed
Co-surgeon allowed

Reduction for Multiple Procedures
Subject to 50% reduction

Bilateral Surgery Payment
N/A

Applicable Medicare Policies

Relative Value Units (RVUs)

Work RVUs	5.15
Non-Facility Total	12.15
Facility Total	8.65

Coding Assistance

57155 includes:

- Positioning and prepping patient
- Examination of site after anesthesia
- Operative services, including inspections around site and closure
- Placement of catheter
- Examination under anesthesia
- Vaginal packing
- Cervical and vaginal dilation
- Cervical dilation (57800)
- Sounding of uterus for size
- Insertion of uterine tandem
- Placement of vaginal ovoids
- Securing of implants

Abbreviated Case Note Example:

- A 55-year-old female patient with stage IIB cervical cancer completed radiation and chemotherapy. She is scheduled for tandems and ovoids for brachytherapy.
- Procedure: Appropriately curved uterine tandem is selected based on the patient anatomy and the flange marker on the tandem is adjusted to match the desired insertion depth. The tandem (hollow tube) is inserted into the uterus taking care to avoid perforation. The other end of the tandem is left protruding through the vaginal introitus. A right and left ovoid (or comparable ring apparatus) are then are placed in the vaginal fornices and tested for optimal fit. The cap size is modified to correctly match the patient's anatomy. The final ovoid assembly is reinserted and fixed to the tandem (and tenaculum) using a central locking mechanism. A posterior vaginal paddle (rectal displacement retractor) may be inserted and attached to the tandem and ovoids..

Additional Notes

- Report 57155 for placement of cervical sleeve for cervical cancer brachytherapy
- For placement of needles or catheters into pelvic organs and/or genitalia for interstitial radioelement application, report 55920 instead

SURGERY

CPT® CODE 57156

Insertion of a vaginal radiation afterloading apparatus for clinical brachytherapy

POLICY INDICATORS

Global Period
0 day post-op period

Assistants at Surgery
Submit reason for assistant

Co-Surgeons Allowed
No co-surgeon

Reduction for Multiple Procedures
Subject to 50% reduction

Bilateral Surgery Payment
N/A

Applicable Medicare Policies

Relative Value Units (RVUs)

Work RVUs	2.69
Non-Facility Total	6.95
Facility Total	4.59

Coding Assistance

57156 includes:

- Positioning and prepping patient
- Examination of site after anesthesia
- Operative services, including inspections around site and closure

Abbreviated Case Note Example:

- A 56-year-old female patient presents with history of hysterectomy present with stage IB adenocarcinoma of the endometrium, grade 3 with lower uterine segment involvement. Patient received radiation and is scheduled for intravaginal insertion of the radiation.
- Procedure: The largest possible size device is determined. A vaginal cylinder, or other multichannel device, is selected and assembled, inserted into the vagina, and assessed for fit and stability. Device modifications may be required depending on this fit, or packing may be required if vaginal ovoids are used.

CPT® CODE 57160

Fitting and insertion of pessary or other intravaginal support device

POLICY INDICATORS

Global Period
0 day post-op period

Assistants at Surgery
No assistant

Co-Surgeons Allowed
No co-surgeon

Reduction for Multiple Procedures
Subject to 50% reduction

Bilateral Surgery Payment
N/A

Applicable Medicare Policies

Relative Value Units (RVUs)

Work RVUs	0.89
Non-Facility Total	2.23
Facility Total	1.38

Coding Assistance

57160 includes:

- Positioning and prepping patient
- Examination of site after anesthesia
- Operative services, including inspections around site and closure
- Insertion of pessary including determination of proper size and type
- Catherization or catheter insertion

Abbreviated Case Note Example:

- A 64-year-old postmenopausal female patient with history of chronic obstructive pulmonary disease (COPD) presents with cystocele and uterine prolapse.
- Procedure: Insert the fitting pessary into the vagina and assess the prolapse reduction. Perform provocative maneuvers for reduction and pain. Then assess the prolapse reduction and confirm the patient has achieved proper placement.

Additional Notes

- The pessary supply is not included. Bill separately 99070, A4561, or A4562 dependent on payer
- Use the appropriate E/M for the follow-up visits to remove, clean, and reinsert pessary
- It is important to note this is a Medicare 0 global day procedure so follow up care other than hospital visit(s) to assess patient status are not included and should be coded separately

SURGERY

CPT® CODE 57170

Diaphragm or cervical cap fitting with instructions

POLICY INDICATORS

Global Period
0 day post-op period

Assistants at Surgery
Submit reason for assistant

Co-Surgeons Allowed
No co-surgeon

Reduction for Multiple Procedures
Subject to 50% reduction

Bilateral Surgery Payment
N/A

Applicable Medicare Policies

Relative Value Units (RVUs)

Work RVUs	0.91
Non-Facility Total	2.32
Facility Total	1.42

Coding Assistance

57170 includes:

- Positioning and prepping patient
- Examination of site after anesthesia
- Operative services, including inspections around site and closure
- Fitting of diaphragm or cervical cap including determination of proper size and type

Additional Notes

- The diaphragm or cervical cap is not included. Bill separately 99070, A4561, or A4562 dependent on payer
- It is important to note this is a Medicare 0 global day procedure so follow up care other than hospital visit(s) to assess patient status are not included and should be coded separately

CPT® CODE 57180

Introduction of any hemostatic agent or pack for spontaneous or traumatic nonobstetrical vaginal hemorrhage (separate procedure)

POLICY INDICATORS

Global Period
10 day post-op period

Assistants at Surgery
No assistant

Co-Surgeons Allowed
No co-surgeon

Reduction for Multiple Procedures
Subject to 50% reduction

Bilateral Surgery Payment
N/A

Applicable Medicare Policies

Relative Value Units (RVUs)

Work RVUs	1.63
Non-Facility Total	5.88
Facility Total	3.65

Coding Assistance

57180 includes:

- Positioning and prepping patient
- Examination of site after anesthesia
- Operative services, including inspections around site and closure
- Appropriate post-op E/M visit(s)
- Removal of hemostatic pack or agent
- Insertion of hemostatic agent or pack

Additional Notes

- If vaginal laceration(s) are sutured, report 57200 instead
- Use the appropriate E/M with a 57 modifier to determine the need for surgery
- This is a CPT separate procedure code. It is usually considered an integral part of a total service and not reported separately. If it is carried out independently report with modifier 59

CPT® CODE 57200

Colporrhaphy, suture of injury of vagina (nonobstetrical)

POLICY INDICATORS

Global Period
90 day post-op period

Assistants at Surgery
Assistant allowed

Co-Surgeons Allowed
Submit reason for co-surgeon

Reduction for Multiple Procedures
Subject to 50% reduction

Bilateral Surgery Payment
N/A

Applicable Medicare Policies

Relative Value Units (RVUs)

Work RVUs	4.42
Non-Facility Total	Only valued for facility
Facility Total	10.04

Coding Assistance

57200 includes:

- Positioning and prepping patient
- Examination of site after anesthesia
- Operative services, including inspections around site and closure
- Appropriate post-op E/M visit(s)
- Photodocumentation
- Introduction of substance
- Repair of injury and/or correction of defect
- Catheter insertion
- Hemostasis
- Wound closure
- Injection of local anesthesia

Additional Notes

- If repair of traumatic injury to the vagina and perineum is performed, report 57210 instead

SURGERY

CPT® CODE 57210

Colpoperineorrhaphy, suture of injury of vagina and/or perineum (nonobstetrical)

POLICY INDICATORS

Global Period
90 day post-op period

Assistants at Surgery
Assistant allowed

Co-Surgeons Allowed
Submit reason for co-surgeon

Reduction for Multiple Procedures
Subject to 50% reduction

Bilateral Surgery Payment
N/A

Applicable Medicare Policies

Relative Value Units (RVUs)

Work RVUs	5.71
Non-Facility Total	Only valued for facility
Facility Total	11.86

Coding Assistance

57210 includes:

- Positioning and prepping patient
- Examination of site after anesthesia
- Operative services, including inspections around site and closure
- Appropriate post-op E/M visit(s)
- Photodocumentation
- Catheter insertion
- Repair of injury and/or correction of defect
- Hemostasis
- Wound closure
- Injection of local anesthesia

Abbreviated Case Note Example:

- Procedure: The physician inserts a speculum into the vagina and identifies the extent of the vaginal laceration or wound that is not related to childbirth or pregnancy. Usually, a local anesthetic is used; however, some instances may require general anesthesia. The wound is closed with absorbable sutures. In 57210, after the speculum is removed, the perineal laceration is closed in layers with sutures.

CPT® CODE 57220

Plastic operation on urethral sphincter, vaginal approach (eg, Kelly urethral plication)

POLICY INDICATORS

Global Period
90 day post-op period

Assistants at Surgery
Assistant allowed

Co-Surgeons Allowed
Submit reason for co-surgeon

Reduction for Multiple Procedures
Subject to 50% reduction

Bilateral Surgery Payment
N/A

Applicable Medicare Policies

Relative Value Units (RVUs)

Work RVUs	4.85
Non-Facility Total	Only valued for facility
Facility Total	10.48

Coding Assistance

57220 includes:

- Positioning and prepping patient
- Examination of site after anesthesia
- Operative services, including inspections around site and closure
- Appropriate post-op E/M visit(s)
- Photodocumentation
- Vaginal wall incision
- Placement of plication sutures
- Hemostasis
- Wound closure
- Injection of local anesthesia
- Catheter insertion

Additional Notes

- If anterior colporrhaphy with Kelly plication is performed, report 57240 instead

CPT® CODE 57230

Plastic repair of urethrocele

POLICY INDICATORS

Global Period
90 day post-op period

Assistants at Surgery
Assistant allowed

Co-Surgeons Allowed
Submit reason for co-surgeon

Reduction for Multiple Procedures
Subject to 50% reduction

Bilateral Surgery Payment
N/A

Applicable Medicare Policies

Relative Value Units (RVUs)

Work RVUs	6.30
Non-Facility Total	Only valued for facility
Facility Total	12.61

Coding Assistance

57230 includes:

- Positioning and prepping patient
- Examination of site after anesthesia
- Operative services, including inspections around site and closure
- Appropriate post-op E/M visit(s)
- Photodocumentation
- Vaginal biopsy
- Catheter insertion
- Vaginal wall incision
- Repair of urethrocele
- Hemostasis
- Wound closure
- Injection of local anesthesia

Additional Notes

- If posterior colporrhaphy is performed, report 57260 instead
- If posterior colporrhaphy plus enterocele repair is performed, report 57265 instead

CPT® CODE 57240

Anterior colporrhaphy, repair of cystocele with or without repair of urethrocele, including cystourethroscopy, when performed

POLICY INDICATORS

Global Period
90 day post-op period

Assistants at Surgery
Assistant allowed

Co-Surgeons Allowed
Submit reason for co-surgeon

Reduction for Multiple Procedures
Subject to 50% reduction

Bilateral Surgery Payment
N/A

Applicable Medicare Policies

Relative Value Units (RVUs)

Work RVUs	10.08
Non-Facility Total	Only valued for facility
Facility Total	18.50

Coding Assistance

57240 includes:

- Positioning and prepping patient
- Examination of site after anesthesia
- Operative services, including inspections around site and closure
- Appropriate post-op E/M visit(s)
- Photodocumentation
- Plastic operation on urethral sphincter, eg, Kelly urethral plication (57220)
- With or without repair of urethrocele
- Vaginal procedures
- Catheterization of catheter insertion
- Incision of vaginal mucosa
- Repair of anterior fascial defect
- Repair of cystocele
- Injection of local anesthesia

Abbreviated Case Note Example:

- A 67-year-old female patient presents with complaints of vaginal pressure. Symptoms are worse when coughing, standing, or lifting. No stress urinary incontinence; diagnosis is anterior compartment defect that protrudes just beyond the introitus with Valsalva maneuver.
- Procedure: Hydrodissection. Full-thickness incision through the vaginal mucosa is made to expose the space from the urethrovesical junction to the vaginal apex; sharp and blunt dissection is used to mobilize the vaginal tissue laterally. Plicating sutures are placed at the level of the urethrovesical junction. Lateral, paravaginal defects, if identified, are individually repaired. Midline plication of the deep vaginal tissue is performed and redundant vaginal epithelium is excised. Hemostasis is obtained.

Additional Notes

- If posterior colporrhaphy is also performed, report 57260 instead
- If posterior colporrhaphy plus enterocele repair is performed, report 57265 instead
- If paravaginal defect repair is performed, report 57285 instead

CPT® CODE 57250

Posterior colporrhaphy, repair of rectocele with or without perineorrhaphy

POLICY INDICATORS

Global Period
90 day post-op period

Assistants at Surgery
Assistant allowed

Co-Surgeons Allowed
Submit reason for co-surgeon

Reduction for Multiple Procedures
Subject to 50% reduction

Bilateral Surgery Payment
N/A

Applicable Medicare Policies

Relative Value Units (RVUs)

Work RVUs	10.08
Non-Facility Total	Only valued for facility
Facility Total	18.56

Coding Assistance

57250 includes:

- Positioning and prepping patient
- Examination of site after anesthesia
- Operative services, including inspections around site and closure
- Appropriate post-op E/M visit(s)
- Photodocumentation
- Perineoplasty
- Catheter insertion
- Repair of posterior vaginal wall
- Repair of rectocele
- Repair of perineum
- Repair of injury and/or correction of defect
- Bladder drainage
- Hemostasis
- Wound closure
- Injection of local anesthesia

Abbreviated Case Note Example:

- A 73-year-old female patient with history of hysterectomy presents with a bulging mass and difficulty completely evacuating with defecation, worsening over time. She is diagnosed with posterior midline defect, which protrudes past the introitus with Valsalva. Recommend a posterior colporrhaphy.
- Procedure: Hydrodissection. Incision is extended into the posterior vaginal epithelium and full-thickness dissection of vaginal epithelium from underlying rectovaginal septum is accomplished to the vaginal apex and medial margins of the levator musculature. Rectal examination. A triangular strip of full-thickness vaginal wall is removed. Apical detachments, if present, are corrected. Repair and plication of the perirectal and rectovaginal fascia are performed from the vaginal apex to the vaginal introitus. Puborectalis and levator ani are plicated distal to the rectovaginal space. Perineal body is reconstructed by plicating the superficial and deep perineal muscles. Distal rectovaginal septum is reattached to the perineal body. Hemostasis is obtained.

Additional Notes

- If anterior colporrhaphy is also performed, report 57260 instead
- If repair of rectocele without posterior colporrhaphy is performed, report 45560 instead

CPT® CODE 57260

Combined anteroposterior colporrhaphy, including cystourethroscopy, when performed

POLICY INDICATORS

Global Period
90 day post-op period

Assistants at Surgery
Assistant allowed

Co-Surgeons Allowed
Submit reason for co-surgeon

Reduction for Multiple Procedures
Subject to 50% reduction

Bilateral Surgery Payment
N/A

Applicable Medicare Policies

Relative Value Units (RVUs)

Work RVUs	13.25
Non-Facility Total	Only valued for facility
Facility Total	23.44

Coding Assistance

57260 includes:

- Positioning and prepping patient
- Examination of site after anesthesia
- Operative services, including inspections around site and closure
- Appropriate post-op E/M visit(s)
- Photodocumentation
- Catheter insertion
- Vaginal procedures

Abbreviated Case Note Example:

- A 65-year-old female patient presents with vulvar pressure and a mass that protrudes from the vagina, which is worse with coughing or standing. No stress urinary incontinence, but incomplete emptying of bowel and bladder. Diagnosis is distal defects in the anterior and posterior compartments that are to the introitus with Valsalva maneuver. Recommend an anterior and posterior colporrhaphy.
- Procedure: Hydrodissection may be performed. Lateral, paravaginal defects, if identified, are individually repaired. Midline plication, suture correction of vaginal defects, and excessive vaginal epithelium is excised. Cystoscopy may be performed. A triangular incision is made on the perineal body, repair and plication of the perirectal and recto-vaginal fascia are performed. Hemostasis is obtained.

Additional Notes

- If enterocele is also performed, report 57265 instead

CPT® CODE 57265

Combined anteroposterior colporrhaphy, including cystourethroscopy, when performed; with enterocele repair

POLICY INDICATORS

Global Period
90 day post-op period

Assistants at Surgery
Assistant allowed

Co-Surgeons Allowed
Submit reason for co-surgeon

Reduction for Multiple Procedures
Subject to 50% reduction

Bilateral Surgery Payment
N/A

Applicable Medicare Policies

Relative Value Units (RVUs)

Work RVUs	15.00
Non-Facility Total	Only valued for facility
Facility Total	26.21

Coding Assistance

57265 includes:

- Positioning and prepping patient
- Examination of site after anesthesia
- Operative services, including inspections around site and closure
- Appropriate post-op E/M visit(s)
- Photodocumentation
- Perineoplasty
- Vaginal procedures
- Catheterization or catheter insertion
- Plastic repair of anterior and posterior vaginal wall
- Repair of rectocele and cystocele
- Repair of enterocele
- Remove of excess vaginal mucosa
- Hemostasis
- Wound closure
- Injection of local anesthesia

Abbreviated Case Note Example:

- A 55-year-old female patient with history of hysterectomy presents with mass protuding from the vagina, worse with coughing or standing. No stress incontinence, but incomplete emptying of bowel and bladder. Diagnosis is anterior compartment defect, a posterior compartment defect, apical descent with ballooning of the apex extending down the upper posterior wall; enterocoele on recto-vaginal exam. Recommend an anterior posterior colporrhaphy with enterocele repair.
- Procedure: Hydrodissection may be performed. Midline plication of the deep vaginal tissue is performed. Excessive vaginal epithelium is excised. Cystoscopy is performed. Bladder mucosal integrity and bilateral ureteral patency are confirmed. Vaginal incision is closed. Full-thickness dissection of vaginal epithelium from underlying recto-vaginal septum is accomplished; further dissection is performed above the vaginal apex to delineate the enterocele sac. The posterior vaginal wall is dissected from the enterocele sac, anterior rectal wall, and rectovaginal septum through sharp and blunt dissection. Small bowel and omental adhesions, if present, are dissected to the level of the neck of the enterocele. Cystoscopy is performed. The anterior and posterior portions of the mucosal apex are reapproximated. Rectal examination is performed to identify rectovaginal fascial defects, laterally, superiorly, and at the perineal body. Portions of full-thickness vaginal wall are removed. Repair and plication of the perirectal and rectovaginal fascia are performed from the vaginal apex to the vaginal introitus. Puborectalis and levator ani are plicated distal to the rectovaginal space. Perineal body is reconstructed by plicating the superficial and deep perineal muscles. Distal rectovaginal septum is reattached to the perineal body. Hemostasis is obtained.

Additional Notes

- 57283 should not be reported with 57265

CPT® CODE 57267

Insertion of mesh or other prosthesis for repair of pelvic floor defect, each site (anterior, posterior compartment), vaginal approach
(List separately in addition to code for primary procedure)

POLICY INDICATORS

Global Period
Global for primary procedure applies

Assistants at Surgery
Assistant allowed

Co-Surgeons Allowed
Submit reason for co-surgeon

Reduction for Multiple Procedures
Not subject to multiple surgery reduction

Bilateral Surgery Payment
N/A

Applicable Medicare Policies

Relative Value Units (RVUs)

Work RVUs	4.88
Non-Facility Total	Only valued for facility
Facility Total	7.47

Coding Assistance

57267 includes:

- Positioning and prepping patient
- Examination of site after anesthesia
- Operative services, including inspections around site and closure
- Appropriate post-op E/M visit(s)
- Catheter insertion
- Prep of surgical graft
- Dissection deep into pelvis
- Attachment of graft
- Resection or irrigation of excess vaginal epithelium
- Hemostasis
- Wound closure
- Injection of local anesthesia
- Photodocumentation

Add-On Code:

- Follow Primary Code Policies

Additional Notes

- CPT add-on code can only be reported when a vaginal repair code (45560, 52740-57265, 57285) is also reported. No modifier 51 is needed.

CPT® CODE 57268

Repair of enterocele, vaginal approach (separate procedure)

POLICY INDICATORS

Global Period
90 day post-op period

Assistants at Surgery
Assistant allowed

Co-Surgeons Allowed
Submit reason for co-surgeon

Reduction for Multiple Procedures
Subject to 50% reduction

Bilateral Surgery Payment
N/A

Applicable Medicare Policies

Relative Value Units (RVUs)

Work RVUs	7.57
Non-Facility Total	Only valued for facility
Facility Total	15.30

Coding Assistance

57268 includes:

- Positioning and prepping patient
- Examination of site after anesthesia
- Operative services, including inspections around site and closure
- Appropriate post-op E/M visit(s)
- Introduction of hemostatic pack (57180)
- Perineoplasty
- Catheter insertion
- Destruction, excision or biopsy of vaginal lesions, any method
- Irrigation and placement of drain
- Hemostasis
- Wound closure
- Injection of local anesthesia

Additional Notes

- This is a CPT separate procedure code, usually part of a total service and not reported separately. If it is independently carried out, report with modifier 59, or other submodifier per payer policy
- Applying a -59 modifier to 57268 may be required by payers for this procedure to be separately reimbursed.

CPT® CODE 57270

Repair of enterocele, abdominal approach (separate procedure)

POLICY INDICATORS

Global Period
90 day post-op period

Assistants at Surgery
Assistant allowed

Co-Surgeons Allowed
Submit reason for co-surgeon

Reduction for Multiple Procedures
Subject to 50% reduction

Bilateral Surgery Payment
N/A

Applicable Medicare Policies
Inpatient-only list

Relative Value Units (RVUs)

Work RVUs	13.67
Non-Facility Total	Only valued for facility
Facility Total	24.44

Coding Assistance

57270 includes:

- Positioning and prepping patient
- Examination of site after anesthesia
- Operative services, including inspections around site and closure
- Appropriate post-op E/M visit(s)
- Introduction of hemostatic pack
- Biopsy of vaginal mucosa
- Catheter insertion
- Enterolysis
- Exploratory laparotomy, retroperitoneal exploration or biopsy
- Pelvic examination under anesthesia
- Abdominal incision
- Repair of enterocele
- Irrigation and placement of drain
- Hemostasis
- Wound closure
- Injection of local anesthesia

Abbreviated Care Note Example:

- A 65-year-old female with history of hysterectomy presents with a bulge in the vaginal area. Diagnosed with an enterocele; undergoes a repair by abdominal approach.
- Procedure: The enterocele defect is located in the pelvis. The defect is repaired by several techniques that obliterate the cul-de-sac. Oftentimes, excision of the enterocele sac is necessary. Hemostasis is secured.

Additional Notes

- This is a CPT separate procedure code, usually part of a total service and not reported separately. If it is independently carried out, report with modifier 59, or other submodifier per payer policy

CPT® CODE 57280

Colpopexy, abdominal approach

POLICY INDICATORS

Global Period
90 day post-op period

Assistants at Surgery
Assistant allowed

Co-Surgeons Allowed
Submit reason for co-surgeon

Reduction for Multiple Procedures
Subject to 50% reduction

Bilateral Surgery Payment
N/A

Applicable Medicare Policies
Inpatient-only list

Relative Value Units (RVUs)

Work RVUs	16.72
Non-Facility Total	Only valued for facility
Facility Total	29.04

Coding Assistance

57280 includes:

- Positioning and prepping patient
- Examination of site after anesthesia
- Operative services, including inspections around site and closure
- Appropriate post-op E/M visit(s)
- Application of allograft
- Enterocele repair
- Catheter insertion
- Enterolysis
- Exploratory laparotomy, retroperitoneal exploration or biopsy

Abbreviated Case Note Example:

- A 70-year-old female patient with a history of leiomyomatosis and repair of cystocele and rectocele. Diagnosed with prolapse of the vaginal vault through the introitus and good anterior and posterior support.
- Procedure: Using an abdominal incision, the bladder is dissected off the anterior vaginal wall and the posterior wall is freed. The peritoneal overlying the sacrum is incised and the periosteum cleared. Using a variety of techniques, the vagina is secured to the periosteum of the sacral promontory. Edges of the "sling" are assessed to prevent internal hernia formation..

Additional Notes

- If performed laparoscopically, report 57425 instead

CPT® CODE 57282

Colpopexy, vaginal; extra-peritoneal approach (sacrospinous, iliococcygeus)

POLICY INDICATORS

Global Period
90 day post-op period

Assistants at Surgery
Assistant allowed

Co-Surgeons Allowed
Submit reason for co-surgeon

Reduction for Multiple Procedures
Subject to 50% reduction

Bilateral Surgery Payment
N/A

Applicable Medicare Policies

Relative Value Units (RVUs)

Work RVUs	11.63
Non-Facility Total	Only valued for facility
Facility Total	20.89

Coding Assistance

57282 includes:

- Positioning and prepping patient
- Examination of site after anesthesia
- Operative services, including inspections around site and closure
- Appropriate post-op E/M visit(s)
- Photodocumentation

Abbreviated Case Note Example:

- A 55-year-old female patient presents with worsening pelvic pressure; diagnosed with apical prolapse of the vagina greater than or equal to 4 cm.
- Procedure: Dissect through the subepithelial tissues and enter the pararectal space. Deflect the rectum, identify the ischial spine digitally, create visualization of the sacrospinous ligament-iliococcygeus muscle complex. Place the permanent fixation sutures. Repeat this deep dissection on the contralateral side. Using a Mayo needle, secure the tagged fixation sutures from each side to the apical endopelvic fascia and vaginal muscularis. Utilizing a pulley knot arrangement, tension the sutures to return the vaginal apex to normal anatomic position high in the pelvis and tie the sutures. Ensure hemostasis. Perform a cystoscopy to ensure no trauma to the bladder.

Additional Notes

- If intro-peritoneal approach is used, report 57283 instead

CPT® CODE 57283

Colpopexy, vaginal; intra-peritoneal approach (uterosacral, levator myorrhaphy)

POLICY INDICATORS

Global Period
90 day post-op period

Assistants at Surgery
Assistant allowed

Co-Surgeons Allowed
Submit reason for co-surgeon

Reduction for Multiple Procedures
Subject to 50% reduction

Bilateral Surgery Payment
N/A

Applicable Medicare Policies

Relative Value Units (RVUs)

Work RVUs	11.66
Non-Facility Total	Only valued for facility
Facility Total	21.06

Coding Assistance

57283 includes:

- Positioning and prepping patient
- Examination of site after anesthesia
- Operative services, including inspections around site and closure
- Appropriate post-op E/M visit(s)
- Photodocumentation

Abbreviated Case Note Example:

- A 65-year-old female patient presents with vaginal bulging; diagnosed with inversion of the vaginal apex 2 cm beyond the hymen; enterocele at the vaginal apex. She consents to intraperitoneal vaginal colpopexy.
- Procedure: Incise the apical vaginal wall, dissect through the subepithelial tissues, and identify the peritoneum. Identify the uterosacral ligaments, place a delayed absorbable suture through the uterosacral ligament distally on one side and through a portion of the posterior peritoneum wall medially. Place a second suture through the uterosacral ligament and place a minimum of three sutures in this same fashion. Repeat. Perform cystoscopy and survey the bladder for abnormality or trauma. Confirm ureteral patency, from cephalad to caudal position; tension each of the suture pairs previously placed. Confirm viscous safety and hemostasis. Fix the sutures to the vaginal mucosae and endopelvic fascia. Ensure retroperitoneal hemostasis.

Additional Notes

- Use this code to report a high uterosacral suspension or a McCall type culdoplasty
- If extra-peritoneal approach is used, report 57282 instead

CPT® CODE 57284

Paravaginal defect repair (including repair of cystocele, if performed); open abdominal approach

POLICY INDICATORS

Global Period
90 day post-op period

Assistants at Surgery
Assistant allowed

Co-Surgeons Allowed
Co-surgeon allowed

Reduction for Multiple Procedures
Subject to 50% reduction

Bilateral Surgery Payment
N/A

Applicable Medicare Policies

Relative Value Units (RVUs)

Work RVUs	14.33
Non-Facility Total	Only valued for facility
Facility Total	25.21

Coding Assistance

57284 includes:

- Positioning and prepping patient
- Examination of site after anesthesia
- Operative services, including inspections around site and closure
- Appropriate post-op E/M visit(s)
- Introduction of hemostatic pack
- Biopsy of vaginal mucosa
- Catheter insertion
- Anterior vesicourtethropexy or urethropexy (Marshall-Marchetti-Krantz/Burch procedure)
- Pelvic examination under anesthesia

Abbreviated Case Note Example:

- A 45-year-old female patient with history of hysterectomy presents with vaginal pressure and heaviness; anterior vaginal wall relaxation reveals a cystocele arising from paravaginal defects. Recommend abdominal paravaginal defect repair.
- Procedure: Make incision in the abdominal wall and access the Retzius space transperitoneally. Extend the dissection to expose the arcus tendineus fascia pelvis (ATFP) bilaterally. Several permanent sutures are passed along the anterior lateral vaginal sulcus (on each side) through the pubocervical fascia. These sutures are then brought through the obturator internus muscle, just above the ATFP, along its full length from the underside of the pubic symphysis down to the ischial spine. This is performed bilaterally. All sutures are tied to obliterate the defect.

Additional Notes

- If repair is performed vaginally, report 57285 instead
- if repair is performed laparoscopically, report 57423 instead
- If abdominal hysterectomy with colpo-urethocystopexy is performed, report 58152 or 58267

CPT® CODE 57285

Paravaginal defect repair (including repair of cystocele, if performed); vaginal approach

POLICY INDICATORS

Global Period
90 day post-op period

Assistants at Surgery
Assistant allowed

Co-Surgeons Allowed
Co-surgeon allowed

Reduction for Multiple Procedures
Subject to 50% reduction

Bilateral Surgery Payment
N/A

Applicable Medicare Policies

Relative Value Units (RVUs)

Work RVUs	11.60
Non-Facility Total	Only valued for facility
Facility Total	20.86

Coding Assistance

57285 includes:

- Positioning and prepping patient
- Examination of site after anesthesia
- Operative services, including inspections around site and closure
- Appropriate post-op E/M visit(s)
- Introduction of hemostatic pack (57180)
- Biopsy of vaginal mucosa
- Catheter insertion
- Colporrhaphy
- Pelvic examination under anesthesia

Abbreviated Case Note Example:

- A 47-year-old female patient presents with cystocele arising from paravaginal defects. Perform a vaginal paravaginal defect repair.
- Procedure: Vaginal access to the space of Retzius is obtained by opening the anterior vaginal wall and dissecting the bladder from the vaginal epithelium. The dissection is extended to expose the arcus tendineus fascia pelvis (ATFP) bilaterally. Several permanent sutures are passed along the anterior lateral vaginal sulcus (on each side) through the pubocervical fascia. These sutures are then brought through the obturator internus muscle, just above the ATFP, along its full length from the underside of the pubic symphysis down to the ischial spine. This is performed bilaterally. Sutures are tied to obliterate the defect.

Additional Notes

- If repair is performed abdominally, report 57284 instead
- If repair is performed laparoscopically, report 57423 instead
- If hysterectomy with colpo-urethocystopexy is performed, report 58182 or 58267 instead

CPT® CODE 57287

Removal or revision of sling for stress incontinence (eg, fascia or synthetic)

POLICY INDICATORS

Global Period
90 day post-op period

Assistants at Surgery
Assistant allowed

Co-Surgeons Allowed
Submit reason for co-surgeon

Reduction for Multiple Procedures
Subject to 50% reduction

Bilateral Surgery Payment
N/A

Applicable Medicare Policies

Relative Value Units (RVUs)

Work RVUs	11.15
Non-Facility Total	Only valued for facility
Facility Total	22.34

Coding Assistance

57287 includes:

- Positioning and prepping patient
- Examination of site after anesthesia
- Operative services, including inspections around site and closure
- Appropriate post-op E/M visit(s)
- Photodocumentation

Abbreviated Case Note Example:

- A 65-year-old female patient with history of a transvaginal sling procedure utilizing synthetic material, presents with urinary retention, and sling removal is recommended.
- Procedure: A left vaginal incision is performed in the anterior vaginal vault lateral to the urethra, and carried down to the graft material. The graft material is dissected bilaterally and graft is removed. Irrigate incision sites and ensure hemostasis. Close the abdominal and vaginal incisions. Perform a cystoscopy.

Additional Notes

- Medicare will not reimburse the primary surgeon to treat a complication during surgery (eg, bladder or small bowel repair)

CPT® CODE 57288

Sling operation for stress incontinence (eg, fascia or synthetic)

POLICY INDICATORS

Global Period
90 day post-op period

Assistants at Surgery
Assistant allowed

Co-Surgeons Allowed
Submit reason for co-surgeon

Reduction for Multiple Procedures
Subject to 50% reduction

Bilateral Surgery Payment
N/A

Applicable Medicare Policies

Relative Value Units (RVUs)

Work RVUs	12.13
Non-Facility Total	Only valued for facility
Facility Total	22.44

Coding Assistance

57288 includes:

- Positioning and prepping patient
- Examination of site after anesthesia
- Operative services, including inspections around site and closure
- Appropriate post-op E/M visit(s)
- Photodocumentation
- Removal of urethral or suprapubic catheter

Abbreviated Case Note Example:

- A 56-year-old female patient presents with urinary incontinence and urethral dysfunction. She is scheduled for a sling operation for stress incontinence.
- Procedure: Make a vaginal incision and resect bilaterally to develop the perivesical space. Perform bilateral perforation on the diaphragm/endopelvic fascia in the retropubic space. Then make a suprapubic incision(s), place and position the sling. Suture the sling in place. Copiously irrigate incision sites and ensure hemostasis. Close and perform cystoscopy.

Additional Notes

- Use this code to report tension-free vaginal tape (TVT) and transobturator tape (TOT) sling procedures
- If this procedure is performed laparoscopically, report 51992 instead

CPT® CODE 57289

Pereyra procedure, including anterior colporrhaphy

POLICY INDICATORS

Global Period
90 day post-op period

Assistants at Surgery
Assistant allowed

Co-Surgeons Allowed
Submit reason for co-surgeon

Reduction for Multiple Procedures
Subject to 50% reduction

Bilateral Surgery Payment
N/A

Applicable Medicare Policies

Relative Value Units (RVUs)

Work RVUs	12.80
Non-Facility Total	Only valued for facility
Facility Total	23.86

Coding Assistance

57289 includes:

- Positioning and prepping patient
- Examination of site after anesthesia
- Operative services, including inspections around site and closure
- Appropriate post-op E/M visit(s)
- Photodocumentation
- Destruction, excision, or biopsy of vaginal lesions

Abbreviated Case Note Example:

- A 70-year-old female patient presents with symptoms of stress urinary incontinence; diagnosed with a large cystocele with loss of urethrovesical support.
- Procedure: Through two small lower abdominal incisions, a suture is placed retropubically and looped around the neck of the bladder where it joins the urethra, anchored to the abdominal wall fascia, thus suspending the urethrovesical angle (Pereyra procedure). The perivesicle fascia is plicated midline, and vaginal mucosa is re-approximated, thus completing the anterior colporrhaphy.

CPT® CODE 57291

Construction of artificial vagina; without graft

POLICY INDICATORS

Global Period
90 day post-op period

Assistants at Surgery
Assistant allowed

Co-Surgeons Allowed
No co-surgeon

Reduction for Multiple Procedures
Subject to 50% reduction

Bilateral Surgery Payment
N/A

Applicable Medicare Policies

Relative Value Units (RVUs)

Work RVUs	8.64
Non-Facility Total	Only valued for facility
Facility Total	16.59

Coding Assistance

57291 includes:

- Positioning and prepping patient
- Examination of site after anesthesia
- Operative services, including inspections around site and closure
- Appropriate post-op E/M visit(s)
- Photodocumentation
- Introduction of hemostatic agent or pack
- Irrigation of vagina

Additional Notes

- If a graft is used, report 57292 instead
- If mold or obturator is removed and replaced in the postoperative period, use 57410 with modifier 78
- For a postoperative counseling visit about sexual function, use the appropriate E/M with modifier 24

CPT® CODE 57292

Construction of artificial vagina; with graft

POLICY INDICATORS

Global Period
90 day post-op period

Assistants at Surgery
Assistant allowed

Co-Surgeons Allowed
Submit reason for co-surgeon

Reduction for Multiple Procedures
Subject to 50% reduction

Bilateral Surgery Payment
N/A

Applicable Medicare Policies

Relative Value Units (RVUs)

Work RVUs	14.01
Non-Facility Total	Only valued for facility
Facility Total	24.91

Coding Assistance

57292 includes:

- Positioning and prepping patient
- Examination of site after anesthesia
- Operative services, including inspections around site and closure
- Appropriate post-op E/M visit(s)
- Photodocumentation
- Introduction of hemostatic agent or pack
- Irrigation of vagina

Additional Notes

- If a graft is used, report 57292 instead
- If mold or obturator is removed and replaced in the postoperative period, use 57410 with modifier 78
- For a postoperative counseling visit about sexual function, use the appropriate E/M with modifier 24

CPT® CODE 57295

Revision (including removal) of prosthetic vaginal graft; vaginal approach

POLICY INDICATORS

Global Period
90 day post-op period

Assistants at Surgery
Assistant allowed

Co-Surgeons Allowed
Submit reason for co-surgeon

Reduction for Multiple Procedures
Subject to 50% reduction

Bilateral Surgery Payment
N/A

Applicable Medicare Policies

Relative Value Units (RVUs)

Work RVUs	7.82
Non-Facility Total	Only valued for facility
Facility Total	15.14

Coding Assistance

57295 includes:

- Positioning and prepping patient
- Examination of site after anesthesia
- Operative services, including inspections around site and closure
- Appropriate post-op E/M visit(s)
- Photodocumentation
- Vaginal biopsy
- Repair of urethrocele
- Plastic operation on urethral sphincter

Abbreviated Case Note Example:

- A 60-year-old female patient with a history of abdominal sacral colpopexy with mesh presents with mesh eroding through the vagina apex. Recommend excision via the vaginal route.
- Procedure: Dissect the vaginal epithelium sharply around the eroding mesh circumferentially about 2 cm. Grasp the eroding mesh and excised sharply all eroding material. Complete excision and close the vaginal epithelium in layers.

Additional Notes

- If performed using an abdominal approach, report 57296 instead
- 57240 is separately billable in connection with 57295 with distinct ICD-10-CM diagnosis code.

CPT® CODE 57296

Revision (including removal) of prosthetic vaginal graft; open abdominal approach

POLICY INDICATORS

Global Period
90 day post-op period

Assistants at Surgery
Assistant allowed

Co-Surgeons Allowed
Submit reason for co-surgeon

Reduction for Multiple Procedures
Subject to 50% reduction

Bilateral Surgery Payment
N/A

Applicable Medicare Policies
Inpatient-only list

Relative Value Units (RVUs)

Work RVUs	16.56
Non-Facility Total	Only valued for facility
Facility Total	28.82

Coding Assistance

57296 includes:

- Positioning and prepping patient
- Examination of site after anesthesia
- Operative services, including inspections around site and closure
- Appropriate post-op E/M visit(s)
- Photodocumentation

Abbreviated Case Note Example:

- A 55-year-old female patient with history of abdominal sacral colpopexy presents with mesh eroding through the apex of the vagina. Recommend excision of the mesh via the abdominal route.
- Procedure: Access the pelvis via laparotomy. Identify the graft and sharply dissect at the area of graft attachment to the vagina. Vaginal epithelium around the eroding mesh is dissected, eroding material is excised and remaining edges of the endopelvic fascia are re-approximated. Repeat dissection and remove the graft. Skin wounds and vaginal mucosa are re-approximated.

Additional Notes

- If performed using an abdominal approach, report 57295 instead

SURGERY

CPT® CODE 57300

Closure of rectovaginal fistula; vaginal or transanal approach

POLICY INDICATORS

Global Period
90 day post-op period

Assistants at Surgery
Assistant allowed

Co-Surgeons Allowed
Submit reason for co-surgeon

Reduction for Multiple Procedures
Subject to 50% reduction

Bilateral Surgery Payment
N/A

Applicable Medicare Policies

Relative Value Units (RVUs)

Work RVUs	8.71
Non-Facility Total	Only valued for facility
Facility Total	18.46

Coding Assistance

57300 includes:

- Positioning and prepping patient
- Examination of site after anesthesia
- Operative services, including inspections around site and closure
- Appropriate post-op E/M visit(s)
- Photodocumentation

Additional Notes

- If colostomy is performed, use 57307 instead
- If performed using an abdominal approach, report 57305 instead
- If performed using a transperineal approach, use 57308 instead

CPT® CODE 57305

Closure of rectovaginal fistula; abdominal approach

POLICY INDICATORS

Global Period
90 day post-op period

Assistants at Surgery
Assistant allowed

Co-Surgeons Allowed
Submit reason for co-surgeon

Reduction for Multiple Procedures
Subject to 50% reduction

Bilateral Surgery Payment
N/A

Applicable Medicare Policies
Inpatient-only list

Relative Value Units (RVUs)

Work RVUs	15.35
Non-Facility Total	Only valued for facility
Facility Total	29.29

Coding Assistance

57305 includes:

- Positioning and prepping patient
- Examination of site after anesthesia
- Operative services, including inspections around site and closure
- Appropriate post-op E/M visit(s)
- Photodocumentation
- Exploratory laparotomy

Abbreviated Case Note Example:

- A 55-year-old female patient with history of total abdominal hysterectomy with bilateral salpingo-oophorectomy presents with leaking stool from vagina; diagnosed with rectovaginal fistula at approximately 15 cm in the rectosigmoid.
- Procedure: Abdominal cavity is explored; the sigmoid is mobilized. The rectovaginal septum is entered and the vagina is bluntly and sharply dissected from the rectum. The fistula is identified and excised. The defect in the rectosigmoid is closed; the defect in the vagina is closed.

Additional Notes

- If colostomy is performed, use 57307 instead
- If performed using vaginal or transanal approach, report 57300 instead
- If performed using a transperineal approach, use 57308 instead

CPT® CODE 57307

Closure of rectovaginal fistula; abdominal approach, with concomitant colostomy

POLICY INDICATORS

Global Period
90 day post-op period

Assistants at Surgery
Assistant allowed

Co-Surgeons Allowed
Submit reason for co-surgeon

Reduction for Multiple Procedures
Subject to 50% reduction

Bilateral Surgery Payment
N/A

Applicable Medicare Policies
Inpatient-only list

Relative Value Units (RVUs)

Work RVUs	17.17
Non-Facility Total	Only valued for facility
Facility Total	32.46

Coding Assistance

57307 includes:

- Positioning and prepping patient
- Examination of site after anesthesia
- Operative services, including inspections around site and closure
- Appropriate post-op E/M visit(s)
- Photodocumentation
- Exploratory laparotomy

Abbreviated Case Note Example:

- A 55-year-old female patient presents with stool leakage from vaginal post total abdominal hysterectomy; diagnosed with a rectovaginal fistula at approximately 15 cm in the rectosigmoid.
- Procedure: Abdominal cavity is explored; the sigmoid is mobilized. The rectovaginal septum is entered and the vagina is bluntly and sharply dissected from the rectum. The fistula is identified and excised. The defect in the rectosigmoid is closed; the defect in the vagina is closed. Diverting colostomy is needed to ensure primary closure of the fistula. A separate skin incision is made for the colostomy. A fascial incision is created and the loop of large bowel is brought out of the abdomen through this opening. It is fixed in place with sutures.

Additional Notes

- If concomitant colostomy is not performed, report 57305 instead
- If performed using vaginal or transanal approach, report 57300 instead
- If performed using a transperineal approach, use 57308 instead

CPT® CODE 57308

Closure of rectovaginal fistula; transperineal approach, with perineal body reconstruction, with or without levator plication

POLICY INDICATORS

Global Period
90 day post-op period

Assistants at Surgery
Assistant allowed

Co-Surgeons Allowed
Submit reason for co-surgeon

Reduction for Multiple Procedures
Subject to 50% reduction

Bilateral Surgery Payment
N/A

Applicable Medicare Policies
Inpatient-only list

Relative Value Units (RVUs)

Work RVUs	10.59
Non-Facility Total	Only valued for facility
Facility Total	20.07

Coding Assistance

57308 includes:

- Positioning and prepping patient
- Examination of site after anesthesia
- Operative services, including inspections around site and closure
- Appropriate post-op E/M visit(s)
- Photodocumentation
- Perineoplasty

Abbreviated Case Note Example:

- A 40-year-old female patient developed a rectovaginal fistula following childbirth; failed prior vaginal repair. A transperineal repair is planned.
- Procedure: Make a semicircular incision in the anterior perineum, and place a probe in the fistula. Separate and dissect the tract from the sphincter; excise the vaginal and rectal mucosa and perform an overlapping sphincter repair. Cover the sphincter with soft tissue, and suture the vaginal mucosa. Perform a perineoplasty with a Y-plasty or X-Z plasty.

Additional Notes

- If performed using vaginal or transanal approach, report 57300 instead
- If performed using an abdominal approach, report 57305 or 57307 instead

SURGERY

CPT® CODE 57310

Closure of urethrovaginal fistula

POLICY INDICATORS

Global Period
90 day post-op period

Assistants at Surgery
Assistant allowed

Co-Surgeons Allowed
Submit reason for co-surgeon

Reduction for Multiple Procedures
Subject to 50% reduction

Bilateral Surgery Payment
N/A

Applicable Medicare Policies

Relative Value Units (RVUs)

Work RVUs	7.65
Non-Facility Total	Only valued for facility
Facility Total	14.90

Coding Assistance

57310 includes:

- Positioning and prepping patient
- Examination of site after anesthesia
- Operative services, including inspections around site and closure
- Appropriate post-op E/M visit(s)
- Photodocumentation

CPT® CODE 57311

Closure of urethrovaginal fistula; with bulbocavernosus transplant

POLICY INDICATORS

Global Period
90 day post-op period

Assistants at Surgery
Assistant allowed

Co-Surgeons Allowed
Submit reason for co-surgeon

Reduction for Multiple Procedures
Subject to 50% reduction

Bilateral Surgery Payment
N/A

Applicable Medicare Policies
Inpatient-only list

Relative Value Units (RVUs)

Work RVUs	8.91
Non-Facility Total	Only valued for facility
Facility Total	16.78

Coding Assistance

57311 includes:

- Positioning and prepping patient
- Examination of site after anesthesia
- Operative services, including inspections around site and closure
- Appropriate post-op E/M visit(s)
- Photodocumentation
- Introduction of hemostatic agent or pack

CPT® CODE 57320

Closure of vesicovaginal fistula; vaginal approach

POLICY INDICATORS

Global Period
90 day post-op period

Assistants at Surgery
Assistant allowed

Co-Surgeons Allowed
Submit reason for co-surgeon

Reduction for Multiple Procedures
Subject to 50% reduction

Bilateral Surgery Payment
N/A

Applicable Medicare Policies

Relative Value Units (RVUs)

Work RVUs	8.88
Non-Facility Total	Only valued for facility
Facility Total	17.01

Coding Assistance

57320 includes:

- Positioning and prepping patient
- Examination of site after anesthesia
- Operative services, including inspections around site and closure
- Appropriate post-op E/M visit(s)
- Photodocumentation

Additional Notes

- For concomitant cystostomy, see codes 51020-51040, 51101-51102

CPT® CODE 57330

Closure of vesicovaginal fistula; transvesical and vaginal approach

POLICY INDICATORS

Global Period
90 day post-op period

Assistants at Surgery
Assistant allowed

Co-Surgeons Allowed
Submit reason for co-surgeon

Reduction for Multiple Procedures
Subject to 50% reduction

Bilateral Surgery Payment
N/A

Applicable Medicare Policies

Relative Value Units (RVUs)

Work RVUs	13.21
Non-Facility Total	Only valued for facility
Facility Total	23.09

Coding Assistance

57330 includes:

- Positioning and prepping patient
- Examination of site after anesthesia
- Operative services, including inspections around site and closure
- Appropriate post-op E/M visit(s)
- Photodocumentation

Additional Notes

- If performed using an abdominal approach, report 51900 instead

CPT® CODE 57335

Vaginoplasty for intersex state

POLICY INDICATORS

Global Period
90 day post-op period

Assistants at Surgery
Assistant allowed

Co-Surgeons Allowed
Submit reason for co-surgeon

Reduction for Multiple Procedures
Subject to 50% reduction

Bilateral Surgery Payment
N/A

Applicable Medicare Policies

Relative Value Units (RVUs)

Work RVUs	20.02
Non-Facility Total	Only valued for facility
Facility Total	35.36

Coding Assistance

57335 includes:

- Positioning and prepping patient
- Examination of site after anesthesia
- Operative services, including inspections around site and closure
- Appropriate post-op E/M visit(s)
- Photodocumentation

Abbreviated Case Note Example:

- Infant with ambiguous genitalia, enlarged phallic structure. Karyotype analysis demonstrates 46,XX and an ultrasound of the abdomen demonstrates ovarian structures lateral to the uterus.
- Procedure: Cystoscopy confirms that the perineal approach. Surgical repair is based on labial and posterior perineal flaps. The development of flaps provides an open perineal vestibule for the posteriority based perineal flap, which is advanced and sutured to ensure an adequate vaginal opening at the introitus. The labial flaps are also advanced laterally creating an open introitus with no injury to the urethra or rectum.

SURGERY

CPT® CODE 57400

Dilation of vagina under anesthesia (other than local)

POLICY INDICATORS

Global Period
0 day post-op period

Assistants at Surgery
Submit reason for assistant

Co-Surgeons Allowed
No co-surgeon

Reduction for Multiple Procedures
Subject to 50% reduction

Bilateral Surgery Payment
N/A

Applicable Medicare Policies

Relative Value Units (RVUs)

Work RVUs	2.27
Non-Facility Total	Only valued for facility
Facility Total	3.92

Coding Assistance

57400 includes:

- Positioning and prepping patient
- Examination of site after anesthesia
- Operative services, including inspections around site and closure

Abbreviated Case Note Example:

- A 50-year-old female patient with history of total abdominal hysterectomy with bilateral salpingo-oophorectomy, and radiation, presents with stenotic vaginal opening.
- Procedure: Under general anesthesia, examine the pelvic , and introduce a series of progressively larger dilators through the introitus to dilate the vagina.

SURGERY

CPT® CODE 57410

Pelvic examination under anesthesia (other than local)

POLICY INDICATORS

Global Period
0 day post-op period

Assistants at Surgery
No assistant

Co-Surgeons Allowed
No co-surgeon

Reduction for Multiple Procedures
Subject to 50% reduction

Bilateral Surgery Payment
N/A

Applicable Medicare Policies

Relative Value Units (RVUs)

Work RVUs	1.75
Non-Facility Total	Only valued for facility
Facility Total	3.19

Coding Assistance

57410 includes:

- Positioning and prepping patient
- Examination of site after anesthesia
- Operative services, including inspections around site and closure

Abbreviated Case Note Example:

- A 40-year-old female patient with oligomenorrhea and severe mental retardation presents for gynecologic evaluation. She is combative and cannot cooperate with having a pelvic exam.
- Procedure: Under general anesthesia, which is necessary, a pelvic examination and Pap smear are performed.

Additional Notes

- This code may be bundled into other procedures; check with payer before reporting separately

CPT® CODE 57415

Removal of impacted vaginal foreign body (separate procedure) under anesthesia (other than local)

POLICY INDICATORS

Global Period
10 day post-op period

Assistants at Surgery
Submit reason for assistant

Co-Surgeons Allowed
No co-surgeon

Reduction for Multiple Procedures
Subject to 50% reduction

Bilateral Surgery Payment
N/A

Applicable Medicare Policies

Relative Value Units (RVUs)

Work RVUs	2.49
Non-Facility Total	Only valued for facility
Facility Total	5.29

Coding Assistance

57415 includes:

- Positioning and prepping patient
- Examination of site after anesthesia
- Operative services, including inspections around site and closure
- Appropriate post-op E/M visit(s)
- Irrigation of vagina with medicament
- Introduction of hemostatic agent or pack

Abbreviated Case Note Example:

- An infant with a foreign body lodged in her vagina; there are unsuccessful attempts to remove the foreign body.
- Procedure: Under general anesthesia, the foreign body is removed, and the vagina vault is lavaged. Simple suturing is necessary.

Additional Notes

- Use the appropriate E/M code if removed without anesthesia

CPT® CODE 57420

Colposcopy of the entire vagina, with cervix if present

POLICY INDICATORS

Global Period
0 day post-op period

Assistants at Surgery
No assistant

Co-Surgeons Allowed
No co-surgeon

Reduction for Multiple Procedures
Subject to 50% reduction

Bilateral Surgery Payment
N/A

Applicable Medicare Policies

Relative Value Units (RVUs)

Work RVUs	1.60
Non-Facility Total	4.01
Facility Total	2.71

Coding Assistance

57420 includes:

- Positioning and prepping patient
- Examination of site after anesthesia
- Operative services, including inspections around site and closure

Abbreviated Case Note Example:

- A 47-year-old female patient with Pap smear test; result shows atypical cells of undetermined significance; cannot rule out dysplasia.
- Procedure: Apply acetic acid to the entire vagina, and evaluate with a colposcope. There is no evidence of neoplastic or preneoplastic changes; the result is interpreted as due to radiation effect.

Additional Notes

- If additional vaginal or cervical procedures are performed using colposcope, do not report this code. See 57421, 57455, and 57456

SURGERY

CPT® CODE 57421

Colposcopy of the entire vagina, with cervix if present; with biopsy(s) of vagina/cervix

POLICY INDICATORS

Global Period
0 day post-op period

Assistants at Surgery
No assistant

Co-Surgeons Allowed
No co-surgeon

Reduction for Multiple Procedures
Subject to 50% reduction

Bilateral Surgery Payment
N/A

Applicable Medicare Policies

Relative Value Units (RVUs)

Work RVUs	2.20
Non-Facility Total	5.35
Facility Total	3.67

Coding Assistance

57421 includes:

- Positioning and prepping patient
- Examination of site after anesthesia
- Operative services, including inspections around site and closure

Abbreviated Case Note Example:

- A 43-year-old female patient presents with a history of radical hysterectomy for squamous cell carcinoma; Pap smear shows high-grade squamous intraepithelial lesion.
- Procedure: Acetic acid is applied to the entire vagina; evaluation with colposcope at several magnifications is performed. Suspect lesion areas are injected with local anesthetic, biopsies are taken, and bleeding is controlled.

Additional Notes

- If additional cervical procedures are performed using colposcope, do not report this code. See 57456, 57460, and 57461

CPT® CODE 57423

Paravaginal defect repair (including repair of cystocele, if performed), laparoscopic approach

POLICY INDICATORS

Global Period
90 day post-op period

Assistants at Surgery
Assistant allowed

Co-Surgeons Allowed
Co-surgeon allowed

Reduction for Multiple Procedures
Subject to 50% reduction

Bilateral Surgery Payment
N/A

Applicable Medicare Policies

Relative Value Units (RVUs)

Work RVUs	16.08
Non-Facility Total	Only valued for facility
Facility Total	27.88

Coding Assistance

57423 includes:

- Positioning and prepping patient
- Examination of site after anesthesia
- Operative services, including inspections around site and closure
- Appropriate post-op E/M visit(s)
- Photodocumentation
- Introduction of hemostatic pack
- Catheter insertion
- Colporrhaphy
- Anterior vesicourethropexy or urethropexy (Marshall-Marchetti-Krantz/Burch procedure)

Abbreviated Case Note Example:

- A 55-year-old female patient presents with complaints of vaginal pressure and heaviness associated with prolonged standing. Inspection of the anterior vaginal wall relaxation reveals a cystocele arising from paravaginal defects. Recommend a laparoscopic paravaginal defect repair.
- Procedure: Laparoscopic access to the space of Retzius is obtained transperitoneally. The dissection is extended to expose the arcus tendineus fascia pelvis (ATFP) bilaterally. Several permanent sutures are passed along the anterior lateral vaginal sulcus through the pubocervical fascia and then through the obturator internus muscle, just above the ATFP, along its full length down to the ischial spine. This is performed bilaterally. Sutures are tied sequentially to obliterate the defect.

Additional Notes

- A diagnostic laparoscopy is included in this procedure
- If report is performed abdominally, report 57284 instead
- If repair is peformed vaginally, report 57285 instead
- If hysterectomy with colpo-urethrocystopexy is performed, report 58152 or 58167 instead

SURGERY

CPT® CODE 57425

Laparoscopy, surgical, colpopexy (suspension of vaginal apex)

POLICY INDICATORS

Global Period
90 day post-op period

Assistants at Surgery
Assistant allowed

Co-Surgeons Allowed
Submit reason for co-surgeon

Reduction for Multiple Procedures
Subject to 50% reduction

Bilateral Surgery Payment
N/A

Applicable Medicare Policies

Relative Value Units (RVUs)

Work RVUs	17.03
Non-Facility Total	Only valued for facility
Facility Total	29.25

Coding Assistance

57425 includes:

- Positioning and prepping patient
- Examination of site after anesthesia
- Operative services, including inspections around site and closure
- Appropriate post-op E/M visit(s)
- Photodocumentation
- Application of allograft
- Catheter insertion
- Enterolysis
- Enterocele repair

Abbreviated Case Note Example:

- A 60-year-old female patient with history of vaginal hysterectomy with native tissue repairs, presents with a recurrent, symptomatic anterior and apical prolapse; diagnosed with prolapse of the vaginal vault through the introitus with adequate distal support. Recommend a laparoscopic sacral colpopexy.
- Procedure: Place a laparoscopic camera. Incise the peritoneum near the vaginal apex. Dissect distally to the urethral-vesical neck, laterally in the anterior compartment; perform recto-vaginal septum dissection. Continue peritoneal dissection from the promontory dissection. Change back the surgical field to the deep pelvis and place the graft. Change back the surgical field to visualization of the sacral promontory. Place two sutures through the cephalad arm of the mesh and through the anterior longitudinal ligament. Perform irrigation and confirm hemostasis. Perform reperitonealization of the cephalad, anterior and posterior arms.

Additional Notes

- A diagnostic laparoscopy is included in this procedure
- Use this code for suspending the vagina to the sacrum via mesh, graft or sutures. Do not use this code to report prophylactic re-attachment of the uterosacral ligaments or uteroscaral plication to the vagina

CPT® CODE 57426

Revision (including removal) of prosthetic vaginal graft, laparoscopic approach

POLICY INDICATORS

Global Period
90 day post-op period

Assistants at Surgery
Assistant allowed

Co-Surgeons Allowed
Submit reason for co-surgeon

Reduction for Multiple Procedures
Subject to 50% reduction

Bilateral Surgery Payment
N/A

Applicable Medicare Policies

Relative Value Units (RVUs)

Work RVUs	14.30
Non-Facility Total	Only valued for facility
Facility Total	26.29

Coding Assistance

57426 includes:

- Positioning and prepping patient
- Examination of site after anesthesia
- Operative services, including inspections around site and closure
- Appropriate post-op E/M visit(s)

Abbreviated Case Note Example:

- A 57-year-old female patient with past history of sacral colpopexy using mesh presents with vaginal discharge, discomfort, and painful intercourse; diagnosed with mesh eroding through the vagina apex. Recommend excision via the laparoscopic route.
- Procedure: Access the pelvis laparoscopically and sharply dissect the vaginal epithelium around the eroding mesh. Excise the eroding material, re-approximate the remaining edges of the endopelvic fascia, and close the vagina.

Additional Notes

- If performed using an abdominal approach, report 57296 instead
- If performed vaginally, report 57295 instead

CPT® CODE 57452

Colposcopy of the cervix including upper/adjacent vagina

POLICY INDICATORS

Global Period
0 day post-op period

Assistants at Surgery
No assistant

Co-Surgeons Allowed
No co-surgeon

Reduction for Multiple Procedures
Subject to 50% reduction

Bilateral Surgery Payment
N/A

Applicable Medicare Policies

Relative Value Units (RVUs)

Work RVUs	1.50
Non-Facility Total	3.80
Facility Total	2.74

Coding Assistance

57452 includes:

- Positioning and prepping patient
- Examination of site after anesthesia
- Operative services, including inspections around site and closure

Abbreviated Case Note Example:

- A 35-year-old female patient with a mildly abnormal Pap smear result is advised to undergo colposcopic visualization of the cervix.
- Procedure: After acetic acid is applied, examine the cervix and vaginal fornices with colposcope at several magnifications.

Additional Notes

- If additional vaginal or cervical procedures are performed using colposcope, do not report this code. See 57421 and 57454-57461

CPT® CODE 57454

Colposcopy of the cervix including upper/adjacent vagina; with biopsy(s) of the cervix and endocervical curettage

POLICY INDICATORS

Global Period
0 day post-op period

Assistants at Surgery
No assistant

Co-Surgeons Allowed
No co-surgeon

Reduction for Multiple Procedures
Endoscopy payment rules apply

Bilateral Surgery Payment
N/A

Applicable Medicare Policies

Relative Value Units (RVUs)

Work RVUs	2.33
Non-Facility Total	5.07
Facility Total	4.02

Coding Assistance

57454 includes:

- Positioning and prepping patient
- Examination of site after anesthesia
- Operative services, including inspections around site and closure
- Destruction of vaginal and vulvar lesions
- Endometrial biopsy

Abbreviated Case Note Example:

- A 25-year-old female patient with abnormal Pap smear; recommend a colposcopic visualization of the cervix.
- Procedure: After acetic acid is applied, examine the cervix and vaginal fornices with colposcope at several magnifications. Visualize the transformation zone, perform an endocervical curettage and cervical biopsy.

Additional Notes

- If not all of the components of this code are performed, report 57455 or 57456 instead

CPT® CODE 57455

Colposcopy of the cervix including upper/adjacent vagina; with biopsy(s) of the cervix

POLICY INDICATORS

Global Period
0 day post-op period

Assistants at Surgery
No assistant

Co-Surgeons Allowed
No co-surgeon

Reduction for Multiple Procedures
Endoscopy payment rules apply

Bilateral Surgery Payment
N/A

Applicable Medicare Policies

Relative Value Units (RVUs)

Work RVUs	1.99
Non-Facility Total	4.86
Facility Total	3.27

Coding Assistance

57455 includes:

- Positioning and prepping patient
- Examination of site after anesthesia
- Operative services, including inspections around site and closure
- Destruction of vaginal and vulvar lesions
- Endometrial biopsy

Abbreviated Case Note Example:

- A 30-year-old female patient presents with a Pap smear test result of epithelial cell abnormality; ASCUS, possible HPV, dysplasia; low-grade squamous intraepithelial lesion encompassing HPV, mild dysplasia, CIN I; any reference to moderate or high-grade dysplasia, CIN III, or invasive carcinoma.
- Procedure: After acetic acid is applied, examine the cervix and vaginal fornices with colposcope at several magnifications. An area of mosaicism is identified and a cervical biopsy is obtained under colposcopic guidance.

Additional Notes

- If cervical dilation is also performed, report 58120 in addition
- If endocervical curettage is also performed, report 57454 instead

SURGERY

CPT® CODE 57456

Colposcopy of the cervix including upper/adjacent vagina; with endocervical curettage

POLICY INDICATORS

Global Period
0 day post-op period

Assistants at Surgery
No assistant

Co-Surgeons Allowed
No co-surgeon

Reduction for Multiple Procedures
Endoscopy payment rules apply

Bilateral Surgery Payment
N/A

Applicable Medicare Policies

Relative Value Units (RVUs)

Work RVUs	1.85
Non-Facility Total	4.55
Facility Total	3.01

Coding Assistance

57456 includes:

- Positioning and prepping patient
- Examination of site after anesthesia
- Operative services, including inspections around site and closure
- Destruction of vaginal and vulvar lesions
- Endometrial biopsy

Abbreviated Case Note Example:

- A 34-year-old female patient with a Pap smear test result of epithelial cell abnormality; ASCUS, possible HPV, dysplasia; low-grade squamous intraepithelial lesion encompassing HPV, mild dysplasia, CIN I; any reference to moderate or high-grade dysplasia, CIN III, or invasive carcinoma.
- Procedure: After acetic acid is applied, examine the cervix and vaginal fornices with colposcope at several magnifications. A suspicious lesion is noted in the endocervical canal and an endocervical curettage is done under direct colposcopic visualization.

Additional Notes

- If cervical dilation is also performed, report 58120 in addition
- If endocervical curettage is also performed, report 57454 instead

SURGERY

CPT® CODE 57460

Colposcopy of the cervix including upper/adjacent vagina; with loop electrode biopsy(s) of the cervix

POLICY INDICATORS

Global Period
0 day post-op period

Assistants at Surgery
No assistant

Co-Surgeons Allowed
No co-surgeon

Reduction for Multiple Procedures
Endoscopy payment rules apply

Bilateral Surgery Payment
N/A

Applicable Medicare Policies

Relative Value Units (RVUs)

Work RVUs	2.83
Non-Facility Total	9.24
Facility Total	4.81

Coding Assistance

57460 includes:

- Positioning and prepping patient
- Examination of site after anesthesia
- Operative services, including inspections around site and closure
- Endometrial biopsy

Abbreviated Case Note Example:

- A 30-year-old female patient with abnormal Pap smear; advise to undergo colposcopic visualization of the cervix.
- Procedure: After acetic acid is applied, examine the cervix and vaginal fornices with colposcope at several magnifications. A suspicious lesion is noted in the endocervical canal and an endocervical curettage is done under direct colposcopic visualization.

Additional Notes

- If loop electrode conization is performed, report 57461 instead

CPT® CODE 57461

Colposcopy of the cervix including upper/adjacent vagina; with loop electrode conization of the cervix

POLICY INDICATORS

Global Period
0 day post-op period

Assistants at Surgery
No assistant

Co-Surgeons Allowed
No co-surgeon

Reduction for Multiple Procedures
Endoscopy payment rules apply

Bilateral Surgery Payment
N/A

Applicable Medicare Policies

Relative Value Units (RVUs)

Work RVUs	3.43
Non-Facility Total	10.34
Facility Total	5.50

Coding Assistance

57461 includes:

- Positioning and prepping patient
- Examination of site after anesthesia
- Operative services, including inspections around site and closure
- Endometrial biopsy

Abbreviated Case Note Example:

- A 40-year-old female patient presents with a class IV Pap smear, confirmed CIN III, extending into the endocervix.
- Procedure: After acetic acid is applied, examine the cervix and vaginal fornices with colposcope at several magnifications; determine the size of the lesion. Loop electrode is then used to ensure excision of the lesion on the ectocervix with adequate margins. A second loop is then utilized to remove the involved portion of the endocervix. Homeostasis is achieved.

Additional Notes

- If colposcopy with loop electrode biopsy is performed, report 57460 instead
- If no colposcopy is performed, report 57522 instead

CPT® CODE 57465

Computer-aided mapping of cervix uteri during colposcopy, including optical dynamic spectral imaging and algorithmic quantification of the acetowhitening effect
(List separately in addition to code for primary procedure)

POLICY INDICATORS

Global Period
Global for primary procedure applies

Assistants at Surgery
Submit reason for assistant

Co-Surgeons Allowed
No co-surgeon

Reduction for Multiple Procedures
Not subject to multiple surgery reduction

Bilateral Surgery Payment
N/A

Applicable Medicare Policies

Relative Value Units (RVUs)

Work RVUs	0.81
Non-Facility Total	1.65
Facility Total	1.28

Coding Assistance

57465 includes:

- Positioning and prepping patient
- Examination of site after anesthesia
- Operative services, including inspections around site and closure
- Appropriate post-op E/M visit(s)

Abbreviated Case Note Example:

- A 40-year-old female patient presents with a Pap smear; HPV-positive test and requires colposcopy (reported separately).
- Procedure: Identify abnormal areas for biopsy sites localization using a spectral imaging for mapping of the cervix.

CPT® CODE 57500

Biopsy of cervix, single or multiple, or local excision of lesion, with or without fulguration (separate procedure)

POLICY INDICATORS

Global Period
0 day post-op period

Assistants at Surgery
No assistant

Co-Surgeons Allowed
No co-surgeon

Reduction for Multiple Procedures
Subject to 50% reduction

Bilateral Surgery Payment
N/A

Applicable Medicare Policies

Relative Value Units (RVUs)

Work RVUs	1.20
Non-Facility Total	4.52
Facility Total	2.27

Coding Assistance

57500 includes:

- Positioning and prepping patient
- Examination of site after anesthesia
- Operative services, including inspections around site and closure
- Endometrial biopsy
- Vaginal colposcopy
- Vaginal or vulvar biopsies
- Dilation and curettage
- Endocervical curettage

Abbreviated Case Note Example:

- A 47-year-old female patient presents with postcoital bleeding; Pap smear taken from the cervix and lesions seen on the cervix. Recommend a biopsy.
- Procedure: The cervix is visualized; a biopsy of cervical lesion(s) is performed. Hemostasis is achieved.

Additional Notes

- If cervical colposcopy is also performed, report 57455 instead
- 57500 is the appropriate code for the removal of a cervical polyp or a polypectomy. This code can only be billed one time (ie, with one unit); it includes multiple biopsies or excisions.

CPT® CODE 57505

Endocervical curettage (not done as part of a dilation and curettage)

POLICY INDICATORS

Global Period
10 day post-op period

Assistants at Surgery
No assistant

Co-Surgeons Allowed
No co-surgeon

Reduction for Multiple Procedures
Subject to 50% reduction

Bilateral Surgery Payment
N/A

Applicable Medicare Policies

Relative Value Units (RVUs)

Work RVUs	1.19
Non-Facility Total	4.59
Facility Total	3.30

Coding Assistance

57505 includes:

- Positioning and prepping patient
- Examination of site after anesthesia
- Operative services, including inspections around site and closure
- Vulvar or vaginal colposcopy
- Cervical, vaginal, or vulvar biopsies

Additional Notes

- If cervical colposcopy is also performed, report 57456 instead
- 57505 does not include or require dilation. If a D&C occurs, 57505 is bundled into the D&C procedure.
- 57522 and 57505 are not bundled in the Correct Coding Initiative (CCI) edits. Payers have bundled them because of the language found in code descriptions. Bundling is not consistent with coding policy.

SURGERY

CPT® CODE 57510

Cautery of cervix; electro or thermal

POLICY INDICATORS

Global Period
10 day post-op period

Assistants at Surgery
No assistant

Co-Surgeons Allowed
No co-surgeon

Reduction for Multiple Procedures
Subject to 50% reduction

Bilateral Surgery Payment
N/A

Applicable Medicare Policies

Relative Value Units (RVUs)

Work RVUs	1.90
Non-Facility Total	4.96
Facility Total	3.40

Coding Assistance

57510 includes:

- Positioning and prepping patient
- Examination of site after anesthesia
- Operative services, including inspections around site and closure
- Appropriate post-op E/M visit(s)

CPT® CODE 57511

Cautery of cervix; cryocautery, initial or repeat

POLICY INDICATORS

Global Period
10 day post-op period

Assistants at Surgery
No assistant

Co-Surgeons Allowed
No co-surgeon

Reduction for Multiple Procedures
Subject to 50% reduction

Bilateral Surgery Payment
N/A

Applicable Medicare Policies

Relative Value Units (RVUs)

Work RVUs	1.95
Non-Facility Total	5.94
Facility Total	4.45

Coding Assistance

57511 includes:

- Positioning and prepping patient
- Examination of site after anesthesia
- Operative services, including inspections around site and closure
- Appropriate post-op E/M visit(s)

CPT® CODE 57513

Cautery of cervix; laser ablation

POLICY INDICATORS

Global Period
10 day post-op period

Assistants at Surgery
No assistant

Co-Surgeons Allowed
No co-surgeon

Reduction for Multiple Procedures
Subject to 50% reduction

Bilateral Surgery Payment
N/A

Applicable Medicare Policies

Relative Value Units (RVUs)

Work RVUs	1.95
Non-Facility Total	6.11
Facility Total	4.43

Coding Assistance

57513 includes:

- Positioning and prepping patient
- Examination of site after anesthesia
- Operative services, including inspections around site and closure
- Appropriate post-op E/M visit(s)

CPT® CODE 57520

Conization of cervix, with or without fulguration, with or without dilation and curettage, with or without repair; cold knife or laser

POLICY INDICATORS

Global Period
90 day post-op period

Assistants at Surgery
No assistant

Co-Surgeons Allowed
No co-surgeon

Reduction for Multiple Procedures
Subject to 50% reduction

Bilateral Surgery Payment
N/A

Applicable Medicare Policies

Relative Value Units (RVUs)

Work RVUs	4.11
Non-Facility Total	10.62
Facility Total	8.99

Coding Assistance

57520 includes:

- Positioning and prepping patient
- Examination of site after anesthesia
- Operative services, including inspections around site and closure
- Appropriate post-op E/M visit(s)

Additional Notes

- Medicare will not reimburse for regional anesthesia administered by the surgeon
- Dilation and curettage
- Used for endocervical excisions (eg, Fischer cone biopsy excisor).

CPT® CODE 57522

Conization of cervix, with or without fulguration, with or without dilation and curettage, with or without repair; loop electrode excision

POLICY INDICATORS

Global Period
90 day post-op period

Assistants at Surgery
No assistant

Co-Surgeons Allowed
No co-surgeon

Reduction for Multiple Procedures
Subject to 50% reduction

Bilateral Surgery Payment
N/A

Applicable Medicare Policies

Relative Value Units (RVUs)

Work RVUs	3.67
Non-Facility Total	9.10
Facility Total	7.73

Coding Assistance

57522 includes:

- Positioning and prepping patient
- Examination of site after anesthesia
- Operative services, including inspections around site and closure
- Appropriate post-op E/M visit(s)

Abbreviated Case Note Example:

- A 32-year-old female patient presents with abnormal Pap smear; colposcopic examination reveals a lesion on the anterior cervix consistent with cervical intraepithelial neoplasia-2 (CIN 2). The limits of the lesion cannot be seen.
- Procedure: After injecting the cervix, a conization of the cervix using a loop electrode excision is performed. The endocervical portion and ectocervical portion of the cervix are removed using a loop electrode.

Additional Notes

- If a colposcopy is also performed, report 57461 instead
- Medicare will not reimburse for regional anesthesia administered by the surgeon
- Dilation and curettage

CPT® CODE 57530

Trachelectomy (cervicectomy), amputation of cervix (separate procedure)

POLICY INDICATORS

Global Period
90 day post-op period

Assistants at Surgery
Assistant allowed

Co-Surgeons Allowed
Submit reason for co-surgeon

Reduction for Multiple Procedures
Subject to 50% reduction

Bilateral Surgery Payment
N/A

Applicable Medicare Policies
Inpatient-only list

Relative Value Units (RVUs)

Work RVUs	5.27
Non-Facility Total	Only valued for facility
Facility Total	11.33

Coding Assistance

57530 includes:

- Positioning and prepping patient
- Examination of site after anesthesia
- Operative services, including inspections around site and closure
- Appropriate post-op E/M visit(s)
- Cervical procedures

Abbreviated Case Note Example:

- A 40-year-old female patient presents with a stage II pelvic organ prolapse; desired uterine preservation.
- Procedure: After induction of anesthesia, the uterosacral pedicles are crossed on the cervical remnant, and sutures are placed bilaterally. The cervix is amputated; 2 Sturmdorf are performed to bring the mucosa of the vaginal wall into the cervix canal. Hemostasis is confirmed.

Additional Notes

- For a Manchester Fothergill procedure, report 57240 or 57260 with this code
- Photodocumentation

CPT® CODE 57531

Radical trachelectomy, with bilateral total pelvic lymphadenectomy and para-aortic lymph node sampling biopsy, with or without removal of tube(s), with or without removal of ovary(s)

POLICY INDICATORS

Global Period
90 day post-op period

Assistants at Surgery
Assistant allowed

Co-Surgeons Allowed
Submit reason for co-surgeon

Reduction for Multiple Procedures
Subject to 50% reduction

Bilateral Surgery Payment
Bilateral surgery

Applicable Medicare Policies
Inpatient-only list

Relative Value Units (RVUs)

Work RVUs	29.95
Non-Facility Total	Only valued for facility
Facility Total	55.06

Coding Assistance

57531 includes:

- Positioning and prepping patient
- Examination of site after anesthesia
- Operative services, including inspections around site and closure
- Appropriate post-op E/M visit(s)
- Exploratory procedures
- Lymph node procedures
- Ureterolysis for fibrosis/scarring
- Vaginectomy, partial

Abbreviated Case Note Example:

- A 65-year-old female patient with past history of subtotal hysterectomy presents with a biopsy-proven invasive squamous cell carcinoma, stage IB cancer of the cervical stump.
- Procedure: An exploration of the abdominal and pelvic cavities is performed. The cervix and upper one-third of the vagina are excised, and removed by dissecting the ureter from the parametria. A radical bilateral pelvic lymphadenectomy is performed along with the radical excision of the cervix. The pelvic lymphadenectomy skeletonizes the common external, hypogastric, and obturator vessels. A selected para-aortic lymph node sampling is performed. The peritoneal cavity is irrigated. Closed suction drains may be used. Local anesthesia is administered when indicated.

Additional Notes

- If 57520 is also reported, use modifier 58 to designate staged procedure
- For a postoperative counseling visit about chemotherapy or radiation therapy, use the appropriate E/M with modifier 24

SURGERY

CPT® CODE 57540

Excision of cervical stump, abdominal approach

POLICY INDICATORS

Global Period
90 day post-op period

Assistants at Surgery
Assistant allowed

Co-Surgeons Allowed
Submit reason for co-surgeon

Reduction for Multiple Procedures
Subject to 50% reduction

Bilateral Surgery Payment
N/A

Applicable Medicare Policies
Inpatient-only list

Relative Value Units (RVUs)

Work RVUs	13.29
Non-Facility Total	Only valued for facility
Facility Total	23.83

Coding Assistance

57540 includes:

- Positioning and prepping patient
- Examination of site after anesthesia
- Operative services, including inspections around site and closure
- Appropriate post-op E/M visit(s)
- Colpopexy, abdominal
- Repair of enterocele, abdominal
- Urinary bladder procedures

Abbreviated Case Note Example:

- A 50-year-old female patient with history of subtotal hysterectomy for fibroids; diagnosed with extensive cervical carcinoma in situ. Recommend excision of cervical stump via an abdominal approach.
- Procedure: The bladder, sigmoid, and rectum are carefully dissected off of the cervix. The vessels are clamped, cut, and suture ligated. The cervix is removed by clamping across the vaginal cuff. The abdomen is closed in layers and dressings applied. Drains may be used.

Additional Notes

- If pelvic floor repair is also performed, report 57545 instead
- Do not report this code when completing a hysterectomy at a single operative session

CPT® CODE 57545

Excision of cervical stump, abdominal approach; with pelvic floor repair

POLICY INDICATORS

Global Period
90 day post-op period

Assistants at Surgery
Assistant allowed

Co-Surgeons Allowed
Submit reason for co-surgeon

Reduction for Multiple Procedures
Subject to 50% reduction

Bilateral Surgery Payment
N/A

Applicable Medicare Policies
Inpatient-only list

Relative Value Units (RVUs)

Work RVUs	14.10
Non-Facility Total	Only valued for facility
Facility Total	25.08

Coding Assistance

57545 includes:

- Positioning and prepping patient
- Examination of site after anesthesia
- Operative services, including inspections around site and closure
- Appropriate post-op E/M visit(s)
- Anterior vescourethropexy (Marshall-Marchetti-Krantz/Burch procedure) or urethropexy
- Pereyra procedure
- Sling operation

Abbreviated Case Note Example:

- A 55-year-old female patient presents with a diagnosis of extensive cervical carcinoma in situ with symptomatic enterocele with pelvic pressure and dyspareunia. Recommend excision of cervical stump with a repair of the enterocele.
- Procedure: The bladder, sigmoid, and rectum are carefully dissected off of the cervix. The vessels are clamped, cut, and suture ligated. The cervix is removed by clamping across the vaginal cuff. Following removal of the cervix, the pelvic floor is repaired by obliterating the cul-de-sac with sutures placed anterior to posterior or circumferentially from the vaginal vault to the rectosigmoid. The abdomen is closed in layers and dressings applied. Drains may be used.

Additional Notes

- Do not report this code when completing a hysterectomy at a single operative session

SURGERY

CPT® CODE 57550

Excision of cervical stump, vaginal approach

POLICY INDICATORS

Global Period
90 day post-op period

Assistants at Surgery
Assistant allowed

Co-Surgeons Allowed
Submit reason for co-surgeon

Reduction for Multiple Procedures
Subject to 50% reduction

Bilateral Surgery Payment
N/A

Applicable Medicare Policies

Relative Value Units (RVUs)

Work RVUs	6.34
Non-Facility Total	Only valued for facility
Facility Total	13.01

Coding Assistance

57550 includes:

- Positioning and prepping patient
- Examination of site after anesthesia
- Operative services, including inspections around site and closure
- Appropriate post-op E/M visit(s)
- Pereyra procedure
- Sling operation
- Vaginal or vulvar colposcopy

Additional Notes

- If an anterior or posterior colporrhaphy or enterocele repair is performed, report 57555 or 57556 instead
- Do not report this code when completing a hysterectomy at a single operative session
- This code is not a laparoscopic code.

SURGERY

CPT® CODE 57555

Excision of cervical stump, vaginal approach; with anterior and/or posterior repair

POLICY INDICATORS

Global Period
90 day post-op period

Assistants at Surgery
Assistant allowed

Co-Surgeons Allowed
Submit reason for co-surgeon

Reduction for Multiple Procedures
Subject to 50% reduction

Bilateral Surgery Payment
N/A

Applicable Medicare Policies

Relative Value Units (RVUs)

Work RVUs	9.94
Non-Facility Total	Only valued for facility
Facility Total	18.66

Coding Assistance

57555 includes:

- Positioning and prepping patient
- Examination of site after anesthesia
- Operative services, including inspections around site and closure
- Appropriate post-op E/M visit(s)
- Photodocumentation
- Biopsy of vaginal mucosa
- Introduction of hemostasis agent or pack
- Vaginectomy

Additional Notes

- Do not report this code when completing a hysterectomy at a single operative session

CPT® CODE 57556

Excision of cervical stump, vaginal approach; with repair of enterocele

POLICY INDICATORS

Global Period
90 day post-op period

Assistants at Surgery
Assistant allowed

Co-Surgeons Allowed
Submit reason for co-surgeon

Reduction for Multiple Procedures
Subject to 50% reduction

Bilateral Surgery Payment
N/A

Applicable Medicare Policies

Relative Value Units (RVUs)

Work RVUs	9.36
Non-Facility Total	Only valued for facility
Facility Total	17.72

Coding Assistance

57556 includes:

- Positioning and prepping patient
- Examination of site after anesthesia
- Operative services, including inspections around site and closure
- Appropriate post-op E/M visit(s)
- Introduction of hemostasis agent or pack

Additional Notes

- Do not report this code when completing a hysterectomy at a single operative session

CPT® CODE 57558

Dilation and curettage of cervical stump

POLICY INDICATORS

Global Period
10 day post-op period

Assistants at Surgery
No assistant

Co-Surgeons Allowed
No co-surgeon

Reduction for Multiple Procedures
Subject to 50% reduction

Bilateral Surgery Payment
N/A

Applicable Medicare Policies

Relative Value Units (RVUs)

Work RVUs	1.72
Non-Facility Total	4.73
Facility Total	3.87

Coding Assistance

57558 includes:

- Positioning and prepping patient
- Examination of site after anesthesia
- Operative services, including inspections around site and closure
- Appropriate post-op E/M visit(s)
- Introduction of hemostasis agent or pack

CPT® CODE 57700

Cerclage of uterine cervix, nonobstetrical

POLICY INDICATORS

Global Period
90 day post-op period

Assistants at Surgery
Submit reason for assistant

Co-Surgeons Allowed
No co-surgeon

Reduction for Multiple Procedures
Subject to 50% reduction

Bilateral Surgery Payment
N/A

Applicable Medicare Policies

Relative Value Units (RVUs)

Work RVUs	4.35
Non-Facility Total	Only valued for facility
Facility Total	10.73

Coding Assistance

57700 includes:

- Positioning and prepping patient
- Examination of site after anesthesia
- Operative services, including inspections around site and closure
- Appropriate post-op E/M visit(s)

CPT® CODE 57720

Trachelorrhaphy, plastic repair of uterine cervix, vaginal approach

POLICY INDICATORS

Global Period
90 day post-op period

Assistants at Surgery
Assistant allowed

Co-Surgeons Allowed
No co-surgeon

Reduction for Multiple Procedures
Subject to 50% reduction

Bilateral Surgery Payment
N/A

Applicable Medicare Policies

Relative Value Units (RVUs)

Work RVUs	4.61
Non-Facility Total	Only valued for facility
Facility Total	10.11

Coding Assistance

57720 includes:

- Positioning and prepping patient
- Examination of site after anesthesia
- Operative services, including inspections around site and closure
- Appropriate post-op E/M visit(s)
- Photodocumentation
- Cervical biopsy

Abbreviated Case Note Example:

- A 30-year-old female patient status post cold knife conization, found to have postoperative cervical conization bleeding along with bleeding on the left ascending cervical vessel.
- Procedure: The vagina is irrigated and the cervical bed is evaluated. Bleeding is noted; hemostatic ligature of Vicryl is placed; bleeding and needle sites are treated with Monsel's. Irrigation performed and noted no active bleeding.

Additional Notes

- If conization is performed, report 57520 instead

CPT® CODE 57800

Dilation of cervical canal, instrumental (separate procedure)

POLICY INDICATORS

Global Period
0 day post-op period

Assistants at Surgery
No assistant

Co-Surgeons Allowed
No co-surgeon

Reduction for Multiple Procedures
Subject to 50% reduction

Bilateral Surgery Payment
N/A

Applicable Medicare Policies

Relative Value Units (RVUs)

Work RVUs	0.77
Non-Facility Total	2.32
Facility Total	1.45

Coding Assistance

57800 includes:

- Positioning and prepping patient
- Examination of site after anesthesia
- Operative services, including inspections around site and closure

Additional Notes

- If a dilation and curettage is also performed, report only 58120
- If cervical dilation is required to access the uterine cavity to obtain a uterine biopsy, report 58120 instead
- Medicare will not reimburse for regional anesthesia administered by the surgeon
- This code should not be used with obstetric patients
- This code must include the use of instruments
- Dilation is not included as a component part of an IUD insertion, and therefore, 57800 for patients with significant cervical stenosis may also be reported

CPT® CODE 58100

Endometrial sampling (biopsy) with or without endocervical sampling (biopsy), without cervical dilation, any method (separate procedure)

POLICY INDICATORS

Global Period
0 day post-op period

Assistants at Surgery
No assistant

Co-Surgeons Allowed
No co-surgeon

Reduction for Multiple Procedures
Subject to 50% reduction

Bilateral Surgery Payment
N/A

Applicable Medicare Policies

Relative Value Units (RVUs)

Work RVUs	1.21
Non-Facility Total	3.01
Facility Total	1.89

Coding Assistance

58100 includes:

- Positioning and prepping patient
- Examination of site after anesthesia
- Operative services, including inspections around site and closure
- Endocervical curettage

Abbreviated Case Note Example:

- A 53-year-old female patient presents with occurrences of unexplained vaginal bleeding; scheduled for endometrial and endocervical sampling.
- Procedure: Local anesthesia may or may not be applied prior. A disposable Pipelle biopsy instrument, or similar biopsy instrument, is passed through the cervical os into the endometrial cavity until the uterine fundus is encountered. Obtain a biopsy specimen.

Additional Notes

- If cervical dilation is performed, report 58120 instead
- If only endocervical curettage is performed, report 57505 instead
- This code is the reason endometrial biopsy should not be an included service in the colposcopy codes

CPT® CODE 58110

Endometrial sampling (biopsy) performed in conjunction with colposcopy
(List separately in addition to code for primary procedure)

POLICY INDICATORS

Global Period
Global for primary procedure applies

Assistants at Surgery
Submit reason for assistant

Co-Surgeons Allowed
No co-surgeon

Reduction for Multiple Procedures
Not subject to multiple surgery reduction

Bilateral Surgery Payment
N/A

Applicable Medicare Policies

Relative Value Units (RVUs)

Work RVUs	0.77
Non-Facility Total	1.50
Facility Total	1.21

Coding Assistance

58110 includes:

- Positioning and prepping patient
- Examination of site after anesthesia
- Operative services, including inspections around site and closure
- Appropriate post-op E/M visit(s)

Add-On Code:

- Follow Primary Code Policies

CPT® CODE 58120

Dilation and curettage, diagnostic and/or therapeutic (nonobstetrical)

POLICY INDICATORS

Global Period
10 day post-op period

Assistants at Surgery
No assistant

Co-Surgeons Allowed
No co-surgeon

Reduction for Multiple Procedures
Subject to 50% reduction

Bilateral Surgery Payment
N/A

Applicable Medicare Policies

Relative Value Units (RVUs)

Work RVUs	3.59
Non-Facility Total	8.94
Facility Total	7.05

Coding Assistance

58120 includes:

- Positioning and prepping patient
- Examination of site after anesthesia
- Operative services, including inspections around site and closure
- Endocervical curettage

Abbreviated Case Note Example:

- A 60-year-old female postmenopausal patient with a failed endometrial biopsy due to rigid stenotic cervix, undergoes a dilation and curettage.
- Procedure: An endocervical curettage with the dilatation of the cervix is performed, followed by an endometrial curettage.

Additional Notes

- If a diagnostic hysteroscopy is also performed, report 58558 instead
- For obstetric patients, see 59160 and 59812-59841
- Medicare will not reimburse for regional anesthesia administered by the surgeon
- Document medical necessity and reported related diagnosis.

CPT® CODE 58140

Myomectomy, excision of fibroid tumor(s) of uterus, 1 to 4 intramural myoma(s) with total weight of 250 g or less and/or removal of surface myomas; abdominal approach

POLICY INDICATORS

Global Period
90 day post-op period

Assistants at Surgery
Assistant allowed

Co-Surgeons Allowed
Submit reason for co-surgeon

Reduction for Multiple Procedures
Subject to 50% reduction

Bilateral Surgery Payment
N/A

Applicable Medicare Policies
Inpatient-only list

Relative Value Units (RVUs)

Work RVUs	15.79
Non-Facility Total	Only valued for facility
Facility Total	27.71

Coding Assistance

58140 includes:

- Positioning and prepping patient
- Examination of site after anesthesia
- Operative services, including inspections around site and closure
- Appropriate post-op E/M visit(s)
- Photodocumentation
- Uterine or hypogastric artery ligation
- Exploratory laparotomy

Abbreviated Case Note Example:

- A 40-year-old female patient with history of failed dilatation and curettage presents with abnormal uterine bleeding; ultrasonography is performed and reveals multiple intramural and subserosal myomata ranging from 1 to 8 cm in size. Recommend myomectomy via an abdominal approach.
- Procedure: An exploratory laparotomy is performed and incision is made. The fibroid(s) are removed and myometrial defects closed.

Additional Notes

- If vaginal approach is used, report 58145 instead

CPT® CODE 58145

Myomectomy, excision of fibroid tumor(s) of uterus, 1 to 4 intramural myoma(s) with total weight of 250 g or less and/or removal of surface myomas; vaginal approach

POLICY INDICATORS

Global Period
90 day post-op period

Assistants at Surgery
Assistant allowed

Co-Surgeons Allowed
Submit reason for co-surgeon

Reduction for Multiple Procedures
Subject to 50% reduction

Bilateral Surgery Payment
N/A

Applicable Medicare Policies

Relative Value Units (RVUs)

Work RVUs	8.91
Non-Facility Total	Only valued for facility
Facility Total	16.95

Coding Assistance

58145 includes:

- Positioning and prepping patient
- Examination of site after anesthesia
- Operative services, including inspections around site and closure
- Appropriate post-op E/M visit(s)
- Photodocumentation
- Colpoperineorrhaphy, suture of injury of vagina

Additional Notes

- If a hysteroscope is used to resect any or all of the fibroid, report 58561 instead
- If an abdominal approach is used, report 58140 instead
- Medicare will not reimburse for regional anesthesia administered by the surgeon
- 58145 is the excision of the fibroid without an hysteroscope. If the purpose of the encounter was to remove a fibroid and the cyst was removed in the process, the removal of the cyst would be considered incidental to the removal of the fibroid. If this was done via a hysteroscope, it would be reported with 58561.

SURGERY

CPT® CODE 58146

Myomectomy, excision of fibroid tumor(s) of uterus, 5 or more intramural myomas and/or intramural myomas with total weight greater than 250 g, abdominal approach

POLICY INDICATORS

Global Period
90 day post-op period

Assistants at Surgery
Assistant allowed

Co-Surgeons Allowed
Submit reason for co-surgeon

Reduction for Multiple Procedures
Subject to 50% reduction

Bilateral Surgery Payment
N/A

Applicable Medicare Policies
Inpatient-only list

Relative Value Units (RVUs)

Work RVUs	20.34
Non-Facility Total	Only valued for facility
Facility Total	34.69

Coding Assistance

58146 includes:

- Positioning and prepping patient
- Examination of site after anesthesia
- Operative services, including inspections around site and closure
- Appropriate post-op E/M visit(s)
- Photodocumentation
- Uterine or hypogastric artery ligation
- Exploratory laparotomy

Abbreviated Case Note Example:

- A 45-year-old female patient with complaint of menorrhagia with anemia. Ultrasonography confirmed a 15-cm uterus with multiple fibroids distorting the endometrium. Because of her desire to have children and keep her uterus, she consents to an abdominal myomectomy.
- Procedure: An abdominal incision is made; the myoma(s) is dissected from the surrounding myometrium and removed. Uterine incision is repaired and closed. Hemostasis is achieved.

SURGERY

CPT® CODE 58150

Total abdominal hysterectomy (corpus and cervix), with or without removal of tube(s), with or without removal of ovary(s)

POLICY INDICATORS

Global Period
90 day post-op period

Assistants at Surgery
Assistant allowed

Co-Surgeons Allowed
Submit reason for co-surgeon

Reduction for Multiple Procedures
Subject to 50% reduction

Bilateral Surgery Payment
N/A

Applicable Medicare Policies
Inpatient-only list

Relative Value Units (RVUs)

Work RVUs	17.31
Non-Facility Total	Only valued for facility
Facility Total	30.70

Coding Assistance

58150 includes:

- Positioning and prepping patient
- Examination of site after anesthesia
- Operative services, including inspections around site and closure
- Appropriate post-op E/M visit(s)
- Myomectomy, abdominal
- Exploratory laparotomy

Abbreviated Case Note Example:

- A 55-year-old female patient presents with bilateral endometriomas densely adherent to the pelvic side walls and total cul-de-sac obliteration, as well as myomata enlarging the uterus to 10- to 12-week size. Scheduled for a total abdominal hysterectomy and bilateral salpingo-oophorectomy.
- Procedure: Total abdominal hysterectomy; bilateral salpingo-oophorectomy is performed. The supporting pedicles containing the tubes, ligaments, and arteries are clamped and cut free. The uterus and cervix are removed along with a narrow rim or cuff of vaginal lining. Vaginal defect is sutured, and incision is closed.

Additional Notes

- If a colpo-urethrocystopexy is also performed, report 58152 instead
- If a hysterectomy is performed for malignancy, report 58951, 58953-58954, or 58956-58958 instead
- If lymph node sampling and partial vaginectomy are also performed, report 58200 instead
- If there is a significant amount of work for enterolysis, report this code with a modifier 22
- If there is a significant amount of work due to grossly distorted, fibrotic, diseased tissue, severe endometriosis to ensure it is not transected and/or to identify and isolate the uterine artery, report this code with modifier 22
- Medicare will not reimburse for the intra-operative repair of injuries to the bowel or urinary bladder when performed by the surgeon

SURGERY

CPT® CODE 58152

Total abdominal hysterectomy (corpus and cervix), with or without removal of tube(s), with or without removal of ovary(s); with colpo-urethrocystopexy (eg, Marshall-Marchetti-Krantz, Burch)

POLICY INDICATORS

Global Period
90 day post-op period

Assistants at Surgery
Assistant allowed

Co-Surgeons Allowed
Submit reason for co-surgeon

Reduction for Multiple Procedures
Subject to 50% reduction

Bilateral Surgery Payment
N/A

Applicable Medicare Policies
Inpatient-only list

Relative Value Units (RVUs)

Work RVUs	21.86
Non-Facility Total	Only valued for facility
Facility Total	37.19

Coding Assistance

58152 includes:

- Positioning and prepping patient
- Examination of site after anesthesia
- Operative services, including inspections around site and closure
- Appropriate post-op E/M visit(s)
- Photodocumentation
- Myomectomy, abdominal
- Exploratory laparotomy

Abbreviated Case Note Example:

- A 47-year-old female patient diagnosed with symptomatic uterine leiomyoma, no evidence of hyperplasia or adenocarcinoma, documented hypermobility of the bladder neck with stress urinary incontinence. Consent for an abdominal hysterectomy with a Burch retropubic colposuspension.
- Procedure: Excision of uterus (corpus and cervix) with removal of tube(s) and ovary(ies). Colpourethrocystopexy, peritoneal cavity irrigation, placement of drain are performed. Hemostasis is achieved.

Additional Notes

- If a colpo-urethrocystopexy is not performed, report 58150 instead
- If a hysterectomy is performed for malignancy, report 58951, 58953-58954, or 58956-58958 instead
- If lymph node sampling and partial vaginectomy are also performed, report 58200 instead
- If there is a significant amount of work for enterolysis, report this code with a modifier 22
- If there is a significant amount of work due to grossly distorted, fibrotic, diseased tissue, severe endometriosis to ensure it is not transected and/or to identify and isolate the uterine artery, report this code with modifier 22
- Medicare will not reimburse for the intra-operative repair of injuries to the bowel or urinary bladder when performed by the surgeon

CPT® CODE 58180

Supracervical abdominal hysterectomy (subtotal hysterectomy), with or without removal of tube(s), with or without removal of ovary(s)

POLICY INDICATORS

Global Period
90 day post-op period

Assistants at Surgery
Assistant allowed

Co-Surgeons Allowed
Submit reason for co-surgeon

Reduction for Multiple Procedures
Subject to 50% reduction

Bilateral Surgery Payment
N/A

Applicable Medicare Policies
Inpatient-only list

Relative Value Units (RVUs)

Work RVUs	16.60
Non-Facility Total	Only valued for facility
Facility Total	28.97

Coding Assistance

58180 includes:

- Positioning and prepping patient
- Examination of site after anesthesia
- Operative services, including inspections around site and closure
- Appropriate post-op E/M visit(s)
- Myomectomy, abdominal
- Exploratory laparotomy

Abbreviated Case Note Example:

- A 45-year-old female patient is assessed for a large pelvic mass; ultrasound reveals bilateral endometriomas densely adherent to the pelvic side walls and total cul-de-sac obliteration, as well as myomata enlarging the uterus to 10- to 12-week size.
- Procedure: Excessive bleeding and dense pelvic adhesions make removal of the uterine cervix very difficult. Because the patient is not tolerating her anesthetic very well, a decision is made to perform a supracervical hysterectomy. Uterine fundus is removed by excision at the level of the internal cervical os. This area is oversewn and hemostasis is achieved.

Additional Notes

- If performed using a laparoscopy, report 58541-58544 instead
- If there is a significant amount of work for enterolysis, report this code with a modifier 22
- If there is a significant amount of work due to grossly distorted, fibrotic, diseased tissue, severe endometriosis to ensure it is not transected and/or to identify and isolate the uterine artery, report this code with modifier 22
- Medicare will not reimburse for the intra-operative repair of injuries to the bowel or urinary bladder when performed by the surgeon

CPT® CODE 58200

Total abdominal hysterectomy, including partial vaginectomy, with para-aortic and pelvic lymph node sampling, with or without removal of tube(s), with or without removal of ovary(s)

POLICY INDICATORS

Global Period
90 day post-op period

Assistants at Surgery
Assistant allowed

Co-Surgeons Allowed
Submit reason for co-surgeon

Reduction for Multiple Procedures
Subject to 50% reduction

Bilateral Surgery Payment
N/A

Applicable Medicare Policies
Inpatient-only list

Relative Value Units (RVUs)

Work RVUs	23.10
Non-Facility Total	Only valued for facility
Facility Total	40.73

Coding Assistance

58200 includes:

- Positioning and prepping patient
- Examination of site after anesthesia
- Operative services, including inspections around site and closure
- Appropriate post-op E/M visit(s)
- Myomectomy, abdominal
- Exploratory laparotomy
- Exploration of retroperitoneum
- Limited lymphadenectomy
- Colpectomy, partial

Abbreviated Case Note Example:

- A 65-year-old female patient with comorbid conditions undergoes dilatation and curettage, revealing a 10-week-size uterus and a large amount of neoplastic-appearing tissue. Pathology reveals a moderately differentiated endometrial adenocarcinoma.
- Procedure: Exploratory laparotomy, total abdominal hysterectomy with bilateral salpingo-oophorectomy with partial vaginectomy, selected bilateral pelvic lymphadenectomy and selected periaortic lymphadenectomy, cytologic washings, and subdiaphragmatic cytologic scrapings. Extrafascial hysterectomy and bilateral salpingo-oophorectomy. A lymph node dissection is dictated by the grade of the tumor and depth of myometrial invasion.

Additional Notes

- If a hysterectomy with pelvic lymphadenectomy is performed, report 58210 instead
- If a hysterectomy is performed for ovarian malignancy, report 58951, 58953-58954, or 58956-58958 instead

CPT® CODE 58210

Radical abdominal hysterectomy, with bilateral total pelvic lymphadenectomy and para-aortic lymph node sampling (biopsy), with or without removal of tube(s), with or without removal of ovary(s)

POLICY INDICATORS

Global Period
90 day post-op period

Assistants at Surgery
Assistant allowed

Co-Surgeons Allowed
Submit reason for co-surgeon

Reduction for Multiple Procedures
Subject to 50% reduction

Bilateral Surgery Payment
Bilateral surgery

Applicable Medicare Policies
Inpatient-only list

Relative Value Units (RVUs)

Work RVUs	30.91
Non-Facility Total	Only valued for facility
Facility Total	54.88

Coding Assistance

58210 includes:

- Positioning and prepping patient
- Examination of site after anesthesia
- Operative services, including inspections around site and closure
- Appropriate post-op E/M visit(s)
- Myomectomy, abdominal
- Exploratory laparotomy
- Exploration of retroperitoneum
- Limited lymphadenectomy
- Colpectomy, partial

Abbreviated Case Note Example:

- A 40-year-old female patient presents with cervical lesion approximately 2 cm in largest diameter, which is confined to the cervix. A biopsy reveals a well-differentiated squamous cell cancer. Scheduled for a radical abdominal hysterectomy with bilateral total pelvic lymphadenectomy and selected periaortic lymph node sampling.
- Procedure: Abdominal and pelvic cavities are explored, and lymph nodes are sent for frozen section. Radical bilateral pelvic lymphadenectomy is performed, either before or after the radical hysterectomy. Abdomen is closed.

Additional Notes

- If 57461 or 57520 is also reported, use modifier 58 to designate staged procedure
- If a hysterectomy is performed for ovarian malignancy, report 58951, 58953-58954, or 58956-58958 instead
- If there is a significant amount of work for enterolysis, report this code with a modifier 22
- If there is a significant amount of work due to grossly distorted, fibrotic, diseased tissue, severe endometriosis to ensure it is not transected and/or to identify and isolate the uterine artery, report this code with modifier 22
- Medicare will not reimburse for the intra-operative repair of injuries to the bowel or urinary bladder when performed by the surgeon
- For a postoperative counseling visit about chemotherapy or radiation therapy, use the appropriate E/M with modifier 24

CPT® CODE 58240

Pelvic exenteration for gynecologic malignancy, with total abdominal hysterectomy or cervicectomy, with or without removal of tube(s), with or without removal of ovary(s), with removal of bladder and ureteral transplantations, and/or abdominoperineal resection of rectum and colon and colostomy, or any combination thereof

POLICY INDICATORS

Global Period
90 day post-op period

Assistants at Surgery
Assistant allowed

Co-Surgeons Allowed
Submit reason for co-surgeon

Reduction for Multiple Procedures
Subject to 50% reduction

Bilateral Surgery Payment
N/A

Applicable Medicare Policies
Inpatient-only list

Relative Value Units (RVUs)

Work RVUs	49.33
Non-Facility Total	Only valued for facility
Facility Total	88.40

Coding Assistance

58240 includes:

- Positioning and prepping patient
- Examination of site after anesthesia
- Operative services, including inspections around site and closure
- Appropriate post-op E/M visit(s)
- Myomectomy, abdominal
- Colostomy
- Exploratory laparotomy
- Exploration of retroperitoneum
- Colpectomy, complete
- Cystectomy (with or without ureteral conduit)

Abbreviated Case Note Example:

- A 40-year-old patient with post-radiation therapy for a stage IB squamous cell cervical carcinoma, recurrence in 2 years. Biopsy is consistent with the primary tumor. Planned for a pelvic exenteration with total abdominal hysterectomy, removal of bladder and ureteral reimplantation, and resection of the rectum and colostomy creation.
- Procedure: Explore the abdominal and pelvic cavities; perform bilateral ureterolysis to prepare for the urinary conduit. A perineal phase is carried out to remove the pelvic disease, a segment of the ileum is harvested, and the ureteral stent is placed. An ostomy for the urinary conduit and sigmoid colostomy is performed.

Additional Notes

- For a postoperative counseling visit about chemotherapy or radiation therapy, use the appropriate E/M with modifier 24
- For a postoperative counseling visit about sexual function, use the appropriate E/M with modifier 24

CPT® CODE 58260

Vaginal hysterectomy, for uterus 250 g or less

POLICY INDICATORS

Global Period
90 day post-op period

Assistants at Surgery
Assistant allowed

Co-Surgeons Allowed
Submit reason for co-surgeon

Reduction for Multiple Procedures
Subject to 50% reduction

Bilateral Surgery Payment
N/A

Applicable Medicare Policies

Relative Value Units (RVUs)

Work RVUs	14.15
Non-Facility Total	Only valued for facility
Facility Total	25.26

Coding Assistance

58260 includes:

- Positioning and prepping patient
- Examination of site after anesthesia
- Operative services, including inspections around site and closure
- Appropriate post-op E/M visit(s)
- Photodocumentation
- Introduction of hemostatic agent or pack

Abbreviated Case Note Example:

- A 40-year-old patient presents with failed oral contraceptives and nonsteroidal anti-inflammatory drugs, and uterus 6-8 weeks in size and boggy. Scheduled for vaginal hysterectomy without removal of adnexae.
- Procedure: The cervix is visualized; excision of the uterus and cervix is performed. Hemostasis is achieved.

Additional Notes

- If a salpingectomy and/or oophorectomy is performed, report 58262 instead
- If an enterocele repair is performed, report 58270 or 58263 instead
- Documentation of a "high" suspension supports the billing of hysterectomy codes with CPT code 57283. The prophylactic suspension of the vagina is considered a component part of the hysterectomy procedure. If billing with 57283, use the -59 modifier to indicate a vaginal hysterectomy to treat a prolapse when a high suspension is performed.

CPT® CODE 58262

Vaginal hysterectomy, for uterus 250 g or less; with removal of tube(s), and/or ovary(s)

POLICY INDICATORS

Global Period
90 day post-op period

Assistants at Surgery
Assistant allowed

Co-Surgeons Allowed
Co-surgeon allowed

Reduction for Multiple Procedures
Subject to 50% reduction

Bilateral Surgery Payment
N/A

Applicable Medicare Policies

Relative Value Units (RVUs)

Work RVUs	15.94
Non-Facility Total	Only valued for facility
Facility Total	27.92

Coding Assistance

58262 includes:

- Positioning and prepping patient
- Examination of site after anesthesia
- Operative services, including inspections around site and closure
- Appropriate post-op E/M visit(s)
- Photodocumentation
- Introduction of hemostatic agent or pack

Abbreviated Case Note Example:

- A 32-year-old female patient with family history of cancer presents with menorrhagia and dysmenorrhea; failed medical management. Consents to a bilateral salpingo-oophorectomy with hysterectomy.
- Procedure: Excise the uterus and cervix; perform excision of one or both tubes and/or one or both ovaries. Achieve hemostasis.

Additional Notes

- If an enterocele repair is performed, report 58263 instead
- Documentation of a "high" suspension supports the billing of hysterectomy codes with CPT code 57283. The prophylactic suspension of the vagina is considered a component part of the hysterectomy procedure. If billing with 57283, use the -59 modifier to indicate a vaginal hysterectomy to treat a prolapse when a high suspension is performed. Documentation should clearly indicate uterus size, a high uterosacral ligament suspension was performed, or a McCall-type culdoplasty was performed.

CPT® CODE 58263

Vaginal hysterectomy, for uterus 250 g or less; with removal of tube(s), and/or ovary(s), with repair of enterocele

POLICY INDICATORS

Global Period
90 day post-op period

Assistants at Surgery
Assistant allowed

Co-Surgeons Allowed
Co-surgeon allowed

Reduction for Multiple Procedures
Subject to 50% reduction

Bilateral Surgery Payment
N/A

Applicable Medicare Policies

Relative Value Units (RVUs)

Work RVUs	17.23
Non-Facility Total	Only valued for facility
Facility Total	29.95

Coding Assistance

58263 includes:

- Positioning and prepping patient
- Examination of site after anesthesia
- Operative services, including inspections around site and closure
- Appropriate post-op E/M visit(s)
- Photodocumentation
- Introduction of hemostatic agent or pack
- Colpopexy, vaginal

Abbreviated Case Note Example:

- A 50-year-old postmenopausal patient presents with uterine prolapse with enterocele. Scheduled for vaginal hysterectomy with bilateral salpingo-oophorectomy with repair of enterocele transvaginally.
- Procedure: Excision of the uterus and cervix, together with one or both tubes and/or one or both ovaries, is performed. The enterocele is repaired, and hemostasis is achieved.

CPT® CODE 58267

Vaginal hysterectomy, for uterus 250 g or less; with colpo-urethrocystopexy (Marshall-Marchetti-Krantz type, Pereyra type) with or without endoscopic control

POLICY INDICATORS

Global Period
90 day post-op period

Assistants at Surgery
Assistant allowed

Co-Surgeons Allowed
Submit reason for co-surgeon

Reduction for Multiple Procedures
Subject to 50% reduction

Bilateral Surgery Payment
N/A

Applicable Medicare Policies
Inpatient-only list

Relative Value Units (RVUs)

Work RVUs	18.36
Non-Facility Total	Only valued for facility
Facility Total	32.16

Coding Assistance

58267 includes:

- Positioning and prepping patient
- Examination of site after anesthesia
- Operative services, including inspections around site and closure
- Appropriate post-op E/M visit(s)
- Photodocumentation
- Introduction of hemostatic agent or pack
- Pereyra procedure
- Cystotomy with suprapubic catheter
- Anterior vesicourethropexy (Marshall-Marchetti-Krantz/Burch procedure) or urethropexy (Marshall-Marchetti-Krantz/Burch procedure)

Abbreviated Case Note Example:

- A 35-year-old female patient with history of small bowel resection presents with menorrhagia and dysmenorrhea; failed medical management. Recommend a vaginal hysterectomy followed by retropubic urethropexy.
- Procedure: Excise the uterus and cervix; perform a colpourethrocystopexy with or without endoscopic control. Achieve hemostasis.

CPT® CODE 58270

Vaginal hysterectomy, for uterus 250 g or less; with repair of enterocele

POLICY INDICATORS

Global Period
90 day post-op period

Assistants at Surgery
Assistant allowed

Co-Surgeons Allowed
Submit reason for co-surgeon

Reduction for Multiple Procedures
Subject to 50% reduction

Bilateral Surgery Payment
N/A

Applicable Medicare Policies

Relative Value Units (RVUs)

Work RVUs	15.30
Non-Facility Total	Only valued for facility
Facility Total	26.92

Coding Assistance

58270 includes:

- Positioning and prepping patient
- Examination of site after anesthesia
- Operative services, including inspections around site and closure
- Appropriate post-op E/M visit(s)
- Photodocumentation
- Introduction of hemostatic agent or pack
- Colpopexy, vaginal

Abbreviated Case Note Example:

- A 38-year-old presents with uterine prolapse with obvious enterocele; symptoms are consistent with prolapse and enterocele. Consents to a vaginal hysterectomy with repair of enterocele.
- Procedure: Cervix is visualized; excision of the uterus and cervix is performed. The enterocele is repaired, and hemostasis is achieved.

Additional Notes

- If removal of tubes and/or ovaries is also performed, report 58263 instead

CPT® CODE 58275

Vaginal hysterectomy, with total or partial vaginectomy

POLICY INDICATORS

Global Period
90 day post-op period

Assistants at Surgery
Assistant allowed

Co-Surgeons Allowed
Submit reason for co-surgeon

Reduction for Multiple Procedures
Subject to 50% reduction

Bilateral Surgery Payment
N/A

Applicable Medicare Policies
Inpatient-only list

Relative Value Units (RVUs)

Work RVUs	17.03
Non-Facility Total	Only valued for facility
Facility Total	29.86

Coding Assistance

58275 includes:

- Positioning and prepping patient
- Examination of site after anesthesia
- Operative services, including inspections around site and closure
- Appropriate post-op E/M visit(s)
- Photodocumentation
- Introduction of hemostatic agent or pack

Abbreviated Case Note Example:

- A 43-year-old patient presents with carcinoma in situ of the cervix, which involves the entire posterior lip of the cervix and extends onto the posterior fornix; vaginal intraepithelial neoplasia associated with the cervical lesion. Scheduled for vaginal hysterectomy with excision of the the posterior vaginal mucosa with dysplastic process.
- Procedure: The uterus and cervix is excised, and a partial or total excision of the vaginal canal is performed. Hemostasis is achieved. Reparative surgery is performed to avoid shortening and decreased caliber of the vagina.

Additional Notes

- If an enterocele repair is also performed, report 58280 instead
- if a colpocystopexy is also performed, report 58267 or 58294 instead

CPT® CODE 58280

Vaginal hysterectomy, with total or partial vaginectomy; with repair of enterocele

POLICY INDICATORS

Global Period
90 day post-op period

Assistants at Surgery
Assistant allowed

Co-Surgeons Allowed
Submit reason for co-surgeon

Reduction for Multiple Procedures
Subject to 50% reduction

Bilateral Surgery Payment
N/A

Applicable Medicare Policies
Inpatient-only list

Relative Value Units (RVUs)

Work RVUs	18.33
Non-Facility Total	Only valued for facility
Facility Total	31.85

Coding Assistance

58280 includes:

- Positioning and prepping patient
- Examination of site after anesthesia
- Operative services, including inspections around site and closure
- Appropriate post-op E/M visit(s)
- Photodocumentation
- Introduction of hemostatic agent or pack
- Colpopexy, vaginal

Abbreviated Case Note Example:

- A 45-year-old patient presents with carcinoma in situ of the cervix, which extends onto the vaginal fornices; significant uterine prolapse along with an enterocele. Elect to undergo vaginal hysterectomy with excision of the portion of the upper vagina involved with dysplastic process.
- Procedure: The uterus and cervix are excised, enterocele is repaired, and partial or total excision of the vaginal canal is performed. Wound is closed.

CPT® CODE 58285

Vaginal hysterectomy, radical (Schauta type operation)

POLICY INDICATORS

Global Period
90 day post-op period

Assistants at Surgery
Assistant allowed

Co-Surgeons Allowed
Submit reason for co-surgeon

Reduction for Multiple Procedures
Subject to 50% reduction

Bilateral Surgery Payment
N/A

Applicable Medicare Policies
Inpatient-only list

Relative Value Units (RVUs)

Work RVUs	23.38
Non-Facility Total	Only valued for facility
Facility Total	42.92

Coding Assistance

58285 includes:

- Positioning and prepping patient
- Examination of site after anesthesia
- Operative services, including inspections around site and closure
- Appropriate post-op E/M visit(s)

Abbreviated Case Note Example:

- A 33-year-old female patient with invasive squamous cell carcinoma clinically confined to the cervix (stage IBI). Elect for radical vaginal hysterectomy.
- Procedure: Excise the uterus and cervix , along with the upper vagina, paracolpos, and parametria. Perform lateral mobilization of the ureters, close the wound, and suture the vaginal cuff.

Additional Notes

- For a postoperative counseling visit about chemotherapy or radiation therapy, use the appropriate E/M with modifier 24
- For a postoperative counseling visit about sexual function, use the appropriate E/M with modifier 24

CPT® CODE 58290

Vaginal hysterectomy, for uterus greater than 250 g

POLICY INDICATORS

Global Period
90 day post-op period

Assistants at Surgery
Assistant allowed

Co-Surgeons Allowed
Submit reason for co-surgeon

Reduction for Multiple Procedures
Subject to 50% reduction

Bilateral Surgery Payment
N/A

Applicable Medicare Policies

Relative Value Units (RVUs)

Work RVUs	20.27
Non-Facility Total	Only valued for facility
Facility Total	34.58

Coding Assistance

58290 includes:

- Positioning and prepping patient
- Examination of site after anesthesia
- Operative services, including inspections around site and closure
- Appropriate post-op E/M visit(s)
- Photodocumentation
- Introduction of hemostatic agent or pack
- Myomectomy

Abbreviated Case Note Example:

- A 55-year-old female patient is seen for profound menorrhagia with anemia, irregular, mobile, 14-week-size fibroid uterus, multiple uterine fibroids confirmed by ultrasonography, several of which impinge on the endometrium.
- Procedure: Determining the size and configuration of the uterine fibroids greatly limits the surgeon. Enter the anterior and posterior cul-de-sacs. Bisect the uterus in anteroposterior direction with a knife with progressive reposition of tenaculums until the fundus is reached. After the uterine fundus can be delivered into the vagina, remove it in multiple separate pieces. Close the peritoneum and vaginal cuff.

Additional Notes

- If a salpingectomy and/or oophorectomy is performed, report 58291 instead
- If an enterocele repair is performed, report 58292 or 58294 instead

SURGERY

CPT® CODE 58291

Vaginal hysterectomy, for uterus greater than 250 g; with removal of tube(s) and/or ovary(s)

POLICY INDICATORS

Global Period
90 day post-op period

Assistants at Surgery
Assistant allowed

Co-Surgeons Allowed
Co-surgeon allowed

Reduction for Multiple Procedures
Subject to 50% reduction

Bilateral Surgery Payment
N/A

Applicable Medicare Policies

Relative Value Units (RVUs)

Work RVUs	22.06
Non-Facility Total	Only valued for facility
Facility Total	37.34

Coding Assistance

58291 includes:

- Positioning and prepping patient
- Examination of site after anesthesia
- Operative services, including inspections around site and closure
- Appropriate post-op E/M visit(s)
- Photodocumentation
- Introduction of hemostatic agent or pack
- Myomectomy

Additional Notes

- If an enterocele repair is performed, report 58294 instead

CPT® CODE 58292

Vaginal hysterectomy, for uterus greater than 250 g; with removal of tube(s) and/or ovary(s), with repair of enterocele

POLICY INDICATORS

Global Period
90 day post-op period

Assistants at Surgery
Assistant allowed

Co-Surgeons Allowed
Co-surgeon allowed

Reduction for Multiple Procedures
Subject to 50% reduction

Bilateral Surgery Payment
N/A

Applicable Medicare Policies

Relative Value Units (RVUs)

Work RVUs	23.35
Non-Facility Total	Only valued for facility
Facility Total	39.33

Coding Assistance

58292 includes:

- Positioning and prepping patient
- Examination of site after anesthesia
- Operative services, including inspections around site and closure
- Appropriate post-op E/M visit(s)
- Photodocumentation
- Introduction of hemostatic agent or pack
- Myomectomy
- Colpopexy, vaginal

CPT® CODE 58294

Vaginal hysterectomy, for uterus greater than 250 g; with repair of enterocele

POLICY INDICATORS

Global Period
90 day post-op period

Assistants at Surgery
Assistant allowed

Co-Surgeons Allowed
Submit reason for co-surgeon

Reduction for Multiple Procedures
Subject to 50% reduction

Bilateral Surgery Payment
N/A

Applicable Medicare Policies

Relative Value Units (RVUs)

Work RVUs	21.55
Non-Facility Total	Only valued for facility
Facility Total	36.55

Coding Assistance

58294 includes:

- Positioning and prepping patient
- Examination of site after anesthesia
- Operative services, including inspections around site and closure
- Appropriate post-op E/M visit(s)
- Photodocumentation
- Introduction of hemostatic agent or pack
- Myomectomy
- Colpopexy, vaginal

Additional Notes

- If removal of tubes and/or ovaries is also performed, report 58292 instead

CPT® CODE 58300

Insertion of intrauterine device (IUD)

POLICY INDICATORS

Global Period
N/A

Assistants at Surgery
N/A

Co-Surgeons Allowed
N/A

Reduction for Multiple Procedures
N/A

Bilateral Surgery Payment
N/A

Applicable Medicare Policies

Relative Value Units (RVUs)

Work RVUs	1.01
Non-Facility Total	3.25
Facility Total	1.51

Coding Assistance

58300 includes:

- Positioning and prepping patient
- Examination of site after anesthesia
- Operative services, including inspections around site and closure
- Appropriate post-op E/M visit(s)

Abbreviated Case Note Example:

- A 35-year-old female patient presents for a new insertion of a new IUD for menorrhagia.
- Procedure: Cervix is prepped, endometrial cavity is sounded to 8 cm, and the IUD is carefully inserted into the uterus. Inserter is removed from the uterus, and the threads are then cut, leaving 2-3 cm visible outside the cervix. Hemostasis is achieved.

Additional Notes

- The IUD device supply is not included. Use 99070 or the appropriate HCPCS code from your payer
- In general, payers will not separately reimburse physicians for intrauterine contraceptive devices (IUDs) unless there is an IUD insertion procedure (CPT code 58300) reported at the same encounter.
- More information is available at https://www.acog.org/programs/long-acting-reversible-contraception-larc/activities-initiatives/medicaid-reimbursement-for-postpartum-larc.

SURGERY

CPT® CODE 58301

Removal of intrauterine device (IUD)

POLICY INDICATORS

Global Period
0 day post-op period

Assistants at Surgery
Submit reason for assistant

Co-Surgeons Allowed
No co-surgeon

Reduction for Multiple Procedures
Subject to 50% reduction

Bilateral Surgery Payment
N/A

Applicable Medicare Policies

Relative Value Units (RVUs)

Work RVUs	1.27
Non-Facility Total	3.28
Facility Total	1.98

Coding Assistance

58301 includes:

- Positioning and prepping patient
- Examination of site after anesthesia
- Operative services, including inspections around site and closure
- Cervical dilation

Abbreviated Case Note Example:

- A 35-year-old female patient presents for the removal of her intrauterine device (IUD).
- Procedure: The cervix is dilated; single-toothed tenaculum is applied to the anterior lip of the cervix; strings of the IUD are grasped, and the IUD is removed.

SURGERY

CPT® CODE 58321

Artificial insemination; intra-cervical

POLICY INDICATORS

Global Period
0 day post-op period

Assistants at Surgery
Submit reason for assistant

Co-Surgeons Allowed
No co-surgeon

Reduction for Multiple Procedures
Subject to 50% reduction

Bilateral Surgery Payment
N/A

Applicable Medicare Policies

Relative Value Units (RVUs)

Work RVUs	0.92
Non-Facility Total	2.48
Facility Total	1.44

Coding Assistance

58321 includes:

- Positioning and prepping patient
- Examination of site after anesthesia
- Operative services, including inspections around site and closure

CPT® CODE 58322

Artificial insemination; intra-uterine

POLICY INDICATORS

Global Period
0 day post-op period

Assistants at Surgery
Submit reason for assistant

Co-Surgeons Allowed
No co-surgeon

Reduction for Multiple Procedures
Subject to 50% reduction

Bilateral Surgery Payment
N/A

Applicable Medicare Policies

Relative Value Units (RVUs)

Work RVUs	1.10
Non-Facility Total	2.74
Facility Total	1.71

Coding Assistance

58322 includes:

- Positioning and prepping patient
- Examination of site after anesthesia
- Operative services, including inspections around site and closure

CPT® CODE 58323

Sperm washing for artificial insemination

POLICY INDICATORS

Global Period
0 day post-op period

Assistants at Surgery
Submit reason for assistant

Co-Surgeons Allowed
No co-surgeon

Reduction for Multiple Procedures
Subject to 50% reduction

Bilateral Surgery Payment
N/A

Applicable Medicare Policies

Relative Value Units (RVUs)

Work RVUs	0.23
Non-Facility Total	0.44
Facility Total	0.36

Coding Assistance

58323 includes:

- Positioning and prepping patient
- Examination of site after anesthesia
- Operative services, including inspections around site and closure

Additional Notes

- If a semen analysis is also performed, report 89260 or 89261 instead

CPT® CODE 58340

Catheterization and introduction of saline or contrast material for saline infusion sonohysterography (SIS) or hysterosalpingography

POLICY INDICATORS

Global Period
0 day post-op period

Assistants at Surgery
No assistant

Co-Surgeons Allowed
No co-surgeon

Reduction for Multiple Procedures
Subject to 50% reduction

Bilateral Surgery Payment
N/A

Applicable Medicare Policies

Relative Value Units (RVUs)

Work RVUs	0.88
Non-Facility Total	6.98
Facility Total	1.75

Coding Assistance

58340 includes:

- Positioning and prepping patient
- Examination of site after anesthesia
- Operative services, including inspections around site and closure

Abbreviated Case Note Example:

- A 37-year-old female patient who has been trying to conceive for over 2 years, presents for consultation and hysterosalpingogram. She consents to sonohysterography and hysterosalpingogram.
- Procedure: Cervix is dilated to accommodate the infusion catheter, and uterine cavity is injected and reveals a 1.8-cm polyp. FemVue apparatus is then placed on the infusion catheter, with saline and bubbles injected into the cavity. Fluid and bubbles noted to be traveling through the left tube to the pelvis, while the right tube was occlused by intrauterine polyps. Tenaculum is taken off the cervix and infusion catheter removed.

CPT® CODE 58345

Transcervical introduction of fallopian tube catheter for diagnosis and/or re-establishing patency (any method), with or without hysterosalpingography

POLICY INDICATORS

Global Period
10 day post-op period

Assistants at Surgery
Assistant allowed

Co-Surgeons Allowed
Co-surgeon allowed

Reduction for Multiple Procedures
Subject to 50% reduction

Bilateral Surgery Payment
150% paid if bilateral

Applicable Medicare Policies

Relative Value Units (RVUs)

Work RVUs	4.70
Non-Facility Total	Only valued for facility
Facility Total	8.72

Coding Assistance

58345 includes:

- Positioning and prepping patient
- Examination of site after anesthesia
- Operative services, including inspections around site and closure
- Appropriate post-op E/M visit(s)
- Injection procedure for hysterosalpingography

CPT® CODE 58346

Insertion of Heyman capsules for clinical brachytherapy

POLICY INDICATORS

Global Period
90 day post-op period

Assistants at Surgery
No assistant

Co-Surgeons Allowed
No co-surgeon

Reduction for Multiple Procedures
Subject to 50% reduction

Bilateral Surgery Payment
N/A

Applicable Medicare Policies

Relative Value Units (RVUs)

Work RVUs	7.56
Non-Facility Total	Only valued for facility
Facility Total	15.16

Coding Assistance

58346 includes:

- Positioning and prepping patient
- Examination of site after anesthesia
- Operative services, including inspections around site and closure
- Appropriate post-op E/M visit(s)
- Cervical dilation
- Vaginal packing
- Placement of Foley catheter
- Pelvic examination under anesthesia

Abbreviated Case Note Example:

- A 65-year-old female patient with comorbid condition diagnosed with uterine cancer; not a candidate for surgery. Decision to treat with radiation therapy including clinical brachytherapy. Scheduled for insertion of Heyman capsules.
- Procedure: Cervix is dilated using Hegar dilators and Heyman (afterloading) capsules are then inserted into the uterine cavity (for as many as 15 capsules). Consider only work related to placing the Heyman capsules. The work of loading the radioactive elements is captured in another, separately reported code.

Additional Notes

- For placement of needles or catheters into pelvic organs and/or genitalia for interstitial radioelement application, report 55920

CPT® CODE 58350

Chromotubation of oviduct, including materials

POLICY INDICATORS

Global Period
10 day post-op period

Assistants at Surgery
No assistant

Co-Surgeons Allowed
No co-surgeon

Reduction for Multiple Procedures
Subject to 50% reduction

Bilateral Surgery Payment
150% paid if bilateral

Applicable Medicare Policies

Relative Value Units (RVUs)

Work RVUs	1.06
Non-Facility Total	4.52
Facility Total	2.85

Coding Assistance

58350 includes:

- Positioning and prepping patient
- Examination of site after anesthesia
- Operative services, including inspections around site and closure
- Appropriate post-op E/M visit(s)

Additional Notes

- If a transcervical fallopian tube catheter is introduced for diagnosis and/or re-establishing patency, report 58345 instead
- 58350 requires a radiologic imaging service (including dye). 58350 is not specific to the method in which the procedure is completed—either laparoscopic or open.

CPT® CODE 58353

Endometrial ablation, thermal, without hysteroscopic guidance

POLICY INDICATORS

Global Period
10 day post-op period

Assistants at Surgery
No assistant

Co-Surgeons Allowed
Co-surgeon allowed

Reduction for Multiple Procedures
Subject to 50% reduction

Bilateral Surgery Payment
N/A

Applicable Medicare Policies

Relative Value Units (RVUs)

Work RVUs	3.60
Non-Facility Total	26.41
Facility Total	6.95

Coding Assistance

58353 includes:

- Positioning and prepping patient
- Examination of site after anesthesia
- Operative services, including inspections around site and closure
- Appropriate post-op E/M visit(s)
- Photodocumentation

Abbreviated Case Note Example:

- A 45-year-old premenopausal female patient is diagnosed with menorrhagia; normal Pap smear and endometrial biopsy. Rule out submucous fibroids, large polyps, and congenital anomalies. Drug therapy, multiple courses of hormone replacement therapy prove inadequate.
- Procedure: Balloon catheter is inserted and filled to pressure of 160-180 mm Hg and held at stable pressure for a minimum of 30 seconds. The controller is activated to achieve treatment temperature. This cycle may require as much as 4 minutes. The therapy cycle is 8 minutes. At completion of the treatment cycle, fluid is removed from the balloon and balloon is removed from the uterus.

Additional Notes

- If hysteroscopy is also performed during the same session, report 58563 instead
- If endometrial cryoablation and curettage with ultrasonic guidance are performed, report 58356 instead

CPT® CODE 58356

Endometrial cryoablation with ultrasonic guidance, including endometrial curettage, when performed

POLICY INDICATORS

Global Period
10 day post-op period

Assistants at Surgery
Assistant allowed

Co-Surgeons Allowed
Co-surgeon allowed

Reduction for Multiple Procedures
Subject to 50% reduction

Bilateral Surgery Payment
N/A

Applicable Medicare Policies

Relative Value Units (RVUs)

Work RVUs	6.41
Non-Facility Total	47.69
Facility Total	10.57

Coding Assistance

58356 includes:

- Positioning and prepping patient
- Examination of site after anesthesia
- Operative services, including inspections around site and closure
- Appropriate post-op E/M visit(s)
- Photodocumentation
- Dilation and curettage
- Catheterization and introduction of contrast
- Endometrial sampling
- Ultrasound procedures

Abbreviated Case Note Example:

- A 37-year-old premenopausal female patient presents with abnormal uterine bleeding where conservative therapy (hormonal therapy and/or D&C) has failed, and hysterectomy is the next treatment option.
- Procedure: Cervical canal is evaluated and dilated. Suction curettage is typically performed. Ultrasound is used to observe and direct cryoprobe probe. Cryoprobe tip temperature is cooled to −60 °C. The cryozone is monitored on ultrasound to ensure cryozone does not extend beyond the serosa. When this freeze is complete, a heat cycle is initiated in the cryoprobe. Once the tip reaches 20 °C, the probe is repositioned and melts a path to the contralateral cornu. Sterile saline is injected and second freeze is initiated. Typically 2-4 freezes are conducted.

CPT® CODE 58400

Uterine suspension, with or without shortening of round ligaments, with or without shortening of sacrouterine ligaments (separate procedure)

POLICY INDICATORS

Global Period
90 day post-op period

Assistants at Surgery
Assistant allowed

Co-Surgeons Allowed
Submit reason for co-surgeon

Reduction for Multiple Procedures
Subject to 50% reduction

Bilateral Surgery Payment
N/A

Applicable Medicare Policies
Inpatient-only list

Relative Value Units (RVUs)

Work RVUs	7.14
Non-Facility Total	Only valued for facility
Facility Total	13.92

Coding Assistance

58400 includes:

- Positioning and prepping patient
- Examination of site after anesthesia
- Operative services, including inspections around site and closure
- Appropriate post-op E/M visit(s)
- Photodocumentation
- Exploratory laparotomy

Additional Notes

- A diagnostic laparoscopy can be reported if it is performed before the open uterine suspension procedure
- If presacral neurectomy is also performed, report 58410 instead

CPT® CODE 58410

Uterine suspension, with or without shortening of round ligaments, with or without shortening of sacrouterine ligaments; with presacral sympathectomy

POLICY INDICATORS

Global Period
90 day post-op period

Assistants at Surgery
Assistant allowed

Co-Surgeons Allowed
Submit reason for co-surgeon

Reduction for Multiple Procedures
Subject to 50% reduction

Bilateral Surgery Payment
N/A

Applicable Medicare Policies
Inpatient-only list

Relative Value Units (RVUs)

Work RVUs	13.80
Non-Facility Total	Only valued for facility
Facility Total	24.54

Coding Assistance

58410 includes:

- Positioning and prepping patient
- Examination of site after anesthesia
- Operative services, including inspections around site and closure
- Appropriate post-op E/M visit(s)
- Photodocumentation
- Exploratory laparotomy

Abbreviated Case Note Example:

- A 30-year-old female patient previously seen for chronic, severe central pelvic pain and endometriosis, presents with a retro-displaced uterus. Failed all conservative methods of pain management; consents to a uterine suspension and presacral sympathectomy.
- Procedure: Sigmoid colon is mobilized to expose the peritoneum, and sympathetic nerve supply is isolated. Appropriate nerve bundle is ligated bilaterally and divided (presacral sympathectomy). Uterine suspension is performed either through shortening the round ligaments or suspending the uterus; abdomen is closed.

CPT® CODE 58520

Hysterorrhaphy, repair of ruptured uterus (nonobstetrical)

POLICY INDICATORS

Global Period
90 day post-op period

Assistants at Surgery
Assistant allowed

Co-Surgeons Allowed
Submit reason for co-surgeon

Reduction for Multiple Procedures
Subject to 50% reduction

Bilateral Surgery Payment
N/A

Applicable Medicare Policies
Inpatient-only list

Relative Value Units (RVUs)

Work RVUs	13.48
Non-Facility Total	Only valued for facility
Facility Total	24.03

Coding Assistance

58520 includes:

- Positioning and prepping patient
- Examination of site after anesthesia
- Operative services, including inspections around site and closure
- Appropriate post-op E/M visit(s)
- Photodocumentation
- Exploratory laparotomy

Abbreviated Case Note Example:

- A 35-year-old female patient is evaluated for abnormal glandular cells on Pap smear; severely stenotic internal os is identified. While attempting to enter the endometrial cavity for D&C, the uterus is perforated and brisk bleeding ensues.
- Procedure: A laparotomy incision is made and the uterine tear is identified and closed in layers after the internal os is dilated from above and endometrial sampling obtained.

CPT® CODE 58540

Hysteroplasty, repair of uterine anomaly (Strassman type)

POLICY INDICATORS

Global Period
90 day post-op period

Assistants at Surgery
Assistant allowed

Co-Surgeons Allowed
No co-surgeon

Reduction for Multiple Procedures
Subject to 50% reduction

Bilateral Surgery Payment
N/A

Applicable Medicare Policies
Inpatient-only list

Relative Value Units (RVUs)

Work RVUs	15.71
Non-Facility Total	Only valued for facility
Facility Total	27.59

Coding Assistance

58540 includes:

- Positioning and prepping patient
- Examination of site after anesthesia
- Operative services, including inspections around site and closure
- Appropriate post-op E/M visit(s)
- Photodocumentation
- Exploratory laparotomy
- Insertion of intrauterine device

Abbreviated Case Note Example:

- A 30-year-old female patient presents for a repair of congenital uterine anomaly as causing repetitive spontaneous pregnancy losses. Hysterosalpingogram and laparoscopy reveal a bicornuate uterus.
- Procedure: An exploratory laparotomy and bicornuate uterus repair are performed. Bivalved uterus is unified by closing the incision along the anteroposterior axis of the uterus. Myometrial defect is closed in multiple layers and meticulous hemostasis is obtained.

SURGERY

CPT® CODE 58541

Laparoscopy, surgical, supracervical hysterectomy, for uterus 250 g or less

POLICY INDICATORS

Global Period
90 day post-op period

Assistants at Surgery
Assistant allowed

Co-Surgeons Allowed
Co-surgeon allowed

Reduction for Multiple Procedures
Endoscopy payment rules apply

Bilateral Surgery Payment
N/A

Applicable Medicare Policies

Relative Value Units (RVUs)

Work RVUs	12.29
Non-Facility Total	Only valued for facility
Facility Total	22.03

Coding Assistance

58541 includes:

- Positioning and prepping patient
- Examination of site after anesthesia
- Operative services, including inspections around site and closure
- Appropriate post-op E/M visit(s)
- Photodocumentation
- Introduction of hemostatic agent or pack
- Myomectomy
- Colpotomy

Abbreviated Case Note Example:

- A 35-year-old female patient presents with chronic, abnormal uterine bleeding; profound for menorrhagia with anemia. Consents to a laparoscopic supracervical hysterectomy without removal of the adnexae.
- Procedure: Laparoscope is inserted; attachments of the uterus are coagulated or ligated and then transected. Myomectomies of individual fibroids may be performed when necessary to debulk the uterus. Endocervical canal is coagulated, and hemostasis of the cervical stump is obtained. Conduct morcellation of the uterine body and remove the specimen.

Additional Notes

- A diagnostic laparoscopy is included in this procedure
- If the procedure is converted to an abdominal hysterectomy, report the open procedure
- If tubes/ovaries are also removed, report 58542 instead
- If cervix is also removed, report 58570 instead
- Do not report 51040 for catheter placement

SURGERY

CPT® CODE 58542

Laparoscopy, surgical, supracervical hysterectomy, for uterus 250 g or less; with removal of tube(s) and/or ovary(s)

POLICY INDICATORS

Global Period
90 day post-op period

Assistants at Surgery
Assistant allowed

Co-Surgeons Allowed
Co-surgeon allowed

Reduction for Multiple Procedures
Subject to 50% reduction

Bilateral Surgery Payment
N/A

Applicable Medicare Policies

Relative Value Units (RVUs)

Work RVUs	14.16
Non-Facility Total	Only valued for facility
Facility Total	24.98

Coding Assistance

58542 includes:

- Positioning and prepping patient
- Examination of site after anesthesia
- Operative services, including inspections around site and closure
- Appropriate post-op E/M visit(s)
- Photodocumentation
- Introduction of hemostatic agent or pack
- Myomectomy
- Colpotomy
- Laparoscopic ovarian procedures

Abbreviated Case Note Example:

- A 40-year-old female patient, previously gravid, is evaluated for profound menorrhagia with anemia. Consents to a laparoscopic supracervical hysterectomy (LSH) with bilateral salpingo-oophorectomy.
- Procedure: Insert the laparoscope; sequentially coagulate or ligate the attachments of the uterus and transect them. Fibroid myomectomies may be performed when necessary; coagulate the endocervical canal, obtain hemostasis of the cervical stump, and conduct morcellation of the uterine body.

Additional Notes

- A diagnostic laparoscopy is included in this procedure
- If the procedure is converted to an abdominal hysterectomy, report the open procedure
- If tubes/ovaries are also removed, report 58542 instead
- If cervix is also removed, report 58570 instead
- Do not report 51040 for catheter placement

SURGERY

CPT® CODE 58543

Laparoscopy, surgical, supracervical hysterectomy, for uterus greater than 250 g

POLICY INDICATORS

Global Period
90 day post-op period

Assistants at Surgery
Assistant allowed

Co-Surgeons Allowed
Co-surgeon allowed

Reduction for Multiple Procedures
Subject to 50% reduction

Bilateral Surgery Payment
N/A

Applicable Medicare Policies

Relative Value Units (RVUs)

Work RVUs	14.39
Non-Facility Total	Only valued for facility
Facility Total	25.35

Coding Assistance

58543 includes:

- Positioning and prepping patient
- Examination of site after anesthesia
- Operative services, including inspections around site and closure
- Appropriate post-op E/M visit(s)
- Photodocumentation
- Introduction of hemostatic agent or pack
- Myomectomy
- Colpotomy

Additional Notes

- A diagnostic laparoscopy is included in this procedure
- If tubes/ovaries are also removed, report 58544 instead
- If cervix is also removed, report 58572 instead
- Do not report 51040 for catheter placement

CPT® CODE 58544

Laparoscopy, surgical, supracervical hysterectomy, for uterus greater than 250 g; with removal of tube(s) and/or ovary(s)

POLICY INDICATORS

Global Period
90 day post-op period

Assistants at Surgery
Assistant allowed

Co-Surgeons Allowed
Co-surgeon allowed

Reduction for Multiple Procedures
Subject to 50% reduction

Bilateral Surgery Payment
N/A

Applicable Medicare Policies

Relative Value Units (RVUs)

Work RVUs	15.60
Non-Facility Total	Only valued for facility
Facility Total	27.27

Coding Assistance

58544 includes:

- Positioning and prepping patient
- Examination of site after anesthesia
- Operative services, including inspections around site and closure
- Appropriate post-op E/M visit(s)
- Photodocumentation
- Introduction of hemostatic agent or pack
- Myomectomy
- Colpotomy
- Laparoscopic ovarian procedures

Additional Notes

- A diagnostic laparoscopy is included in this procedure
- If the procedure is converted to an abdominal hysterectomy, report the open procedure
- If the cervix is also removed, report 58573 instead
- Do not report 51040 for catheter placement

CPT® CODE 58545

Laparoscopy, surgical, myomectomy, excision; 1 to 4 intramural myomas with total weight of 250 g or less and/or removal of surface myomas

POLICY INDICATORS

Global Period
90 day post-op period

Assistants at Surgery
Assistant allowed

Co-Surgeons Allowed
Co-surgeon allowed

Reduction for Multiple Procedures
Subject to 50% reduction

Bilateral Surgery Payment
N/A

Applicable Medicare Policies

Relative Value Units (RVUs)

Work RVUs	15.55
Non-Facility Total	Only valued for facility
Facility Total	27.15

Coding Assistance

58545 includes:

- Positioning and prepping patient
- Examination of site after anesthesia
- Operative services, including inspections around site and closure
- Appropriate post-op E/M visit(s)
- Photodocumentation
- Application of materials to prevent adhesion formation

Abbreviated Case Note Example:

- A 45-year-old female patient presents with enlarging symptomatic pelvic mass with increasing uterus, causing urinary frequency, nocturia, and dyspareunia. Leiomyomatous uterus with two separate myomas 4 x 5 and 3 x 4 cm. Patient wants to keep uterus for fertility purposes.
- Procedure: After inserting the laparoscope, the myoma is exposed and carefully dissected from the surrounding myometrium. If a pedicle is identified, it is isolated, independently coagulated, and transected. Size of the myoma determines whether it is suture tagged or placed in cul-de-sac for later retrieval. The second, third, and fourth myomas are removed with suture placement for hemostasis, followed by uterine reconstruction. Upon achieving hemostasis and uterine reconstruction, the myomas are retrieved and morcellated.

Additional Notes

- A diagnostic laparoscopy is included in this procedure

CPT® CODE 58546

Laparoscopy, surgical, myomectomy, excision; 5 or more intramural myomas and/or intramural myomas with total weight greater than 250 g

POLICY INDICATORS

Global Period
90 day post-op period

Assistants at Surgery
Assistant allowed

Co-Surgeons Allowed
Co-surgeon allowed

Reduction for Multiple Procedures
Subject to 50% reduction

Bilateral Surgery Payment
N/A

Applicable Medicare Policies

Relative Value Units (RVUs)

Work RVUs	19.94
Non-Facility Total	Only valued for facility
Facility Total	33.46

Coding Assistance

58546 includes:

- Positioning and prepping patient
- Examination of site after anesthesia
- Operative services, including inspections around site and closure
- Appropriate post-op E/M visit(s)
- Photodocumentation
- Application of materials to prevent adhesion formation

Abbreviated Case Note Example:

- A 37-year-old female patient presents with a 16-week-size fibroid uterus, a 15-cm uterus with six distinct intramural myomas distorting the endometrium. Patient wants to keep uterus for fertility purposes. Elects for a laparoscopic myomectomy.
- Procedure: The cervix is dilated, and the uterine manipulator applied. The patient is placed in Trendelenburg position. Once the myoma has been exposed, it is grasped with a specially designed myoma forceps. Careful dissection frees the myoma from surrounding myometrium. If pedicle is identified, it is isolated and independently coagulated and then transected. Upon achieving hemostasis and uterine reconstruction, the myomas are then individually retrieved and morcellated.

Additional Notes

- A diagnostic laparoscopy is included in this procedure

CPT® CODE 58548

Laparoscopy, surgical, with radical hysterectomy, with bilateral total pelvic lymphadenectomy and para-aortic lymph node sampling (biopsy), with removal of tube(s) and ovary(s), if performed

POLICY INDICATORS

Global Period
90 day post-op period

Assistants at Surgery
Assistant allowed

Co-Surgeons Allowed
Co-surgeon allowed

Reduction for Multiple Procedures
Subject to 50% reduction

Bilateral Surgery Payment
Bilateral surgery

Applicable Medicare Policies
Inpatient-only list

Relative Value Units (RVUs)

Work RVUs	31.63
Non-Facility Total	Only valued for facility
Facility Total	56.70

Coding Assistance

58548 includes:

- Positioning and prepping patient
- Examination of site after anesthesia
- Operative services, including inspections around site and closure
- Appropriate post-op E/M visit(s)
- Photodocumentation
- Introduction of hemostatic agent or pack
- Myomectomy
- Colpotomy
- Dilation and curettage of cervical stump
- Laparoscopy hysterectomy and lymph node procedures

Abbreviated Case Note Example:

- A 55-year-old female patient presents with exophytic cervical lesion, biopsy-proven to be an invasive squamous cell cancer confined to the cervix, without parametrial extension. Consents to a laparoscopic radical hysterectomy with laparoscopic pelvic lymphadenectomy and para-aortic node sampling.
- Procedure: Insert the laparoscope, place the patient in a Trendelenburg position, and open the peritoneum lateral to the ovarian vessels from the external iliac to the common iliac vessels. A laparoscopic total pelvic lymphadenectomy is performed.

Additional Notes

- A diagnostic laparoscopy is included in this procedure
- If the procedure is converted to an abdominal hysterectomy, report the open procedure
- If performed abdominally, report 58210 instead
- If performed vaginally, report 58285 instead
- Do not report 51040 for catheter placement

CPT® CODE 58550

Laparoscopy, surgical, with vaginal hysterectomy, for uterus 250 g or less

POLICY INDICATORS

Global Period
90 day post-op period

Assistants at Surgery
Assistant allowed

Co-Surgeons Allowed
Co-surgeon allowed

Reduction for Multiple Procedures
Endoscopy payment rules apply

Bilateral Surgery Payment
N/A

Applicable Medicare Policies

Relative Value Units (RVUs)

Work RVUs	15.10
Non-Facility Total	Only valued for facility
Facility Total	26.60

Coding Assistance

58550 includes:

- Positioning and prepping patient
- Examination of site after anesthesia
- Operative services, including inspections around site and closure
- Appropriate post-op E/M visit(s)
- Photodocumentation
- Introduction of hemostatic agent or pack
- Myomectomy
- Colpotomy

Abbreviated Case Note Example:

- A 50-year-old female patient presents with an irregular, mobile 4- to 6-week-size fibroid uterus. Ultrasound confirms multiple uterine fibroids, several of which impinge on the endometrium. Elect for a laparoscopic assisted vaginal hysterectomy (LAVH).
- Procedure: Under general anesthesia, the cervix is dilated in order to facilitate the Valchev uterine manipulator. Using laparoscopic guidance, the utero-ovarian vasculature is clamped, cauterized and suture ligated; Valchev uterine manipulator is removed. Using Haney clamps, the uterosacral ligaments, cardinal, and broad ligaments are clamped, cut and ligated bilaterally. When completely freed, the uterus is delivered, both ovaries are identified, and hemostasis is achieved.

Additional Notes

- A diagnostic laparoscopy is included in this procedure
- If the procedure is converted to an abdominal hysterectomy, report the open procedure
- If a total laparoscopic hysterectomy is performed (ie, no tissue is removed vaginally), report 58570 instead
- Do not report 51040 for catheter placement

SURGERY

CPT® CODE 58552

Laparoscopy, surgical, with vaginal hysterectomy, for uterus 250 g or less; with removal of tube(s) and/or ovary(s)

POLICY INDICATORS

Global Period
90 day post-op period

Assistants at Surgery
Assistant allowed

Co-Surgeons Allowed
Co-surgeon allowed

Reduction for Multiple Procedures
Subject to 50% reduction

Bilateral Surgery Payment
N/A

Applicable Medicare Policies

Relative Value Units (RVUs)

Work RVUs	16.91
Non-Facility Total	Only valued for facility
Facility Total	29.57

Coding Assistance

58552 includes:

- Positioning and prepping patient
- Examination of site after anesthesia
- Operative services, including inspections around site and closure
- Appropriate post-op E/M visit(s)
- Photodocumentation
- Introduction of hemostatic agent or pack
- Myomectomy
- Colpotomy
- Laparoscopic ovarian procedures

Abbreviated Case Note Example:

- A 50-year-old female patient presents with an irregular, mobile 4- to 6-week-size fibroid uterus; multiple uterine fibroids, several of which impinge on the endometrium.
- Procedure: Cervix is dilated to place a Valchev uterine manipulator. A laparoscope is used for the abdominal portion. A circumferential incision is then made around the cervix and the cervicovesical space is entered anteriorly. Continued intermittent clamping, incising, and suture until the cornual region of the uterus is reached. The uterus, tubes, and ovaries are then removed and handed off the field.

Additional Notes

- A diagnostic laparoscopy is included in this procedure
- If the procedure is converted to an abdominal hysterectomy, report the open procedure
- If a total laparoscopic hysterectomy is performed (ie, no tissue is removed vaginally), report 58571 instead
- Do not report 51040 for catheter placement

CPT® CODE 58553

Laparoscopy, surgical, with vaginal hysterectomy, for uterus greater than 250 g

POLICY INDICATORS

Global Period
90 day post-op period

Assistants at Surgery
Assistant allowed

Co-Surgeons Allowed
Co-surgeon allowed

Reduction for Multiple Procedures
Subject to 50% reduction

Bilateral Surgery Payment
N/A

Applicable Medicare Policies

Relative Value Units (RVUs)

Work RVUs	20.06
Non-Facility Total	Only valued for facility
Facility Total	33.65

Coding Assistance

58553 includes:

- Positioning and prepping patient
- Examination of site after anesthesia
- Operative services, including inspections around site and closure
- Appropriate post-op E/M visit(s)
- Photodocumentation
- Introduction of hemostatic agent or pack
- Myomectomy
- Colpotomy

Abbreviated Case Note Example:

- A 40-year-old female patient presents with an irregular, mobile 12- to 14-week-size fibroid uterus. Ultrasound confirms multiple uterine fibroids, several of which impinge on the endometrium.
- Procedure: Under general anesthesia, the cervix is dilated to place a Valchev uterine manipulator. A laparoscope is used for the abdominal portion. A circumferential incision is then made around the cervix and the cervicovesical space is entered anteriorly. Continued intermittent clamping, incising, and suture until the cornual region of the uterus is reached. The uterus, tubes, and ovaries are then removed and handed off the field.

Additional Notes

- A diagnostic laparoscopy is included in this procedure
- If the procedure is converted to an abdominal hysterectomy, report the open procedure
- If a total laparoscopic hysterectomy is performed (ie, no tissue is removed vaginally), report 58572 instead
- Do not report 51040 for catheter placement

SURGERY

CPT® CODE 58554

Laparoscopy, surgical, with vaginal hysterectomy, for uterus greater than 250 g; with removal of tube(s) and/or ovary(s)

POLICY INDICATORS

Global Period
90 day post-op period

Assistants at Surgery
Assistant allowed

Co-Surgeons Allowed
Co-surgeon allowed

Reduction for Multiple Procedures
Subject to 50% reduction

Bilateral Surgery Payment
N/A

Applicable Medicare Policies

Relative Value Units (RVUs)

Work RVUs	23.11
Non-Facility Total	Only valued for facility
Facility Total	39.19

Coding Assistance

58554 includes:

- Positioning and prepping patient
- Examination of site after anesthesia
- Operative services, including inspections around site and closure
- Appropriate post-op E/M visit(s)
- Photodocumentation
- Introduction of hemostatic agent or pack
- Myomectomy
- Colpotomy
- Laparoscopic ovarian procedures
- Dilation and curettage of cervical stump

Abbreviated Case Note Example:

- A 52-year-old female patient with family history of ovarian cancer presents with irregular, mobile 12- to 14-week-size fibroid uterus. Ultrasound confirms multiple uterine fibroids, several of which impinge on the endometrium.
- Procedure: A Valchev uterine manipulator is placed after the cervix is adequately dilated. The laparoscope is then advanced to perform the abdominal portion. Based on multiple large fibroids and position, a myomectomy must first be performed to allow safe removal of the uterus transvaginally. Each fibroid is removed from the myometrium using careful sharp dissection. Once removed, the fibroids are suture tagged and placed into the posterior cul-de-sac to be removed at the time of the vaginal portion of the hysterectomy.

Additional Notes

- A diagnostic laparoscopy is included in this procedure
- If the procedure is converted to an abdominal hysterectomy, report the open procedure
- If a total laparoscopic hysterectomy is performed (ie, no tissue is removed vaginally), report 58573 instead
- Do not report 51040 for catheter placement

SURGERY

CPT® CODE 58555

Hysteroscopy, diagnostic (separate procedure)

POLICY INDICATORS

Global Period
0 day post-op period

Assistants at Surgery
Submit reason for assistant

Co-Surgeons Allowed
Co-surgeon allowed

Reduction for Multiple Procedures
Subject to 50% reduction

Bilateral Surgery Payment
N/A

Applicable Medicare Policies

Relative Value Units (RVUs)

Work RVUs	2.65
Non-Facility Total	10.17
Facility Total	4.57

Coding Assistance

58555 includes:

- Positioning and prepping patient
- Examination of site after anesthesia
- Operative services, including inspections around site and closure
- Photodocumentation
- Any cervical, vaginal or open laparotomy procedure
- Laparoscopy
- Myomectomy (abdominal)
- Cervical ripening and paracervical block
- Fallopian tube catheter
- Vaginal biopsy

Abbreviated Case Note Example:

- A 50-year-old perimenopausal female patient presents with abnormal uterine bleeding. Recommend diagnostic hysteroscopy.
- Procedure: A bimanual pelvic examination is performed to assess uterine size, position, and mobility. The adnexa and posterior cul-de-sac are palpated for the presence of masses or nodularity. The bladder is drained with a catheter. The cervix is exposed, grasped, and dilated slightly larger than the scope. The uterine sound is passed. The scope is inserted, and the physician confirms proper pressure setting of the pump or gravity flow to adequately distend the endometrial cavity. The entire endometrial cavity is examined, including the anterior, posterior, fundal, and lateral walls. The endocervical canal is examined.

Additional Notes

- If other procedures are performed through the hysteroscopy, report one of 58558-58563 instead
- Medicare will not reimburse for regional anesthesia administered by the surgeon

SURGERY

CPT® CODE 58558

Hysteroscopy, surgical; with sampling (biopsy) of endometrium and/or polypectomy, with or without D&C

POLICY INDICATORS

Global Period
0 day post-op period

Assistants at Surgery
No assistant

Co-Surgeons Allowed
Co-surgeon allowed

Reduction for Multiple Procedures
Endoscopy payment rules apply

Bilateral Surgery Payment
N/A

Applicable Medicare Policies

Relative Value Units (RVUs)

Work RVUs	4.17
Non-Facility Total	37.32
Facility Total	6.94

Coding Assistance

58558 includes:

- Positioning and prepping patient
- Examination of site after anesthesia
- Operative services, including inspections around site and closure
- Photodocumentation

Abbreviated Case Note Example:

- A 45-year-old perimenopausal female patient presents with an endometrial polyp. Elect to perform hysteroscopy with removal of polyp, dilation and curettage.
- Procedure: A bimanual pelvic examination. The bladder is drained with a catheter. The cervix is exposed, grasped, and dilated to accommodate the diagnostic hysteroscope. The endocervical canal is examined. The cervix is further dilated to admit the operative hysteroscope and excise the entire lesion(s). Curettage of the endometrial cavity is performed. The endometrial and endocervical canal is examined; irregular polypoid mass is identified. The cervix is further dilated to admit the operative hysteroscope and excise the entire lesion(s). Curettage of the endometrial cavity is performed.

Additional Notes

- A diagnostic laparoscopy is included in this procedure
- If other procedures are performed through the hysteroscopy, report one of 58559-58562 instead
- Medicare will not reimburse for regional anesthesia administered by the surgeon

SURGERY

CPT® CODE 58559

Hysteroscopy, surgical; with lysis of intrauterine adhesions (any method)

POLICY INDICATORS

Global Period
0 day post-op period

Assistants at Surgery
No assistant

Co-Surgeons Allowed
Co-surgeon allowed

Reduction for Multiple Procedures
Endoscopy payment rules apply

Bilateral Surgery Payment
N/A

Applicable Medicare Policies

Relative Value Units (RVUs)

Work RVUs	5.20
Non-Facility Total	Only valued for facility
Facility Total	8.49

Coding Assistance

58559 includes:

- Positioning and prepping patient
- Examination of site after anesthesia
- Operative services, including inspections around site and closure
- Photodocumentation

Abbreviated Case Note Example:

- A 37-year-old female patient with history of spontaneous abortions, presents with multiple thin irregular filling defects within the endometrial cavity that are suggestive of intrauterine adhesions.
- Procedure: A bimanual pelvic examination is performed, and the bladder is drained with a catheter. The cervix is exposed, grasped, and dilated to accommodate the diagnostic hysteroscope. The entire endometrial cavity is examined, including the anterior, posterior, fundal, and lateral walls and both tubal ostia. The endocervical canal is examined. Inspection of the endometrial cavity confirms the presence of intrauterine adhesions. The cervix is further dilated to admit the operative hysteroscope, and the adhesions are lysed.

Additional Notes

- A diagnostic laparoscopy is included in this procedure
- Medicare will not reimburse for regional anesthesia administered by the surgeon

CPT® CODE 58560

Hysteroscopy, surgical; with division or resection of intrauterine septum (any method)

POLICY INDICATORS

Global Period
0 day post-op period

Assistants at Surgery
Assistant allowed

Co-Surgeons Allowed
Co-surgeon allowed

Reduction for Multiple Procedures
Endoscopy payment rules apply

Bilateral Surgery Payment
N/A

Applicable Medicare Policies

Relative Value Units (RVUs)

Work RVUs	5.75
Non-Facility Total	Only valued for facility
Facility Total	9.35

Coding Assistance

58560 includes:

- Positioning and prepping patient
- Examination of site after anesthesia
- Operative services, including inspections around site and closure
- Photodocumentation

Abbreviated Case Note Example:

- A 40-year-old female patient presents with history of multiple pregnancy losses; evaluation reveals a thick uterine septum.
- Procedure: A bimanual pelvic examination is performed, and the bladder is drained with a catheter. The cervix is exposed, grasped, and dilated to accommodate the diagnostic hysteroscope. The entire endometrial cavity is examined, including the anterior, posterior, fundal, and lateral walls and bilateral tubal ostia. The endocervical canal is examined. The septum is identified and resected.

Additional Notes

- A diagnostic laparoscopy is included in this procedure
- A surgical assistant may be needed for a laparoscopy
- Medicare will not reimburse for regional anesthesia administered by the surgeon

CPT® CODE 58561

Hysteroscopy, surgical; with removal of leiomyomata

POLICY INDICATORS

Global Period
0 day post-op period

Assistants at Surgery
Submit reason for assistant

Co-Surgeons Allowed
Co-surgeon allowed

Reduction for Multiple Procedures
Endoscopy payment rules apply

Bilateral Surgery Payment
N/A

Applicable Medicare Policies

Relative Value Units (RVUs)

Work RVUs	6.60
Non-Facility Total	Only valued for facility
Facility Total	10.70

Coding Assistance

58561 includes:

- Positioning and prepping patient
- Examination of site after anesthesia
- Operative services, including inspections around site and closure
- Photodocumentation
- Endometrial sampling

Abbreviated Case Note Example:

- A 40-year-old female patient with a complaint of menorrhagia; found to have a submucousal leiomyomata. Consents to a hysteroscopy with removal of leiomyomata.
- Procedure: A bimanual pelvic examination is performed, and the bladder is drained with a catheter. The cervix is exposed, grasped, and dilated to accommodate the diagnostic hysteroscope. The entire endometrial cavity is examined, including the anterior, posterior, fundal, and lateral walls and bilateral tubal ostia. The endocervical canal is examined. Hysteroscopy reveals submucous myomas. The myomas are resected.

Additional Notes

- A diagnostic laparoscopy is included in this procedure
- A surgical assistant may be needed for a laparoscopy
- Medicare will not reimburse for regional anesthesia administered by the surgeon

CPT® CODE 58562

Hysteroscopy, surgical; with removal of impacted foreign body

POLICY INDICATORS

Global Period
0 day post-op period

Assistants at Surgery
No assistant

Co-Surgeons Allowed
Co-surgeon allowed

Reduction for Multiple Procedures
Endoscopy payment rules apply

Bilateral Surgery Payment
N/A

Applicable Medicare Policies

Relative Value Units (RVUs)

Work RVUs	4.00
Non-Facility Total	12.23
Facility Total	6.63

Coding Assistance

58562 includes:

- Positioning and prepping patient
- Examination of site after anesthesia
- Operative services, including inspections around site and closure
- Photodocumentation
- Endometrial sampling
- Removal of intrauterine device

Abbreviated Case Note Example:

- A 44-year-old female patient presents with an impacted intrauterine device (IUD); unable to remove in the physician's office. Scheduled for a hysteroscopy with resection of impacted foreign body.
- Procedure: A bimanual pelvic examination is performed, and the bladder is drained with a catheter. The cervix is exposed, grasped, and dilated to accommodate the hysteroscope. The entire endometrial cavity is examined, including the anterior, posterior, fundal, and lateral walls and bilateral tubal ostia. The endocervical canal is examined. The IUD is located, dissected out of the uterine wall, and removed from the uterine cavity.

Additional Notes

- A diagnostic laparoscopy is included in this procedure
- A surgical assistant may be needed for a laparoscopy
- Medicare will not reimburse for regional anesthesia administered by the surgeon

CPT® CODE 58563

Hysteroscopy, surgical; with endometrial ablation (eg, endometrial resection, electrosurgical ablation, thermoablation)

POLICY INDICATORS

Global Period
0 day post-op period

Assistants at Surgery
Submit reason for assistant

Co-Surgeons Allowed
Co-surgeon allowed

Reduction for Multiple Procedures
Endoscopy payment rules apply

Bilateral Surgery Payment
N/A

Applicable Medicare Policies

Relative Value Units (RVUs)

Work RVUs	4.47
Non-Facility Total	59.03
Facility Total	7.36

Coding Assistance

58563 includes:

- Positioning and prepping patient
- Examination of site after anesthesia
- Operative services, including inspections around site and closure
- Photodocumentation
- Endometrial sampling

Abbreviated Case Note Example:

- A 47-year-old female patient presents for management of menorrhagia that is unresponsive to medical management. Consents to a hysteroscopy with endometrial ablation.
- Procedure: A bimanual pelvic examination is performed, and the bladder is drained with a catheter. The cervix is progressively dilated to accommodate the diagnostic hysteroscope. The entire endometrial cavity is examined, including the anterior, posterior, fundal, and lateral walls and bilateral tubal ostia. The endocervical canal is examined. A curettage may be performed. The entire endometrium is ablated.

Additional Notes

- A diagnostic laparoscopy is included in this procedure
- If 58561 is also performed, report it as the primary procedure
- A surgical assistant may be needed for a laparoscopy
- Medicare will not reimburse for regional anesthesia administered by the surgeon

CPT® CODE 58565

Hysteroscopy, surgical; with bilateral fallopian tube cannulation to induce occlusion by placement of permanent implants

POLICY INDICATORS

Global Period
90 day post-op period

Assistants at Surgery
No assistant

Co-Surgeons Allowed
Co-surgeon allowed

Reduction for Multiple Procedures
Endoscopy payment rules apply

Bilateral Surgery Payment
Bilateral surgery

Applicable Medicare Policies

Relative Value Units (RVUs)

Work RVUs	7.12
Non-Facility Total	47.21
Facility Total	13.77

Coding Assistance

58565 includes:

- Positioning and prepping patient
- Examination of site after anesthesia
- Operative services, including inspections around site and closure

Abbreviated Case Note Example:

- A 35-year-old female patient desires permanent sterilization but is a poor candidate for laparoscopy due to several previous abdominal surgical procedures.
- Procedure: A pelvic exam is performed. A perineal/vaginal prep is performed. A paracervical block is performed. The cervix is serially dilated. The operative hysteroscope is introduced. A complete diagnostic survey of the uterine cavity is performed. Each tube is cannulated; microinserts are placed bilaterally, and the hysteroscope is removed from the uterus.

Additional Notes

- A diagnostic laparoscopy is included in this procedure
- If other procedures are performed through the hysteroscopy, report one of 58559-58562 instead

CPT® CODE 58570

Laparoscopy, surgical, with total hysterectomy, for uterus 250 g or less

POLICY INDICATORS

Global Period
90 day post-op period

Assistants at Surgery
Assistant allowed

Co-Surgeons Allowed
Co-surgeon allowed

Reduction for Multiple Procedures
Subject to 50% reduction

Bilateral Surgery Payment
N/A

Applicable Medicare Policies

Relative Value Units (RVUs)

Work RVUs	13.36
Non-Facility Total	Only valued for facility
Facility Total	24.37

Coding Assistance

58570 includes:

- Positioning and prepping patient
- Examination of site after anesthesia
- Operative services, including inspections around site and closure
- Appropriate post-op E/M visit(s)
- Photodocumentation
- Introduction of hemostatic agent or pack
- Myomectomy
- Dilation and curettage of cervical stump
- Pelvic examination under anesthesia

Abbreviated Case Note Example:

- A 45-year-old female patient presents with a chronic abnormal uterine bleeding; desires to keep her ovaries. Scheduled for a total laparoscopic hysterectomy (TLH) without removal of the adnexae.
- Procedure: A Foley catheter is placed transurethrally and a uterine manipulator transcervically. A laparoscopy is performed; the utero-ovarian ligament is sequentially coagulated or ligated, and the uterus and cervix are removed through the vagina. After the specimen has been removed completely, reinsert the occluding device and then reinflate the abdominal cavity. Laparoscopic suture closure of the vaginal cuff is performed, and hemostasis is confirmed.

Additional Notes

- A diagnostic laparoscopy is included in this procedure
- If the procedure is converted to an abdominal hysterectomy, report the open procedure
- If the cervix is not removed, report 58541 instead
- If tubes/ovaries are also removed, report 58571 instead
- Do not report 51040 for catheter placement
- The differentiating characteristic between a total laparoscopic hysterectomy (TLH) and a laparoscopy with vaginal hysterectomy (LAVH) procedure is how the structures are detached.
- TLH includes laparoscopically detaching the entire uterine cervix and body from the surrounding supporting structures and suturing the vaginal cuff. It includes bivalving, coring, or morcellating the excised tissues, as required. The uterus is then removed through either the vagina or abdomen. Removing the uterus vaginally does not change the circumstances for reporting TLH codes.

CPT® CODE 58571

Laparoscopy, surgical, with total hysterectomy, for uterus 250 g or less; with removal of tube(s) and/or ovary(s)

POLICY INDICATORS

Global Period
90 day post-op period

Assistants at Surgery
Assistant allowed

Co-Surgeons Allowed
Co-surgeon allowed

Reduction for Multiple Procedures
Subject to 50% reduction

Bilateral Surgery Payment
N/A

Applicable Medicare Policies

Relative Value Units (RVUs)

Work RVUs	15.00
Non-Facility Total	Only valued for facility
Facility Total	27.38

Coding Assistance

58571 includes:

- Positioning and prepping patient
- Examination of site after anesthesia
- Operative services, including inspections around site and closure
- Appropriate post-op E/M visit(s)
- Photodocumentation
- Introduction of hemostatic agent or pack
- Myomectomy
- Dilation and curettage of cervical stump
- Pelvic examination under anesthesia
- Laparoscopic ovarian procedures

Abbreviated Case Note Example:

- A 37-year-old female patient is evaluated for profound menorrhagia with anemia. Elects to have both her cervix and ovaries removed. Consents to a total laparoscopic hysterectomy (TLH) with bilateral salpingo-oophorectomy.
- Procedure: The laparoscopy is performed, and the bladder peritoneum is opened and dissected off. The attachments of the uterus are sequentially coagulated or ligated; occluding device within the vagina is placed and anterior and posterior colpotomy incision is performed. The uterus and cervix are removed through the vagina; laparoscopic suture closure of the vaginal cuff is performed.

Additional Notes

- A diagnostic laparoscopy is included in this procedure
- If the procedure is converted to an abdominal hysterectomy, report the open procedure
- If the cervix is not removed, report 58542 instead
- If tubes/ovaries are also removed, report 58571 instead
- Do not report 51040 for catheter placement
- Laparoscopic procedures can be identified by terms such as "trocar," "robotic," and "pneumoperitoneum." Any reference to an "open entry technique" is simply an alternative method of inserting the trocars to begin the procedure, due to the patient-specific anatomic issues that were present.

CPT® CODE 58572

Laparoscopy, surgical, with total hysterectomy, for uterus greater than 250 g

POLICY INDICATORS

Global Period
90 day post-op period

Assistants at Surgery
Assistant allowed

Co-Surgeons Allowed
Co-surgeon allowed

Reduction for Multiple Procedures
Subject to 50% reduction

Bilateral Surgery Payment
N/A

Applicable Medicare Policies

Relative Value Units (RVUs)

Work RVUs	17.71
Non-Facility Total	Only valued for facility
Facility Total	31.37

Coding Assistance

58572 includes:

- Positioning and prepping patient
- Examination of site after anesthesia
- Operative services, including inspections around site and closure
- Appropriate post-op E/M visit(s)
- Photodocumentation
- Introduction of hemostatic agent or pack
- Myomectomy
- Dilation and curettage of cervical stump
- Pelvic examination under anesthesia

Additional Notes

- A diagnostic laparoscopy is included in this procedure
- If the procedure is converted to an abdominal hysterectomy, report the open procedure
- If the cervix is not removed, report 58543 instead
- If tubes/ovaries are also removed, report 58573 instead
- Do not report 51040 for catheter placement
- To determine the difference between 58150 and 58572, determine if most of the case was performed laparoscopically. Even if the extension of the incision was done to facilitate completion of the laparoscopic procedure, it would continue to be reported as 58572. The incision extension does not change the fundamental nature of the service. If the incision was enlarged earlier in the procedure and key elements of the procedure were performed directly through that incision, then use 58150.

SURGERY

CPT® CODE 58573

Laparoscopy, surgical, with total hysterectomy, for uterus greater than 250 g; with removal of tube(s) and/or ovary(s)

POLICY INDICATORS

Global Period
90 day post-op period

Assistants at Surgery
Assistant allowed

Co-Surgeons Allowed
Co-surgeon allowed

Reduction for Multiple Procedures
Subject to 50% reduction

Bilateral Surgery Payment
N/A

Applicable Medicare Policies

Relative Value Units (RVUs)

Work RVUs	20.79
Non-Facility Total	Only valued for facility
Facility Total	36.68

Coding Assistance

58573 includes:

- Positioning and prepping patient
- Examination of site after anesthesia
- Operative services, including inspections around site and closure
- Appropriate post-op E/M visit(s)
- Photodocumentation
- Introduction of hemostatic agent or pack
- Myomectomy
- Dilation and curettage of cervical stump
- Pelvic examination under anesthesia
- Laparascopic ovarian procedures

Additional Notes

- A diagnostic laparoscopy is included in this procedure
- If the procedure is converted to an abdominal hysterectomy, report the open procedure
- If the cervix is not removed, report 58544 instead
- If tubes/ovaries are also removed, report 58572 instead
- Do not report 51040 for catheter placement
- The work of the procedure itself accomplished laparoscopically confirms the use of 58573. Documentation must also include the weight of the uterus in the operative report and the structures removed.

CPT® CODE 58575

Laparoscopy, surgical, total hysterectomy for resection of malignancy (tumor debulking), with omentectomy including salpingo-oophorectomy, unilateral or bilateral, when performed

POLICY INDICATORS

Global Period
90 day post-op period

Assistants at Surgery
Assistant allowed

Co-Surgeons Allowed
Co-surgeon allowed

Reduction for Multiple Procedures
Subject to 50% reduction

Bilateral Surgery Payment
Bilateral surgery

Applicable Medicare Policies
Inpatient-only list

Relative Value Units (RVUs)

Work RVUs	32.60
Non-Facility Total	Only valued for facility
Facility Total	58.25

Coding Assistance

58575 includes:

- Positioning and prepping patient
- Examination of site after anesthesia
- Operative services, including inspections around site and closure
- Appropriate post-op E/M visit(s)
- Hysterectomy (abdominal)
- Exploratory laparotomy
- Excision or destruction of intra-abdominal or retroperitoneal tumors, cysts, or endometriomas
- Lymphandectomy and pelvic and para-aortic lymph node dissection
- Omentectomy
- Salping-oophorectomy, unilateral or bilateral

Abbreviated Case Note Example:

- A 60-year-old female patient with advanced stage ovarian cancer with a large malignant pleural effusion. Reassessment after chemotherapy demonstrates a good partial response, with imaging tests that show an enlarged right ovarian mass, peritoneal thickening with an omental tumor, and a 3-cm mesenteric nodule.
- Procedure: A diagnostic laparoscopy is performed. Adhesions from the ovarian cancer are systematically lysed. Biopsies of suspicious lesions are obtained. The bowel is mobilized and dissected out of the pelvis. The ureters are freed from pelvic and peritoneal metastasis. A total laparoscopic hysterectomy with bilateral salpingo-oophorectomy is performed. The uterus and ovaries are removed through the vagina. Extra-ovarian tumor masses are resected in the pelvis, the abdomen, and from the bowel mesentery and diaphragm. An omentectomy is performed. Specimens are removed through the vagina, and vaginal closure is performed.

SURGERY

CPT® CODE 58580

Transcervical ablation of uterine fibroid(s), including intraoperative ultrasound guidance and monitoring, radiofrequency

POLICY INDICATORS

Global Period
10-day post-op period

Assistants at Surgery
Assistant allowed

Co-Surgeons Allowed
No co-surgeon

Reduction for Multiple Procedures
Subject to 50% reduction

Bilateral Surgery Payment
N/A

Applicable Medicare Policies

Relative Value Units (RVUs)

Work RVUs	7.21
Non-Facility Total	80.42
Facility Total	12.17

Coding Assistance

58580 includes:

- Positioning and prepping patient
- Examination of site after anesthesia
- Operative services, including inspections around site and closure
- Appropriate post-op E/M visit(s)
- Diagnostic laparoscopy

Abbreviated Case Note Example:

- A 40-year-old patient presents with heavy menstrual bleeding for 6 months. Examination reveals an 8-week-sized uterus. A human chorionic gonadotropin test performed is negative, and endometrial biopsy is normal. Transvaginal sonogram shows multiple fibroids, the largest of which is a transmural myoma at 5.2 × 4.5 × 4.6 cm.
- Procedure: A cervical dilation is performed, and the transcervical fibroid ablation device is inserted into the uterus. Leiomyomata are visualized with the integrated intrauterine ultrasound (IUUS) probe and mapped in a systematic fashion within the uterus to confirm the number and location of fibroids. After identifying fibroids to treat and articulating the IUUS probe, use the graphical overlay to target and plan ablations in the fibroid. Advance a trocar-tipped introducer into the fibroid under guided IUUS visualization. Confirm the thermal safety border to be within the uterine serosal margin in all adjacent ultrasound planes and activate the radiofrequency energy. Each treated fibroid will receive one or more ellipsoidal ablations to achieve durable symptom relief. Repeat treatment steps to treat any additional fibroids that were previously mapped.

CPT® CODE 58600

Ligation or transection of fallopian tube(s), abdominal or vaginal approach, unilateral or bilateral

POLICY INDICATORS

Global Period
90 day post-op period

Assistants at Surgery
Assistant allowed

Co-Surgeons Allowed
Submit reason for co-surgeon

Reduction for Multiple Procedures
Subject to 50% reduction

Bilateral Surgery Payment
Bilateral surgery

Applicable Medicare Policies

Relative Value Units (RVUs)

Work RVUs	5.91
Non-Facility Total	Only valued for facility
Facility Total	11.20

Coding Assistance

58600 includes:

- Positioning and prepping patient
- Examination of site after anesthesia
- Operative services, including inspections around site and closure
- Appropriate post-op E/M visit(s)
- Hysterectomy (abdominal)
- Exploratory laparotomy
- Colpotomy

Abbreviated Case Note Example:

- A 45-year-old female patient presents for elective sterilization.
- Procedure: Under anesthesia, a colpotomy/mini-laparotomy incision is made and the fallopian tube(s) are doubly ligated; specimen is excised and sent to the pathologist.

SURGERY

CPT® CODE 58605

Ligation or transection of fallopian tube(s), abdominal or vaginal approach, postpartum, unilateral or bilateral, during same hospitalization (separate procedure)

POLICY INDICATORS

Global Period
90 day post-op period

Assistants at Surgery
Assistant allowed

Co-Surgeons Allowed
No co-surgeon

Reduction for Multiple Procedures
Subject to 50% reduction

Bilateral Surgery Payment
Bilateral surgery

Applicable Medicare Policies
Inpatient-only list

Relative Value Units (RVUs)

Work RVUs	5.28
Non-Facility Total	Only valued for facility
Facility Total	10.17

Coding Assistance

58605 includes:

- Positioning and prepping patient
- Examination of site after anesthesia
- Operative services, including inspections around site and closure
- Appropriate post-op E/M visit(s)
- Hysterectomy (abdominal)
- Exploratory laparotomy
- Colpotomy

Abbreviated Case Note Example:

- A 40-year-old post-delivery female patient desires elective sterilization.
- Procedure: Under anesthesia, a colpotomy/mini-laparotomy incision is made and the fallopian tube(s) are doubly ligated; specimen is excised and sent to pathologist.

Additional Notes

- If salpingectomy or salpingo-oophorectomy is performed, report 58700 or 58720 instead
- If performed laparoscopically, report 58670 or 58671 instead, If more extensive procedures are performed at the same time, report this code after them
- Preoperative counseling may be reported separately

CPT® CODE 58611

Ligation or transection of fallopian tube(s) when done at the time of cesarean delivery or intra-abdominal surgery (not a separate procedure) (List separately in addition to code for primary procedure)

POLICY INDICATORS

Global Period
Global for primary procedure applies

Assistants at Surgery
Assistant allowed

Co-Surgeons Allowed
No co-surgeon

Reduction for Multiple Procedures
Not subject to multiple surgery reduction

Bilateral Surgery Payment
N/A

Applicable Medicare Policies
Inpatient-only list

Relative Value Units (RVUs)

Work RVUs	1.45
Non-Facility Total	Only valued for facility
Facility Total	2.25

Coding Assistance

58611 includes:

- Positioning and prepping patient
- Examination of site after anesthesia
- Operative services, including inspections around site and closure
- Appropriate post-op E/M visit(s)

Add-On Code:

- Follow Primary Code Policies

CPT® CODE 58615

Occlusion of fallopian tube(s) by device (eg, band, clip, Falope ring) vaginal or suprapubic approach

POLICY INDICATORS

Global Period
10 day post-op period

Assistants at Surgery
Assistant allowed

Co-Surgeons Allowed
No co-surgeon

Reduction for Multiple Procedures
Subject to 50% reduction

Bilateral Surgery Payment
N/A

Applicable Medicare Policies

Relative Value Units (RVUs)

Work RVUs	3.94
Non-Facility Total	Only valued for facility
Facility Total	7.62

Coding Assistance

58615 includes:

- Positioning and prepping patient
- Examination of site after anesthesia
- Operative services, including inspections around site and closure
- Appropriate post-op E/M visit(s)
- Photodocumentation
- Exploratory laparotomy
- Colpotomy

Additional Notes

- If hysteroscopic tubal cannulation for occlusion is performed, report 58565 instead
- If performed laparoscopically, report 58671 instead

CPT® CODE 58660

Laparoscopy, surgical; with lysis of adhesions (salpingolysis, ovariolysis) (separate procedure)

POLICY INDICATORS

Global Period
90 day post-op period

Assistants at Surgery
Assistant allowed

Co-Surgeons Allowed
Co-surgeon allowed

Reduction for Multiple Procedures
Endoscopy payment rules apply

Bilateral Surgery Payment
N/A

Applicable Medicare Policies

Relative Value Units (RVUs)

Work RVUs	11.59
Non-Facility Total	Only valued for facility
Facility Total	20.70

Coding Assistance

58660 includes:

- Positioning and prepping patient
- Examination of site after anesthesia
- Operative services, including inspections around site and closure
- Appropriate post-op E/M visit(s)
- Photodocumentation

Abbreviated Case Note Example:

- A 37-year-old patient with history of appendectomy, difficulty with conception; found to have peritubal adhesions.
- Procedure: Laparoscopy is performed, which shows multiple layers of filmy and dense adhesion throughout the pelvis. The tubes and ovaries are adherent to each other as well as to the pelvic side wall. There are also adhesions between the posterior uterus and rectum. Chromotubation is performed, which demonstrates bilateral tubal patency. Adhesiolysis is performed, and at the conclusion of the operative session, the tubes, ovaries, and uterus are completely free.

Additional Notes

- A diagnostic laparoscopy is included in this procedure

SURGERY

CPT® CODE 58661

Laparoscopy, surgical; with removal of adnexal structures (partial or total oophorectomy and/or salpingectomy)

POLICY INDICATORS

Global Period
10 day post-op period

Assistants at Surgery
Assistant allowed

Co-Surgeons Allowed
Co-surgeon allowed

Reduction for Multiple Procedures
Endoscopy payment rules apply

Bilateral Surgery Payment
150% paid if bilateral

Applicable Medicare Policies

Relative Value Units (RVUs)

Work RVUs	11.35
Non-Facility Total	Only valued for facility
Facility Total	19.65

Coding Assistance

58661 includes:

- Positioning and prepping patient
- Examination of site after anesthesia
- Operative services, including inspections around site and closure
- Appropriate post-op E/M visit(s)
- Photodocumentation
- 58661 is used in cases for treatment of disease process, sterilization, or for prophylactic removal of the fallopian tubes as a risk-reduction method, but no specific disease process in the tubes is present at the time of the procedure. This includes when laparoscopic sterilization is performed via partial or total salpingectomy, when an oophorectomy and/or salpingectomy is performed to address a disease process (eg, hydrosalpinx, torsion, cystic structures, etc.). See Appendix Z for more information.

Additional Notes

- A diagnostic laparoscopy is included in this procedure
- For laparoscopic aspiration of ovarian cyst, report 49322 instead
- For laparoscopic biopsy of ovary or fallopian tube, report 49321 instead

SURGERY

CPT® CODE 58662

Laparoscopy, surgical; with fulguration or excision of lesions of the ovary, pelvic viscera, or peritoneal surface by any method

POLICY INDICATORS

Global Period
90 day post-op period

Assistants at Surgery
Assistant allowed

Co-Surgeons Allowed
Co-surgeon allowed

Reduction for Multiple Procedures
Endoscopy payment rules apply

Bilateral Surgery Payment
N/A

Applicable Medicare Policies

Relative Value Units (RVUs)

Work RVUs	12.15
Non-Facility Total	Only valued for facility
Facility Total	21.50

Coding Assistance

58662 includes:

- Positioning and prepping patient
- Examination of site after anesthesia
- Operative services, including inspections around site and closure
- Appropriate post-op E/M visit(s)
- Photodocumentation

Abbreviated Case Note Example:

- A 44-year-old patient with severe dysmenorrhea, pelvic pain, and dysparunia; failed medical management.
- Procedure: Laparoscopy is performed, revealing multiple implants of endometriosis; both ovaries are free, but each has surface implants of endometriosis. The lesions of endometriosis are excised, vaporized, or cauterized, and lesions on the ovaries are excised, vaporized, or cauterized. Chromotubation is performed, and meticulous hemostasis is maintained.

Additional Notes

- A diagnostic laparoscopy is included in this procedure

CPT® CODE 58670

Laparoscopy, surgical; with fulguration of oviducts (with or without transection)

POLICY INDICATORS

Global Period
90 day post-op period

Assistants at Surgery
No assistant

Co-Surgeons Allowed
Co-surgeon allowed

Reduction for Multiple Procedures
Endoscopy payment rules apply

Bilateral Surgery Payment
N/A

Applicable Medicare Policies

Relative Value Units (RVUs)

Work RVUs	5.91
Non-Facility Total	Only valued for facility
Facility Total	11.22

Coding Assistance

58670 includes:

- Positioning and prepping patient
- Examination of site after anesthesia
- Operative services, including inspections around site and closure
- Appropriate post-op E/M visit(s)
- Photodocumentation

Abbreviated Case Note Example:

- A 30-year-old female patient requires sterilization.
- Procedure: After inserting the laparoscope, the entire abdomen and pelvis are viewed and pathology noted. Each fallopian tube is identified, and traced to its fimbriated end; midportion of each tube is coagulated and may be transected. Both tubes are fulgurated in the isthmic portion. Meticulous hemostasis is maintained.

Additional Notes

- A diagnostic laparoscopy is included in this procedure

CPT® CODE 58671

Laparoscopy, surgical; with occlusion of oviducts by device (eg, band, clip, or Falope ring)

POLICY INDICATORS

Global Period
90 day post-op period

Assistants at Surgery
No assistant

Co-Surgeons Allowed
Co-surgeon allowed

Reduction for Multiple Procedures
Endoscopy payment rules apply

Bilateral Surgery Payment
N/A

Applicable Medicare Policies

Relative Value Units (RVUs)

Work RVUs	5.91
Non-Facility Total	Only valued for facility
Facility Total	11.22

Coding Assistance

58671 includes:

- Positioning and prepping patient
- Examination of site after anesthesia
- Operative services, including inspections around site and closure
- Appropriate post-op E/M visit(s)
- Photodocumentation

Abbreviated Case Note Example:

- Typical patient presentation: Patient requests sterilization.
- Procedure: 58671 is used when laparoscopic sterilization is performed with a band, clip, or Falope ring, or a similar device. Bimanual pelvic exam is done, and cervix is dilated. The laparoscope is inserted, and the entire abdomen and pelvis are viewed systematically. The mid-portion of each tube is identified and a band or clip placed while making sure that no adjoining structures or bowel are damaged. See Appendix Z.

Additional Notes

- A diagnostic laparoscopy is included in this procedure
- If hysteroscopic tubal cannulation for occlusion is performed, report 58565 instead

CPT® CODE 58672

Laparoscopy, surgical; with fimbrioplasty

POLICY INDICATORS

Global Period
90 day post-op period

Assistants at Surgery
Assistant allowed

Co-Surgeons Allowed
No co-surgeon

Reduction for Multiple Procedures
Endoscopy payment rules apply

Bilateral Surgery Payment
150% paid if bilateral

Applicable Medicare Policies

Relative Value Units (RVUs)

Work RVUs	12.91
Non-Facility Total	Only valued for facility
Facility Total	21.96

Coding Assistance

58672 includes:

- Positioning and prepping patient
- Examination of site after anesthesia
- Operative services, including inspections around site and closure
- Appropriate post-op E/M visit(s)
- Photodocumentation

Abbreviated Case Note Example:

- Typical patient presentation: Hysterosalpingogram shows that the distal tube is dilated; fimbrial adhesions are noted via laparoscopy.
- Procedure: 58672 is used when a laparoscopic procedure is performed to treat disease or disorders of the fimbriae of the fallopian tubes—usually to repair, restore, or enhance fertility. The fimbrial adhesions are meticulously lysed with care not to damage the fimbriae. The distal tube may be "flowered" back or sutured.

Additional Notes

- A diagnostic laparoscopy is included in this procedure

CPT® CODE 58673

Laparoscopy, surgical; with salpingostomy (salpingoneostomy)

POLICY INDICATORS

Global Period
90 day post-op period

Assistants at Surgery
Assistant allowed

Co-Surgeons Allowed
No co-surgeon

Reduction for Multiple Procedures
Endoscopy payment rules apply

Bilateral Surgery Payment
150% paid if bilateral

Applicable Medicare Policies

Relative Value Units (RVUs)

Work RVUs	14.04
Non-Facility Total	Only valued for facility
Facility Total	23.83

Coding Assistance

58673 includes:

- Positioning and prepping patient
- Examination of site after anesthesia
- Operative services, including inspections around site and closure
- Appropriate post-op E/M visit(s)
- Photodocumentation

Abbreviated Case Note Example:

- Typical patient presentation: Hysterosalpingogram shows nonpatent hydrosalpinges; laparoscopy notes right tube completely free and the distal end is completed closed and dilated with no evidence of fimbria.
- Procedure: 58673 is used when an incision is made laparoscopically into the fallopian tube to address a structural issue or disease process, but the tube itself is not removed. The distal right tube is isolated. The avascular planes are identified and cruciate incisions made in the distal tube with either scissors, electrosurgery, or laser. Multiple flaps are created. Meticulous hemostasis is obtained with care not to damage the tubal flaps. Each of these flaps is "flowered" back with the laser or electrosurgery or sewn back to create the new opening in the fallopian tube. This code is used only to address gynecologic issues—not obstetric issues. See Appendix Z.

Additional Notes

- A diagnostic laparoscopy is included in this procedure

CPT® CODE 58674

Laparoscopy, surgical, ablation of uterine fibroid(s) including intraoperative ultrasound guidance and monitoring, radiofrequency

POLICY INDICATORS

Global Period
90 day post-op period

Assistants at Surgery
Assistant allowed

Co-Surgeons Allowed
Co-surgeon allowed

Reduction for Multiple Procedures
Subject to 50% reduction

Bilateral Surgery Payment
N/A

Applicable Medicare Policies

Relative Value Units (RVUs)

Work RVUs	14.08
Non-Facility Total	Only valued for facility
Facility Total	24.47

Coding Assistance

58674 includes:

- Positioning and prepping patient
- Examination of site after anesthesia
- Operative services, including inspections around site and closure
- Appropriate post-op E/M visit(s)

Abbreviated Case Note Example:

- Typical patient presentation: A pelvic sonogram demonstrated multiple uterine fibroids, ranging in size from 1 cm to 7 cm in diameter, that are intramural and submucosal in location.
- Procedure: Using the laparoscopic ultrasound as a guide, the radiofrequency thermal ablation device is placed within the first myoma, and the array is deployed. Radiofrequency energy heats the myoma to 100 °C (monitored by thermocouples within the device), and the temperature is maintained at that level for the number of minutes indicated on the device manufacturer's chart.

CPT® CODE 58700

Salpingectomy, complete or partial, unilateral or bilateral (separate procedure)

POLICY INDICATORS

Global Period
90 day post-op period

Assistants at Surgery
Assistant allowed

Co-Surgeons Allowed
Submit reason for co-surgeon

Reduction for Multiple Procedures
Subject to 50% reduction

Bilateral Surgery Payment
Bilateral surgery

Applicable Medicare Policies
Inpatient-only list

Relative Value Units (RVUs)

Work RVUs	12.95
Non-Facility Total	Only valued for facility
Facility Total	24.21

Coding Assistance

58700 includes:

- Positioning and prepping patient
- Examination of site after anesthesia
- Operative services, including inspections around site and closure
- Appropriate post-op E/M visit(s)
- Exploratory laparotomy

Abbreviated Case Note Example:

- Typical patient presentation: Hysterosalpingogram shows severely damaged tubes with evidence of bilateral salpingitis isthmica nodosa and bilateral nonpatent hydrosalpinges. An exploratory laparotomy is performed which shows large nonpatent hydrosalpinges.
- Procedure: Left and right fallopian tubes are removed.

Additional Notes

- If performed laparoscopically, report 58661 instead
- If oophorectomy is also performed, report 58720 instead
- if salpingectomy is performed for removal of ectopic pregnancy, report 59120 instead

CPT® CODE 58720

Salpingo-oophorectomy, complete or partial, unilateral or bilateral (separate procedure)

POLICY INDICATORS

Global Period
90 day post-op period

Assistants at Surgery
Assistant allowed

Co-Surgeons Allowed
Submit reason for co-surgeon

Reduction for Multiple Procedures
Subject to 50% reduction

Bilateral Surgery Payment
Bilateral surgery

Applicable Medicare Policies
Inpatient-only list

Relative Value Units (RVUs)

Work RVUs	12.16
Non-Facility Total	Only valued for facility
Facility Total	22.96

Coding Assistance

58720 includes:

- Positioning and prepping patient
- Examination of site after anesthesia
- Operative services, including inspections around site and closure
- Appropriate post-op E/M visit(s)
- Exploratory laparotomy

Abbreviated Case Note Example:

- Typical patient presentation: Bilateral ovarian cysts.
- Procedure: The vascular supply of the tubes and ovaries is ligated and divided.

Additional Notes

- Use this code for removal of paratubal cyst

CPT® CODE 58740

Lysis of adhesions (salpingolysis, ovariolysis)

POLICY INDICATORS

Global Period
90 day post-op period

Assistants at Surgery
Assistant allowed

Co-Surgeons Allowed
Submit reason for co-surgeon

Reduction for Multiple Procedures
Subject to 50% reduction

Bilateral Surgery Payment
N/A

Applicable Medicare Policies
Inpatient-only list

Relative Value Units (RVUs)

Work RVUs	14.90
Non-Facility Total	Only valued for facility
Facility Total	27.30

Coding Assistance

58740 includes:

- Positioning and prepping patient
- Examination of site after anesthesia
- Operative services, including inspections around site and closure
- Appropriate post-op E/M visit(s)
- Exploratory laparotomy

Abbreviated Case Note Example:

- Typical patient presentation: Hysterosalpingogram shows patent tubes and loculation of contrast around both tubes suggesting peritubal adhesions.
- Procedure: An exploratory laparotomy shows multiple layers of filmy and dense adhesions throughout the pelvis. The tubes and ovaries are adherent to each other as well as to the pelvic side wall and adhesions between the posterior uterus and rectum. Chromotubation is performed which demonstrates bilateral tubal patency. Meticulous adhesiolysis is performed, and the tubes, ovaries, and uterus are completely free.

Additional Notes

- If performed laparoscopically, report 58660 instead

CPT® CODE 58750

Tubotubal anastomosis

POLICY INDICATORS

Global Period
90 day post-op period

Assistants at Surgery
Assistant allowed

Co-Surgeons Allowed
Submit reason for co-surgeon

Reduction for Multiple Procedures
Subject to 50% reduction

Bilateral Surgery Payment
150% paid if bilateral

Applicable Medicare Policies
Inpatient-only list

Relative Value Units (RVUs)

Work RVUs	15.64
Non-Facility Total	Only valued for facility
Facility Total	27.37

Coding Assistance

58750 includes:

- Positioning and prepping patient
- Examination of site after anesthesia
- Operative services, including inspections around site and closure
- Appropriate post-op E/M visit(s)
- Photodocumentation
- Diagnostic chromotubation

Abbreviated Case Note Example:

- Typical patient presentation: Patient desires fertility post tubal ligation. Laparoscopic evaluation showed 4-cm tube distally on right, 3-cm tube proximally on right.
- Procedure: Exploratory laparotomy is performed. The uterus and tubal segments are elevated with appropriate packing and adhesions are lysed as indicated. The segments are mobilized and the blocked portion of the tube is excised and it is sutured cleanly to the unblocked portion. This is done through the use of an operating microscope.

CPT® CODE 58752

Tubouterine implantation

POLICY INDICATORS

Global Period
90 day post-op period

Assistants at Surgery
Assistant allowed

Co-Surgeons Allowed
No co-surgeon

Reduction for Multiple Procedures
Subject to 50% reduction

Bilateral Surgery Payment
150% paid if bilateral

Applicable Medicare Policies
Inpatient-only list

Relative Value Units (RVUs)

Work RVUs	15.64
Non-Facility Total	Only valued for facility
Facility Total	27.29

Coding Assistance

58752 includes:

- Positioning and prepping patient
- Examination of site after anesthesia
- Operative services, including inspections around site and closure
- Appropriate post-op E/M visit(s)
- Exploratory laparotomy
- Diagnostic chromotubation
- Utero-tubal stent supply

Abbreviated Case Note Example:

- Typical patient presentation: Desires fertility post tubal ligation. Laparoscopic evaluation showed 6-cm tube distally and no proximal tube on the right. The left tube was previously removed.
- Procedure: Adhesions are lysed as indicated. The distal segment is mobilized. The uterine cornu is incised until patency is established. The tubal lumen is approximated via repair of mesosalpinx. The ligated portion of distal tubal segment is excised.

CPT® CODE 58760

Fimbrioplasty

POLICY INDICATORS

Global Period
90 day post-op period

Assistants at Surgery
Assistant allowed

Co-Surgeons Allowed
Submit reason for co-surgeon

Reduction for Multiple Procedures
Subject to 50% reduction

Bilateral Surgery Payment
150% paid if bilateral

Applicable Medicare Policies
Inpatient-only list

Relative Value Units (RVUs)

Work RVUs	13.93
Non-Facility Total	Only valued for facility
Facility Total	24.69

Coding Assistance

58760 includes:

- Positioning and prepping patient
- Examination of site after anesthesia
- Operative services, including inspections around site and closure
- Appropriate post-op E/M visit(s)
- Photodocumentation
- Diagnostic chromotubation
- Exploratory laparotomy

Abbreviated Case Note Example:

- Typical patient presentation: Patient desires fertility post left salpingectomy for ectopic pregnancy, and is noted to have right fimbrial agglutination at that time.
- Procedure: Adhesions are lysed as indicated. The tube is mobilized, dye injected. Areas of fimbrial agglutination are carefully lysed to allow maximal motion of fimbrial segments. Patency established.

Additional Notes

- If performed laparoscopically, report 58672 instead

CPT® CODE 58770

Salpingostomy (salpingoneostomy)

POLICY INDICATORS

Global Period
90 day post-op period

Assistants at Surgery
Assistant allowed

Co-Surgeons Allowed
No co-surgeon

Reduction for Multiple Procedures
Subject to 50% reduction

Bilateral Surgery Payment
150% paid if bilateral

Applicable Medicare Policies

Relative Value Units (RVUs)

Work RVUs	14.77
Non-Facility Total	Only valued for facility
Facility Total	25.91

Coding Assistance

58770 includes:

- Positioning and prepping patient
- Examination of site after anesthesia
- Operative services, including inspections around site and closure
- Appropriate post-op E/M visit(s)
- Photodocumentation
- Diagnostic chromotubation
- Exploratory laparotomy

Abbreviated Case Note Example:

- Typical patient presentation: Patient desires post salpingectomy for an ectopic pregnancy and noted right hydrosalpinx.
- Procedure: Adhesions lysed as indicated. The tube is mobilized, dye injected. Area of tubal occlusion identified. Stellate incision made. Hemostasis obtained. Leaflets inverted, sutured to serosa with 6-0 sutures. Patency established.

Additional Notes

- If performed laparoscopically, report 58673 instead
- If ovarian cystectomy is performed, report code 58925 instead

CPT® CODE 58800

Drainage of ovarian cyst(s), unilateral or bilateral (separate procedure); vaginal approach

POLICY INDICATORS

Global Period
90 day post-op period

Assistants at Surgery
No assistant

Co-Surgeons Allowed
No co-surgeon

Reduction for Multiple Procedures
Subject to 50% reduction

Bilateral Surgery Payment
Bilateral surgery

Applicable Medicare Policies

Relative Value Units (RVUs)

Work RVUs	4.62
Non-Facility Total	10.88
Facility Total	9.56

Coding Assistance

58800 includes:

- Positioning and prepping patient
- Examination of site after anesthesia
- Operative services, including inspections around site and closure
- Appropriate post-op E/M visit(s)
- Photodocumentation
- Colpotomy

Additional Notes

- If performed using an abdominal approach, report 58805 instead

CPT® CODE 58805

Drainage of ovarian cyst(s), unilateral or bilateral (separate procedure); abdominal approach

POLICY INDICATORS

Global Period
90 day post-op period

Assistants at Surgery
Assistant allowed

Co-Surgeons Allowed
Submit reason for co-surgeon

Reduction for Multiple Procedures
Subject to 50% reduction

Bilateral Surgery Payment
Bilateral surgery

Applicable Medicare Policies

Relative Value Units (RVUs)

Work RVUs	6.42
Non-Facility Total	Only valued for facility
Facility Total	12.90

Coding Assistance

58805 includes:

- Positioning and prepping patient
- Examination of site after anesthesia
- Operative services, including inspections around site and closure
- Appropriate post-op E/M visit(s)
- Photodocumentation
- Exploratory laparotomy

Additional Notes

- If performed using an abdominal approach, report 58800 instead

CPT® CODE 58820

Drainage of ovarian abscess; vaginal approach, open

POLICY INDICATORS

Global Period
90 day post-op period

Assistants at Surgery
Assistant allowed

Co-Surgeons Allowed
No co-surgeon

Reduction for Multiple Procedures
Subject to 50% reduction

Bilateral Surgery Payment
150% paid if bilateral

Applicable Medicare Policies

Relative Value Units (RVUs)

Work RVUs	4.70
Non-Facility Total	Only valued for facility
Facility Total	10.25

Coding Assistance

58820 includes:

- Positioning and prepping patient
- Examination of site after anesthesia
- Operative services, including inspections around site and closure
- Appropriate post-op E/M visit(s)
- Photodocumentation

Additional Notes

- If performed using an abdominal approach, report 58822 instead

CPT® CODE 58822

Drainage of ovarian abscess; abdominal approach

POLICY INDICATORS

Global Period
90 day post-op period

Assistants at Surgery
Assistant allowed

Co-Surgeons Allowed
Submit reason for co-surgeon

Reduction for Multiple Procedures
Subject to 50% reduction

Bilateral Surgery Payment
150% paid if bilateral

Applicable Medicare Policies
Inpatient-only list

Relative Value Units (RVUs)

Work RVUs	11.81
Non-Facility Total	Only valued for facility
Facility Total	21.52

Coding Assistance

58822 includes:

- Positioning and prepping patient
- Examination of site after anesthesia
- Operative services, including inspections around site and closure
- Appropriate post-op E/M visit(s)
- Photodocumentation
- Exploratory laparotomy

Abbreviated Case Note Example:

- Typical patient presentation: Severe pelvic pain and high fever. Large right tubo-ovarian abscess. Despite aggressive antibiotic therapy, the patient has remained febrile with little or no clinical improvement. A decision is made to drain the abscesses surgically.
- Procedure: The abscess is localized, incised, and drained. Copious lavage is used. An intra-operative decision is made as to which organs can be preserved. Numerous drains are placed in the area of the abscess and brought out through separate small abdominal incisions.

Additional Notes

- If performed using a vaginal approach, report 58820 instead
- If an ovarian cystectomy is performed, report 58925 instead

CPT® CODE 58825

Transposition, ovary(s)

POLICY INDICATORS

Global Period
90 day post-op period

Assistants at Surgery
Assistant allowed

Co-Surgeons Allowed
Submit reason for co-surgeon

Reduction for Multiple Procedures
Subject to 50% reduction

Bilateral Surgery Payment
N/A

Applicable Medicare Policies
Inpatient-only list

Relative Value Units (RVUs)

Work RVUs	11.78
Non-Facility Total	Only valued for facility
Facility Total	21.36

Coding Assistance

58825 includes:

- Positioning and prepping patient
- Examination of site after anesthesia
- Operative services, including inspections around site and closure
- Appropriate post-op E/M visit(s)
- Exploratory laparotomy

Abbreviated Case Note Example:

- Typical patient presentation: Patient post pelvic and abdominal radiation therapy and wishes to preserve fertility. Bilateral ovarian transposition is recommended to preserve normal ovarian function.
- Procedure: Repositioning of ovaries and securing them in place.

CPT® CODE 58900

Biopsy of ovary, unilateral or bilateral (separate procedure)

POLICY INDICATORS

Global Period
90 day post-op period

Assistants at Surgery
Assistant allowed

Co-Surgeons Allowed
Submit reason for co-surgeon

Reduction for Multiple Procedures
Subject to 50% reduction

Bilateral Surgery Payment
Bilateral surgery

Applicable Medicare Policies

Relative Value Units (RVUs)

Work RVUs	6.59
Non-Facility Total	Only valued for facility
Facility Total	13.18

Coding Assistance

58900 includes:

- Positioning and prepping patient
- Examination of site after anesthesia
- Operative services, including inspections around site and closure
- Appropriate post-op E/M visit(s)
- Photodocumentation
- Exploratory laparotomy

Additional Notes

- If an ovarian cystectomy is performed, report 58925 instead
- If a laparoscopic biopsy of ovary or fallopian tube is performed, report 49321 instead
- If a different procedure is performed on the opposite side, use a 59 modifier on this code

SURGERY

CPT® CODE 58920

Wedge resection or bisection of ovary, unilateral or bilateral

POLICY INDICATORS

Global Period
90 day post-op period

Assistants at Surgery
Assistant allowed

Co-Surgeons Allowed
Submit reason for co-surgeon

Reduction for Multiple Procedures
Subject to 50% reduction

Bilateral Surgery Payment
Bilateral surgery

Applicable Medicare Policies

Relative Value Units (RVUs)

Work RVUs	11.95
Non-Facility Total	Only valued for facility
Facility Total	21.50

Coding Assistance

58920 includes:

- Positioning and prepping patient
- Examination of site after anesthesia
- Operative services, including inspections around site and closure
- Appropriate post-op E/M visit(s)
- Photodocumentation
- Exploratory laparotomy

Abbreviated Case Note Example:

- Typical patient presentation: Adnexal mass believed to be of benign origin. At surgery, the ovarian mass appears suspicious, is biopsied, and malignancy is confirmed. A second operation for the purpose of staging disease is recommended.
- Procedure: A wedge resection of the remaining ovary is performed, and appropriate treatment is carried out.

Additional Notes

- If performed laparoscopically, report 59661 instead

CPT® CODE 58925

Ovarian cystectomy, unilateral or bilateral

POLICY INDICATORS

Global Period
90 day post-op period

Assistants at Surgery
Assistant allowed

Co-Surgeons Allowed
Submit reason for co-surgeon

Reduction for Multiple Procedures
Subject to 50% reduction

Bilateral Surgery Payment
Bilateral surgery

Applicable Medicare Policies

Relative Value Units (RVUs)

Work RVUs	12.43
Non-Facility Total	Only valued for facility
Facility Total	23.22

Coding Assistance

58925 includes:

- Positioning and prepping patient
- Examination of site after anesthesia
- Operative services, including inspections around site and closure
- Appropriate post-op E/M visit(s)
- Exploratory laparotomy

Abbreviated Case Note Example:

- Typical patient presentation: Persistent 6-cm complex adnexal mass.
- Procedure: Ovarian cystectomy, including exploratory laparotomy, analysis of minor adhesions, removal of the ovarian cyst(s), and reconstruction of the ovary. Frozen section is done to confirm that the cyst is benign.

CPT® CODE 58940

Oophorectomy, partial or total, unilateral or bilateral

POLICY INDICATORS

Global Period
90 day post-op period

Assistants at Surgery
Assistant allowed

Co-Surgeons Allowed
Submit reason for co-surgeon

Reduction for Multiple Procedures
Subject to 50% reduction

Bilateral Surgery Payment
Bilateral surgery

Applicable Medicare Policies
Inpatient-only list

Relative Value Units (RVUs)

Work RVUs	8.22
Non-Facility Total	Only valued for facility
Facility Total	16.80

Coding Assistance

58940 includes:

- Positioning and prepping patient
- Examination of site after anesthesia
- Operative services, including inspections around site and closure
- Appropriate post-op E/M visit(s)
- Exploratory laparotomy

Additional Notes

- For oophorectomy with concomitant debulking for ovarian malignancy, report 58952 instead

CPT® CODE 58943

Oophorectomy, partial or total, unilateral or bilateral; for ovarian, tubal or primary peritoneal malignancy, with para-aortic and pelvic lymph node biopsies, peritoneal washings, peritoneal biopsies, diaphragmatic assessments, with or without salpingectomy(s), with or without omentectomy

POLICY INDICATORS

Global Period
90 day post-op period

Assistants at Surgery
Assistant allowed

Co-Surgeons Allowed
Submit reason for co-surgeon

Reduction for Multiple Procedures
Subject to 50% reduction

Bilateral Surgery Payment
N/A

Applicable Medicare Policies
Inpatient-only list

Relative Value Units (RVUs)

Work RVUs	19.52
Non-Facility Total	Only valued for facility
Facility Total	36.26

Coding Assistance

58943 includes:

- Positioning and prepping patient
- Examination of site after anesthesia
- Operative services, including inspections around site and closure
- Appropriate post-op E/M visit(s)
- Exploratory laparotomy
- Limited lymphadenectomy
- Exploration of retroperitoneum

Additional Notes

- For complete pelvic lymphadenectomy and bilateral salpingo-oophorectomy with omentectomy for ovarian cancer, another option is to report 58950 with 38770
- If hysterectomy is performed, report 58951 instead
- If radical dissection is performed, report 58952 instead
- For a postoperative counseling visit about chemotherapy, use the appropriate E/M with modifier 24

CPT® CODE 58950

Resection (initial) of ovarian, tubal or primary peritoneal malignancy with bilateral salpingo-oophorectomy and omentectomy

POLICY INDICATORS

Global Period
90 day post-op period

Assistants at Surgery
Assistant allowed

Co-Surgeons Allowed
Submit reason for co-surgeon

Reduction for Multiple Procedures
Subject to 50% reduction

Bilateral Surgery Payment
Bilateral surgery

Applicable Medicare Policies
Inpatient-only list

Relative Value Units (RVUs)

Work RVUs	18.37
Non-Facility Total	Only valued for facility
Facility Total	34.77

Coding Assistance

58950 includes:

- Positioning and prepping patient
- Examination of site after anesthesia
- Operative services, including inspections around site and closure
- Appropriate post-op E/M visit(s)
- Exploratory laparotomy
- Omentectomy
- Salpingo-oophorectomy, unilateral or bilateral
- Transitional care management

Abbreviated Case Note Example:

- Typical patient presentation: Bilateral pelvic masses.
- Procedure: Exploratory laparotomy confirmed the presence of bilateral ovarian masses. A bilateral salpingo-oophorectomy was performed, and a frozen section obtained intraoperatively confirmed the presence of a well-differentiated mucinous carcinoma. Because of the high risk of occult metastatic disease to the omentum, an omentectomy was also performed.

Additional Notes

- If hysterectomy is performed, report 58951 instead
- If radical dissection is performed, report 58952 instead
- For resection of recurrent malignancy, report 58957 and 58958 instead
- For a postoperative counseling visit about treatment options, use the appropriate E/M with modifier 24

CPT® CODE 58951

Resection (initial) of ovarian, tubal or primary peritoneal malignancy with bilateral salpingo-oophorectomy and omentectomy; with total abdominal hysterectomy, pelvic and limited para-aortic lymphadenectomy

POLICY INDICATORS

Global Period
90 day post-op period

Assistants at Surgery
Assistant allowed

Co-Surgeons Allowed
Submit reason for co-surgeon

Reduction for Multiple Procedures
Subject to 50% reduction

Bilateral Surgery Payment
Bilateral surgery

Applicable Medicare Policies
Inpatient-only list

Relative Value Units (RVUs)

Work RVUs	24.26
Non-Facility Total	Only valued for facility
Facility Total	43.51

Coding Assistance

58951 includes:

- Positioning and prepping patient
- Examination of site after anesthesia
- Operative services, including inspections around site and closure
- Appropriate post-op E/M visit(s)
- Exploratory laparotomy
- Lymphadenectomy
- Exploration of retroperitoneum

Abbreviated Case Note Example

- Typical patient presentation: Fixed pelvic mass and ascites and high probability of ovarian cancer.
- Procedure: Exploratory laparotomy reveals bilateral ovarian cancers with metastasis noted in the omentum. Total abdominal hysterectomy with bilateral salpingo-oophorectomy and omentectomy. This portion of the procedure excised all of the visible tumor. Because of a high risk of occult metastatic disease to the pelvic and/or paraaortic lymph nodes, a bilateral pelvic and limited paraaortic lymphadenectomy was also performed.

Additional Notes

- If radical dissection is performed, report 58952 instead
- For resection of recurrent malignancy, report 58957 and/or 58958 instead
- If malignancy is not present, report 58150, 58152, 58200, or 58210 instead
- If lymphadenectomy is not performed, report 58956 instead
- For a postoperative counseling visit about treatment options, use the appropriate E/M with modifier 24
- If debulking is also performed, see codes 58953-58954 and 58957

CPT® CODE 58952

Resection (initial) of ovarian, tubal or primary peritoneal malignancy with bilateral salpingo-oophorectomy and omentectomy; with radical dissection for debulking (ie, radical excision or destruction, intra-abdominal or retroperitoneal tumors)

POLICY INDICATORS

Global Period
90 day post-op period

Assistants at Surgery
Assistant allowed

Co-Surgeons Allowed
Submit reason for co-surgeon

Reduction for Multiple Procedures
Subject to 50% reduction

Bilateral Surgery Payment
Bilateral surgery

Applicable Medicare Policies
Inpatient-only list

Relative Value Units (RVUs)

Work RVUs	27.29
Non-Facility Total	Only valued for facility
Facility Total	49.61

Coding Assistance

58952 includes:

- Positioning and prepping patient
- Examination of site after anesthesia
- Operative services, including inspections around site and closure
- Appropriate post-op E/M visit(s)
- Exploratory laparotomy
- Lymphadenectomy
- Exploration of retroperitoneum
- Salpingo-oophorectomy, unilateral or bilateral
- Omentectomy
- Excision or destruction of intra-abdominal or retroperitoneal tumors, cysts, or endometriomas

Abbreviated Case Note Example:

- Typical patient presentation: Ascites and a pelvic mass. Evaluation has yielded a presumed diagnosis of ovarian cancer.
- Procedure: A bilateral salpingo-oophorectomy is performed by dissecting the pelvic side walls, ureters, and sigmoid from the adnexal masses. The pelvic peritoneum may need to be removed as part of the radical resection. An omentectomy is performed. An attempt is made to remove all tumor nodules larger than 1 cm in the abdomen and pelvis. An omentectomy is performed.

Additional Notes

- If radical dissection is performed, report 58952 instead
- For resection of recurrent malignancy, report 58957 and/or 58958 instead
- If malignancy is not present, report 58150, 58152, 58200, or 58210 instead
- If lymphadenectomy is not performed, report 58956 instead
- For a postoperative counseling visit about treatment options, use the appropriate E/M with modifier 24
- If debulking is also performed, see codes 58953-58954 and 58957

SURGERY

CPT® CODE 58953

Bilateral salpingo-oophorectomy with omentectomy, total abdominal hysterectomy and radical dissection for debulking

POLICY INDICATORS

Global Period
90 day post-op period

Assistants at Surgery
Assistant allowed

Co-Surgeons Allowed
Submit reason for co-surgeon

Reduction for Multiple Procedures
Subject to 50% reduction

Bilateral Surgery Payment
Bilateral surgery

Applicable Medicare Policies
Inpatient-only list

Relative Value Units (RVUs)

Work RVUs	34.13
Non-Facility Total	Only valued for facility
Facility Total	60.32

Coding Assistance

58953 includes:

- Positioning and prepping patient
- Examination of site after anesthesia
- Operative services, including inspections around site and closure
- Appropriate post-op E/M visit(s)
- Exploratory laparotomy
- Limited lymphadenectomy
- Hysterectomy, abdominal
- Salpingo-oophorectomy, unilateral or bilateral
- Omentectomy
- Excision or destruction of intra-abdominal or retroperitoneal tumors, cysts, or endometriomas

Abbreviated Case Note Example:

- Typical patient presentation: Distended abdomen from ascites with a pelvic mass and a ballotable abdominal mass.
- Procedure: Exploratory laparotomy for a presumed advanced ovarian malignancy revealed bilateral ovarian cancers with extensive pelvic tumor nodularity in the cul-de-sac of the pelvis in addition to extensive omental replacement with metastatic cancer. The patient undergoes a total abdominal hysterectomy with bilateral salpingo-oophorectomy, excision of the pelvic peritoneum with removal of the metastatic implants within the pelvis, and an omentectomy.

Additional Notes

- If hysterectomy is not performed for malignancy, report 58150, 58152, 58200, or 58210 instead
- If lymphadenectomy is not performed, report 58954 instead
- For a postoperative counseling visit about treatment options, use the appropriate E/M with modifier 24

SURGERY

CPT® CODE 58954

Bilateral salpingo-oophorectomy with omentectomy, total abdominal hysterectomy and radical dissection for debulking; with pelvic lymphadenectomy and limited para-aortic lymphadenectomy

POLICY INDICATORS

Global Period
90 day post-op period

Assistants at Surgery
Assistant allowed

Co-Surgeons Allowed
Submit reason for co-surgeon

Reduction for Multiple Procedures
Subject to 50% reduction

Bilateral Surgery Payment
Bilateral surgery

Applicable Medicare Policies
Inpatient-only list

Relative Value Units (RVUs)

Work RVUs	37.13
Non-Facility Total	Only valued for facility
Facility Total	65.28

Coding Assistance

58954 includes:

- Positioning and prepping patient
- Examination of site after anesthesia
- Operative services, including inspections around site and closure
- Appropriate post-op E/M visit(s)
- Exploratory laparotomy
- Lymphadenectomy
- Hysterectomy, abdominal
- Salpingo-oophorectomy, unilateral or bilateral
- Omentectomy
- Excision or destruction of intra-abdominal or retroperitoneal tumors, cysts or endometriomas

Abbreviated Case Note Example:

- Typical patient presentation: Distended abdomen from ascites with a pelvic mass and a ballotable abdominal mass.
- Procedure: Exploratory laparotomy for a presumed advanced ovarian malignancy found to have bilateral ovarian cancers with extensive pelvic tumor nodularity in the cul-de-sac of the pelvis in addition to extensive omental replacement with metastatic cancer. The patient undergoes a total abdominal hysterectomy with bilateral salpingo-oophorectomy, excision of the pelvic peritoneum with removal of the metastatic implants within the pelvis, and an omentectomy. The visible cancer has been resected. Because of a high risk of pelvic or periaortic metastasis a pelvic lymphadenectomy including external iliac, hypogastric, and obturator nodes is done, and the lower periaortic lymph nodes (below the renal vessels) are biopsied or excised.

Additional Notes

- If hysterectomy is not performed for malignancy, report 58150, 58152, 58200, or 58210 instead
- If lymphadenectomy is not performed, report 58953 instead
- For a postoperative counseling visit about treatment options, use the appropriate E/M with modifier 24

CPT® CODE 58956

Bilateral salpingo-oophorectomy with total omentectomy, total abdominal hysterectomy for malignancy

POLICY INDICATORS

Global Period
90 day post-op period

Assistants at Surgery
Assistant allowed

Co-Surgeons Allowed
Submit reason for co-surgeon

Reduction for Multiple Procedures
Subject to 50% reduction

Bilateral Surgery Payment
Bilateral surgery

Applicable Medicare Policies
Inpatient-only list

Relative Value Units (RVUs)

Work RVUs	22.80
Non-Facility Total	Only valued for facility
Facility Total	41.06

Coding Assistance

58956 includes:

- Positioning and prepping patient
- Examination of site after anesthesia
- Operative services, including inspections around site and closure
- Appropriate post-op E/M visit(s)
- Exploratory laparotomy
- Hysterectomy (all approaches)
- Omentectomy
- Salpingo-oophorectomy, unilateral or bilateral
- Ovarian surgery
- Excision or destruction of intra-abdominal or retroperitoneal tumors, cysts or endometriomas

Abbreviated Case Note Example:

- Typical patient presentation: FIGO grade 3 endometrial carcinoma.
- Procedure: Exploratory laparotomy. At the time of surgery there are several 2-cm implants found in the omentum. There is no adenopathy and no peritoneal implants. A total abdominal hysterectomy (TAH) and bilateral salpingo-oophorectomy are performed.

Additional Notes

- If radical dissection is performed, report 58953 instead
- If radical dissection for debulking, pelvic lymphadenectomy and limited para-aortic lymphadenectomy are also performed, report 58954 instead
- For a postoperative counseling visit about treatment options, use the appropriate E/M with modifier 24

SURGERY

CPT® CODE 58958

Resection (tumor debulking) of recurrent ovarian, tubal, primary peritoneal, uterine malignancy (intra-abdominal, retroperitoneal tumors), with omentectomy, if performed; with pelvic lymphadenectomy and limited para-aortic lymphadenectomy

POLICY INDICATORS

Global Period
90 day post-op period

Assistants at Surgery
Assistant allowed

Co-Surgeons Allowed
Submit reason for co-surgeon

Reduction for Multiple Procedures
Subject to 50% reduction

Bilateral Surgery Payment
Bilateral surgery

Applicable Medicare Policies
Inpatient-only list

Relative Value Units (RVUs)

Work RVUs	29.22
Non-Facility Total	Only valued for facility
Facility Total	49.73

Coding Assistance

58958 includes:

- Positioning and prepping patient
- Examination of site after anesthesia
- Operative services, including inspections around site and closure
- Appropriate post-op E/M visit(s)
- Exploratory laparotomy
- Enterolysis
- Omentectomy
- Salpingo-oophorectomy, unilateral or bilateral
- Exploration of retroperitoneum, including excision or destruction of tumors, cysts, and endometriomas
- Lymphadenectomy, pelvic and para-aortic

Abbreviated Case Note Example:

- Typical patient presentation: Previous history of optimally debulked stage IIIC epithelial ovarian cancer and CT scan of the abdomen and pelvic that suggests recurrent tumors involving the pelvis, right paracolic gutter, and right pelvic and para-aortic nodes.
- Procedure: Resection of the recurrent ovarian malignancy, including lymphadenectomy of pelvic and aortic nodal metastases, is performed. A general exploration of the abdomen, pelvis, and viscera found recurrent malignancy. Adhesions of bowel loops from the abdomen and pelvis are lysed. The pelvic side wall mass is approached by opening the retroperitoneum and developing the perirectal and perivesical spaces. The pelvic mass is resected with peritoneal margins. Multiple tumor masses involving the bowel mesentery are excised and fulgurated. Metastatic pelvic lymph nodes over the external iliac vessels and obturator space are resected.

Additional Notes

- If lymphadenectomy is not performed, report 58957 instead
- If reporting excision of initial malignancy, report 58950-58954 instead
- For a postoperative counseling visit about treatment options, use the appropriate E/M with modifier 24

CPT® CODE 58960

Laparotomy, for staging or restaging of ovarian, tubal, or primary peritoneal malignancy (second look), with or without omentectomy, peritoneal washing, biopsy of abdominal and pelvic peritoneum, diaphragmatic assessment with pelvic and limited para-aortic lymphadenectomy

POLICY INDICATORS

Global Period
90 day post-op period

Assistants at Surgery
Assistant allowed

Co-Surgeons Allowed
Submit reason for co-surgeon

Reduction for Multiple Procedures
Subject to 50% reduction

Bilateral Surgery Payment
N/A

Applicable Medicare Policies
Inpatient-only list

Relative Value Units (RVUs)

Work RVUs	15.79
Non-Facility Total	Only valued for facility
Facility Total	30.15

Coding Assistance

58960 includes:

- Positioning and prepping patient
- Examination of site after anesthesia
- Operative services, including inspections around site and closure
- Appropriate post-op E/M visit(s)
- Exploratory laparotomy
- Lymphadenectomy
- Omentectomy
- Exploration of retroperitoneum

Abbreviated Case Note Example:

- Typical patient presentation: Completed 6 cycles of platinum-based chemotherapy following cytoreductive surgery for ovarian cancer.
- Procedure: End-staging laparotomy. Peritoneal washings are taken and subdiaphragmatic scrapings are obtained for cytologic evaluation. Multiple biopsies are taken from the abdominal and pelvic peritoneum. A selected bilateral pelvic and paraaortic lymphadenectomy is performed. An omentectomy is done, if not done at the initial surgery.

Additional Notes

- Use modifier 58 to report as a staged procedure
- For a postoperative counseling visit about treatment options, use the appropriate E/M with modifier 24

CPT® CODE 58970

Follicle puncture for oocyte retrieval, any method

POLICY INDICATORS

Global Period
0 day post-op period

Assistants at Surgery
Submit reason for assistant

Co-Surgeons Allowed
No co-surgeon

Reduction for Multiple Procedures
Subject to 50% reduction

Bilateral Surgery Payment
N/A

Applicable Medicare Policies

Relative Value Units (RVUs)

Work RVUs	3.52
Non-Facility Total	7.22
Facility Total	5.89

Coding Assistance

58970 includes:

- Positioning and prepping patient
- Examination of site after anesthesia
- Operative services, including inspections around site and closure
- Photodocumentation
- Diagnostic laparoscopy

CPT® CODE 58974

Embryo transfer, intrauterine

POLICY INDICATORS

Global Period
0 day post-op period

Assistants at Surgery
Assistant allowed

Co-Surgeons Allowed
Submit reason for co-surgeon

Reduction for Multiple Procedures
Subject to 50% reduction

Bilateral Surgery Payment
N/A

Applicable Medicare Policies

Relative Value Units (RVUs)

Work RVUs	0.00
Non-Facility Total	0.00
Facility Total	0.00

Coding Assistance

58974 includes:

- Positioning and prepping patient
- Examination of site after anesthesia
- Operative services, including inspections around site and closure

CPT® CODE 58976

Gamete, zygote, or embryo intrafallopian transfer, any method

POLICY INDICATORS

Global Period
0 day post-op period

Assistants at Surgery
Assistant allowed

Co-Surgeons Allowed
Submit reason for co-surgeon

Reduction for Multiple Procedures
Subject to 50% reduction

Bilateral Surgery Payment
N/A

Applicable Medicare Policies

Relative Value Units (RVUs)

Work RVUs	3.82
Non-Facility Total	7.73
Facility Total	6.34

Coding Assistance

58976 includes:

- Positioning and prepping patient
- Examination of site after anesthesia
- Operative services, including inspections around site and closure
- Photodocumentation
- Diagnostic laparoscopy or hysteroscopy

CPT® CODE 59000

Amniocentesis; diagnostic

POLICY INDICATORS

Global Period
0 day post-op period

Assistants at Surgery
No assistant

Co-Surgeons Allowed
No co-surgeon

Reduction for Multiple Procedures
Subject to 50% reduction

Bilateral Surgery Payment
N/A

Applicable Medicare Policies

Relative Value Units (RVUs)

Work RVUs	1.30
Non-Facility Total	3.55
Facility Total	2.42

Coding Assistance

59000 includes:

- Positioning and prepping patient
- Examination of site after anesthesia
- Operative services, including inspections around site and closure

CPT® CODE 59001

Amniocentesis; therapeutic amniotic fluid reduction (includes ultrasound guidance)

POLICY INDICATORS

Global Period
0 day post-op period

Assistants at Surgery
No assistant

Co-Surgeons Allowed
No co-surgeon

Reduction for Multiple Procedures
Subject to 50% reduction

Bilateral Surgery Payment
N/A

Applicable Medicare Policies

Relative Value Units (RVUs)

Work RVUs	3.00
Non-Facility Total	Only valued for facility
Facility Total	5.34

Coding Assistance

59001 includes:

- Positioning and prepping patient
- Examination of site after anesthesia
- Operative services, including inspections around site and closure
- Ultrasound guidance

CPT® CODE 59012

Cordocentesis (intrauterine), any method

POLICY INDICATORS

Global Period
0 day post-op period

Assistants at Surgery
Submit reason for assistant

Co-Surgeons Allowed
No co-surgeon

Reduction for Multiple Procedures
Subject to 50% reduction

Bilateral Surgery Payment
N/A

Applicable Medicare Policies

Relative Value Units (RVUs)

Work RVUs	3.44
Non-Facility Total	Only valued for facility
Facility Total	6.03

Coding Assistance

59012 includes:

- Positioning and prepping patient
- Examination of site after anesthesia
- Operative services, including inspections around site and closure

CPT® CODE 59015

Chorionic villus sampling, any method

POLICY INDICATORS

Global Period
0 day post-op period

Assistants at Surgery
Submit reason for assistant

Co-Surgeons Allowed
No co-surgeon

Reduction for Multiple Procedures
Subject to 50% reduction

Bilateral Surgery Payment
N/A

Applicable Medicare Policies

Relative Value Units (RVUs)

Work RVUs	2.20
Non-Facility Total	4.77
Facility Total	3.94

Coding Assistance

59015 includes:

- Positioning and prepping patient
- Examination of site after anesthesia
- Operative services, including inspections around site and closure

CPT® CODE 59020

Fetal contraction stress test

POLICY INDICATORS

Global Period
0 day post-op period

Assistants at Surgery
Submit reason for assistant

Co-Surgeons Allowed
No co-surgeon

Reduction for Multiple Procedures
Not subject to multiple surgery reduction

Bilateral Surgery Payment
N/A

Applicable Medicare Policies

Relative Value Units (RVUs)

Work RVUs	0.66
Non-Facility Total	2.13
Facility Total	Only valued for non-facility

SURGERY

CPT® CODE 59025

Fetal non-stress test

POLICY INDICATORS

Global Period
0 day post-op period

Assistants at Surgery
Submit reason for assistant

Co-Surgeons Allowed
No co-surgeon

Reduction for Multiple Procedures
Not subject to multiple surgery reduction

Bilateral Surgery Payment
N/A

Applicable Medicare Policies

Relative Value Units (RVUs)

Work RVUs	0.53
Non-Facility Total	1.48
Facility Total	Only valued for non-facility

CPT® CODE 59030

Fetal scalp blood sampling

POLICY INDICATORS

Global Period
0 day post-op period

Assistants at Surgery
Submit reason for assistant

Co-Surgeons Allowed
No co-surgeon

Reduction for Multiple Procedures
Subject to 50% reduction

Bilateral Surgery Payment
N/A

Applicable Medicare Policies

Relative Value Units (RVUs)

Work RVUs	1.99
Non-Facility Total	Only valued for facility
Facility Total	3.36

Coding Assistance

59030 includes:

- Positioning and prepping patient
- Examination of site after anesthesia
- Operative services, including inspections around site and closure

Additional Notes

- If additional samplings are performed, use the 76 or 77 modifier

CPT® CODE 59070

Transabdominal amnioinfusion, including ultrasound guidance

POLICY INDICATORS

Global Period
0 day post-op period

Assistants at Surgery
Assistant allowed

Co-Surgeons Allowed
No co-surgeon

Reduction for Multiple Procedures
Subject to 50% reduction

Bilateral Surgery Payment
N/A

Applicable Medicare Policies

Relative Value Units (RVUs)

Work RVUs	5.24
Non-Facility Total	11.96
Facility Total	9.27

Coding Assistance

59070 includes:

- Positioning and prepping patient
- Examination of site after anesthesia
- Operative services, including inspections around site and closure
- Ultrasound guidance

Additional Notes

- For unlisted fetal invasive procedure, report 59897 instead

CPT® CODE 59072

Fetal umbilical cord occlusion, including ultrasound guidance

POLICY INDICATORS

Global Period
0 day post-op period

Assistants at Surgery
No assistant

Co-Surgeons Allowed
No co-surgeon

Reduction for Multiple Procedures
Subject to 50% reduction

Bilateral Surgery Payment
N/A

Applicable Medicare Policies

Relative Value Units (RVUs)

Work RVUs	8.99
Non-Facility Total	Only valued for facility
Facility Total	15.62

Coding Assistance

59072 includes:

- Positioning and prepping patient
- Examination of site after anesthesia
- Operative services, including inspections around site and closure
- Ultrasound guidance

Additional Notes

- For unlisted fetal invasive procedure, report 59897 instead

SURGERY

CPT® CODE 59074

Fetal fluid drainage (eg, vesicocentesis, thoracocentesis, paracentesis), including ultrasound guidance

POLICY INDICATORS

Global Period
0 day post-op period

Assistants at Surgery
Assistant allowed

Co-Surgeons Allowed
No co-surgeon

Reduction for Multiple Procedures
Subject to 50% reduction

Bilateral Surgery Payment
N/A

Applicable Medicare Policies

Relative Value Units (RVUs)

Work RVUs	5.24
Non-Facility Total	11.53
Facility Total	9.27

Coding Assistance

59074 includes:

- Positioning and prepping patient
- Examination of site after anesthesia
- Operative services, including inspections around site and closure
- Ultrasound guidance

Additional Notes

- For unlisted fetal invasive procedure, report 59897 instead

CPT® CODE 59076

Fetal shunt placement, including ultrasound guidance

POLICY INDICATORS

Global Period
0 day post-op period

Assistants at Surgery
Assistant allowed

Co-Surgeons Allowed
No co-surgeon

Reduction for Multiple Procedures
Subject to 50% reduction

Bilateral Surgery Payment
N/A

Applicable Medicare Policies

Relative Value Units (RVUs)

Work RVUs	8.99
Non-Facility Total	Only valued for facility
Facility Total	15.62

Coding Assistance

59076 includes:

- Positioning and prepping patient
- Examination of site after anesthesia
- Operative services, including inspections around site and closure
- Ultrasound guidance

Additional Notes

- For unlisted fetal invasive procedure, report 59897 instead

CPT® CODE 59100

Hysterotomy, abdominal (eg, for hydatidiform mole, abortion)

POLICY INDICATORS

Global Period
90 day post-op period

Assistants at Surgery
Assistant allowed

Co-Surgeons Allowed
Submit reason for co-surgeon

Reduction for Multiple Procedures
Subject to 50% reduction

Bilateral Surgery Payment
N/A

Applicable Medicare Policies

Relative Value Units (RVUs)

Work RVUs	13.37
Non-Facility Total	Only valued for facility
Facility Total	25.88

Coding Assistance

59100 includes:

- Positioning and prepping patient
- Examination of site after anesthesia
- Operative services, including inspections around site and closure
- Appropriate post-op E/M visit(s)
- Exploratory laparotomy

Additional Notes

- If hysterectomy is performed, report 58150 or 58180 instead

CPT® CODE 59120

Surgical treatment of ectopic pregnancy; tubal or ovarian, requiring salpingectomy and/or oophorectomy, abdominal or vaginal approach

POLICY INDICATORS

Global Period
90 day post-op period

Assistants at Surgery
Assistant allowed

Co-Surgeons Allowed
Submit reason for co-surgeon

Reduction for Multiple Procedures
Subject to 50% reduction

Bilateral Surgery Payment
N/A

Applicable Medicare Policies
Inpatient-only list

Relative Value Units (RVUs)

Work RVUs	12.67
Non-Facility Total	Only valued for facility
Facility Total	24.68

Coding Assistance

59120 includes:

- Positioning and prepping patient
- Examination of site after anesthesia
- Operative services, including inspections around site and closure
- Appropriate post-op E/M visit(s)
- Exploratory laparotomy

CPT® CODE 59121

Surgical treatment of ectopic pregnancy; tubal or ovarian, without salpingectomy and/or oophorectomy

POLICY INDICATORS

Global Period
90 day post-op period

Assistants at Surgery
Assistant allowed

Co-Surgeons Allowed
Submit reason for co-surgeon

Reduction for Multiple Procedures
Subject to 50% reduction

Bilateral Surgery Payment
N/A

Applicable Medicare Policies
Inpatient-only list

Relative Value Units (RVUs)

Work RVUs	12.74
Non-Facility Total	Only valued for facility
Facility Total	24.69

Coding Assistance

59121 includes:

- Positioning and prepping patient
- Examination of site after anesthesia
- Operative services, including inspections around site and closure
- Appropriate post-op E/M visit(s)
- Photodocumentation
- Exploratory laparotomy

CPT® CODE 59130

Surgical treatment of ectopic pregnancy; abdominal pregnancy

POLICY INDICATORS

Global Period
90 day post-op period

Assistants at Surgery
Submit reason for assistant

Co-Surgeons Allowed
No co-surgeon

Reduction for Multiple Procedures
Subject to 50% reduction

Bilateral Surgery Payment
N/A

Applicable Medicare Policies
Inpatient-only list

Relative Value Units (RVUs)

Work RVUs	15.08
Non-Facility Total	Only valued for facility
Facility Total	28.64

Coding Assistance

59130 includes:

- Positioning and prepping patient
- Examination of site after anesthesia
- Operative services, including inspections around site and closure
- Appropriate post-op E/M visit(s)
- Photodocumentation
- Exploratory laparotomy

CPT® CODE 59136

Surgical treatment of ectopic pregnancy; interstitial, uterine pregnancy with partial resection of uterus

POLICY INDICATORS

Global Period
90 day post-op period

Assistants at Surgery
Assistant allowed

Co-Surgeons Allowed
No co-surgeon

Reduction for Multiple Procedures
Subject to 50% reduction

Bilateral Surgery Payment
N/A

Applicable Medicare Policies
Inpatient-only list

Relative Value Units (RVUs)

Work RVUs	14.25
Non-Facility Total	Only valued for facility
Facility Total	27.19

Coding Assistance

59136 includes:

- Positioning and prepping patient
- Examination of site after anesthesia
- Operative services, including inspections around site and closure
- Appropriate post-op E/M visit(s)
- Photodocumentation
- Exploratory laparotomy

CPT® CODE 59140

Surgical treatment of ectopic pregnancy; cervical, with evacuation

POLICY INDICATORS

Global Period
90 day post-op period

Assistants at Surgery
Assistant allowed

Co-Surgeons Allowed
No co-surgeon

Reduction for Multiple Procedures
Subject to 50% reduction

Bilateral Surgery Payment
N/A

Applicable Medicare Policies
Inpatient-only list

Relative Value Units (RVUs)

Work RVUs	5.94
Non-Facility Total	Only valued for facility
Facility Total	12.64

Coding Assistance

59140 includes:

- Positioning and prepping patient
- Examination of site after anesthesia
- Operative services, including inspections around site and closure
- Appropriate post-op E/M visit(s)
- Photodocumentation

CPT® CODE 59150

Laparoscopic treatment of ectopic pregnancy; without salpingectomy and/or oophorectomy

POLICY INDICATORS

Global Period
90 day post-op period

Assistants at Surgery
Assistant allowed

Co-Surgeons Allowed
No co-surgeon

Reduction for Multiple Procedures
Subject to 50% reduction

Bilateral Surgery Payment
N/A

Applicable Medicare Policies

Relative Value Units (RVUs)

Work RVUs	12.29
Non-Facility Total	Only valued for facility
Facility Total	23.95

Coding Assistance

59150 includes:

- Positioning and prepping patient
- Examination of site after anesthesia
- Operative services, including inspections around site and closure
- Appropriate post-op E/M visit(s)
- Photodocumentation
- Diagnostic laparotomy

CPT® CODE 59151

Laparoscopic treatment of ectopic pregnancy; with salpingectomy and/or oophorectomy

POLICY INDICATORS

Global Period
90 day post-op period

Assistants at Surgery
Assistant allowed

Co-Surgeons Allowed
No co-surgeon

Reduction for Multiple Procedures
Subject to 50% reduction

Bilateral Surgery Payment
N/A

Applicable Medicare Policies

Relative Value Units (RVUs)

Work RVUs	12.11
Non-Facility Total	Only valued for facility
Facility Total	23.41

Coding Assistance

59151 includes:

- Positioning and prepping patient
- Examination of site after anesthesia
- Operative services, including inspections around site and closure
- Appropriate post-op E/M visit(s)
- Photodocumentation
- Diagnostic laparotomy

CPT® CODE 59160

Curettage, postpartum

POLICY INDICATORS

Global Period
10 day post-op period

Assistants at Surgery
No assistant

Co-Surgeons Allowed
No co-surgeon

Reduction for Multiple Procedures
Subject to 50% reduction

Bilateral Surgery Payment
N/A

Applicable Medicare Policies

Relative Value Units (RVUs)

Work RVUs	2.76
Non-Facility Total	8.11
Facility Total	5.67

Coding Assistance

59160 includes:

- Positioning and prepping patient
- Examination of site after anesthesia
- Operative services, including inspections around site and closure
- Appropriate post-op E/M visit(s)
- Administration of intravenous oxytocin
- Cervical dilation

SURGERY

CPT® CODE 59200

Insertion of cervical dilator (eg, laminaria, prostaglandin) (separate procedure)

POLICY INDICATORS

Global Period
0 day post-op period

Assistants at Surgery
No assistant

Co-Surgeons Allowed
No co-surgeon

Reduction for Multiple Procedures
Subject to 50% reduction

Bilateral Surgery Payment
N/A

Applicable Medicare Policies

Relative Value Units (RVUs)

Work RVUs	1.20
Non-Facility Total	3.98
Facility Total	2.02

Coding Assistance

59200 includes:

- Positioning and prepping patient
- Examination of site after anesthesia
- Operative services, including inspections around site and closure

Additional Notes

- Code 59200 is bundled with all of the delivery codes per CCI edits; it cannot be unbundled, even with a modifier.
- If this service is performed one day or more before delivery, it can be reported separately.
- If cervical dilation is personally performed (or directly supervised) by the billing physician on a calendar date other than the date of delivery, it should be billed with code 59200 and no modifier.

CPT® CODE 59300

Episiotomy or vaginal repair, by other than attending

POLICY INDICATORS

Global Period
0 day post-op period

Assistants at Surgery
Submit reason for assistant

Co-Surgeons Allowed
No co-surgeon

Reduction for Multiple Procedures
Subject to 50% reduction

Bilateral Surgery Payment
N/A

Applicable Medicare Policies

Relative Value Units (RVUs)

Work RVUs	2.41
Non-Facility Total	6.83
Facility Total	4.44

Coding Assistance

59300 includes:

- Positioning and prepping patient
- Examination of site after anesthesia
- Uncomplicated bladder catheterization or catheter insertion
- Injection of anesthetic nerve block (eg, paracervical, pudendal nerve block)
- Operative services, including inspections around site, suturing of incision or vaginal lacerations, hemostasis and closure

Additional Notes

- This code may not be reported by the attending physician

CPT® CODE 59320

Cerclage of cervix, during pregnancy; vaginal

POLICY INDICATORS

Global Period
0 day post-op period

Assistants at Surgery
Submit reason for assistant

Co-Surgeons Allowed
No co-surgeon

Reduction for Multiple Procedures
Subject to 50% reduction

Bilateral Surgery Payment
N/A

Applicable Medicare Policies

Relative Value Units (RVUs)

Work RVUs	2.48
Non-Facility Total	Only valued for facility
Facility Total	4.58

Coding Assistance

59320 includes:

- Positioning and prepping patient
- Examination of site after anesthesia
- Uncomplicated bladder catheterization or catheter insertion
- Injection of anesthetic nerve block (eg, paracervical, pudendal nerve block)
- Operative services, including inspections around site; application of traction device; circumferential placement of one or more sutures around the uterine cervix, anchored into the cervical stroma, and tied; hemostasis and closure

Additional Notes

- This code is used for all vaginal cerclages including suture(s) placed through the cervical epithelium (eg, McDonald) and those buried beneath the cervical epithelium (eg, Shirodkar)

SURGERY

CPT® CODE 59325

Cerclage of cervix, during pregnancy; abdominal

POLICY INDICATORS

Global Period
0 day post-op period

Assistants at Surgery
Submit reason for assistant

Co-Surgeons Allowed
No co-surgeon

Reduction for Multiple Procedures
Subject to 50% reduction

Bilateral Surgery Payment
N/A

Applicable Medicare Policies
Inpatient-only list

Relative Value Units (RVUs)

Work RVUs	4.06
Non-Facility Total	Only valued for facility
Facility Total	7.24

Coding Assistance

59325 includes:

- Positioning and prepping patient
- Examination of site after anesthesia
- Uncomplicated bladder catheterization or catheter insertion
- Injection of anesthetic nerve block (eg, paracervical, pudendal nerve block)
- Operative services, including exploratory laparotomy, inspections around site, placement of cerclage around internal cervical os, hemostasis, and closure

CPT® CODE 59350

Hysterorrhaphy of ruptured uterus

POLICY INDICATORS

Global Period
0 day post-op period

Assistants at Surgery
Assistant allowed

Co-Surgeons Allowed
No co-surgeon

Reduction for Multiple Procedures
Subject to 50% reduction

Bilateral Surgery Payment
N/A

Applicable Medicare Policies
Inpatient-only list

Relative Value Units (RVUs)

Work RVUs	4.94
Non-Facility Total	Only valued for facility
Facility Total	8.34

Coding Assistance

59350 includes:

- Positioning and prepping patient
- Examination of site after anesthesia
- Uncomplicated bladder catheterization or catheter insertion
- Injection of anesthetic nerve block (eg, paracervical, pudendal nerve block)
- Operative services, including exploratory laparotomy, inspections around site, injection of vasopressors, repair of uterine defect, hemostasis and closure

CPT® CODE 59812

Treatment of incomplete abortion, any trimester, completed surgically

POLICY INDICATORS

Global Period
90 day post-op period

Assistants at Surgery
No assistant

Co-Surgeons Allowed
No co-surgeon

Reduction for Multiple Procedures
Subject to 50% reduction

Bilateral Surgery Payment
N/A

Applicable Medicare Policies

Relative Value Units (RVUs)

Work RVUs	4.44
Non-Facility Total	10.92
Facility Total	9.33

Coding Assistance

59812 includes:

- Positioning and prepping patient
- Examination of site after anesthesia
- Uncomplicated bladder catheterization or catheter insertion
- Injection of anesthetic nerve block (eg, paracervical, pudendal nerve block)
- Operative services, including inspections around site, injection of vasopressors, dilation and curettage, repair of any cervical laceration, and hemostasis
- Appropriate post-op E/M visit(s)

Additional Notes

- For the medical treatment of a spontaneous or missed abortion, report the appropriate E/M code

CPT® CODE 59820

Treatment of missed abortion, completed surgically; first trimester

POLICY INDICATORS

Global Period
90 day post-op period

Assistants at Surgery
No assistant

Co-Surgeons Allowed
No co-surgeon

Reduction for Multiple Procedures
Subject to 50% reduction

Bilateral Surgery Payment
N/A

Applicable Medicare Policies

Relative Value Units (RVUs)

Work RVUs	4.84
Non-Facility Total	13.25
Facility Total	11.73

Coding Assistance

59820 includes:

- Positioning and prepping patient
- Examination of site after anesthesia
- Uncomplicated bladder catheterization or catheter insertion
- Injection of anesthetic nerve block (eg, paracervical, pudendal nerve block)
- Operative services, including inspections around site, injection of vasopressors, dilation and curettage, repair of any cervical laceration, and hemostasis
- Appropriate post-op E/M visit(s)

Additional Notes

- For the medical treatment of a spontaneous or missed abortion, report the appropriate E/M code

CPT® CODE 59821

Treatment of missed abortion, completed surgically; second trimester

POLICY INDICATORS

Global Period
90 day post-op period

Assistants at Surgery
Submit reason for assistant

Co-Surgeons Allowed
No co-surgeon

Reduction for Multiple Procedures
Subject to 50% reduction

Bilateral Surgery Payment
N/A

Applicable Medicare Policies

Relative Value Units (RVUs)

Work RVUs	5.09
Non-Facility Total	13.05
Facility Total	11.46

Coding Assistance

59821 includes:

- Positioning and prepping patient
- Examination of site after anesthesia
- Uncomplicated bladder catheterization or catheter insertion
- Injection of anesthetic nerve block (eg, paracervical, pudendal nerve block)
- Operative services, including inspections around site, injection of vasopressors, dilation and curettage or evacuation, repair of any cervical laceration, and hemostasis
- Appropriate post-op E/M visit(s)

Additional Notes

- For the medical treatment of a spontaneous or missed abortion, report the appropriate E/M code

CPT® CODE 59830

Treatment of septic abortion, completed surgically

POLICY INDICATORS

Global Period
90 day post-op period

Assistants at Surgery
Submit reason for assistant

Co-Surgeons Allowed
No co-surgeon

Reduction for Multiple Procedures
Subject to 50% reduction

Bilateral Surgery Payment
N/A

Applicable Medicare Policies
Inpatient-only list

Relative Value Units (RVUs)

Work RVUs	6.59
Non-Facility Total	Only valued for facility
Facility Total	14.03

Coding Assistance

59830 includes:

- Positioning and prepping patient
- Examination of site after anesthesia
- Uncomplicated bladder catheterization or catheter insertion
- Injection of anesthetic nerve block (eg, paracervical, pudendal nerve block)
- Operative services, including inspections around site, injection of vasopressors, dilation and curettage or evacuation, repair of any cervical laceration, and hemostasis
- Appropriate post-op E/M visit(s)

Additional Notes

- For the medical treatment of a spontaneous or missed abortion, report the appropriate E/M code

CPT® CODE 59840

Induced abortion, by dilation and curettage

POLICY INDICATORS

Global Period
10 day post-op period

Assistants at Surgery
Submit reason for assistant

Co-Surgeons Allowed
No co-surgeon

Reduction for Multiple Procedures
Subject to 50% reduction

Bilateral Surgery Payment
N/A

Applicable Medicare Policies

Relative Value Units (RVUs)

Work RVUs	3.01
Non-Facility Total	7.51
Facility Total	6.70

Coding Assistance

59840 includes:

- Positioning and prepping patient
- Examination of site after anesthesia
- Uncomplicated bladder catheterization or catheter insertion
- Injection of anesthetic nerve block (eg, paracervical, pudendal nerve block)
- Operative services, including inspections around site, injection of vasopressors, dilation and curettage, repair of any cervical laceration, and hemostasis
- Appropriate post-op E/M visit(s)

Additional Notes

- For the outpatient medical treatment of an induced abortion (medication abortion), report the appropriate E/M code
- For the inpatient medical treatment of an induced abortion with hospital admission, requiring dilation and curettage, report 59851 or 59856 as appropriate

CPT® CODE 59841

Induced abortion, by dilation and evacuation

POLICY INDICATORS

Global Period
10 day post-op period

Assistants at Surgery
Submit reason for assistant

Co-Surgeons Allowed
No co-surgeon

Reduction for Multiple Procedures
Subject to 50% reduction

Bilateral Surgery Payment
N/A

Applicable Medicare Policies

Relative Value Units (RVUs)

Work RVUs	5.65
Non-Facility Total	12.87
Facility Total	11.30

Coding Assistance

59841 includes:

- Positioning and prepping patient
- Examination of site after anesthesia
- Uncomplicated bladder catheterization or catheter insertion
- Injection of anesthetic nerve block (eg, paracervical, pudendal nerve block)
- Operative services, including inspections around site, injection of vasopressors, dilation and evacuation, repair of any cervical laceration, and hemostasis
- Appropriate post-op E/M visit(s)

Additional Notes

- For the outpatient medical treatment of an induced abortion (medication abortion), report the appropriate E/M code
- For the inpatient medical treatment of an induced abortion with hospital admission, requiring dilation and evacuation, report 59851 or 59856 as appropriate

CPT® CODE 59850

Induced abortion, by 1 or more intra-amniotic injections (amniocentesis-injections), including hospital admission and visits, delivery of fetus and secundines

POLICY INDICATORS

Global Period
90 day post-op period

Assistants at Surgery
Submit reason for assistant

Co-Surgeons Allowed
No co-surgeon

Reduction for Multiple Procedures
Subject to 50% reduction

Bilateral Surgery Payment
N/A

Applicable Medicare Policies
Inpatient-only list

Relative Value Units (RVUs)

Work RVUs	5.90
Non-Facility Total	Only valued for facility
Facility Total	11.90

Coding Assistance

59850 includes:

- Positioning and prepping patient
- Examination of site after anesthesia
- Hospital admission and visits
- Uncomplicated bladder catheterization or catheter insertion
- Injection of anesthetic nerve block (eg, paracervical, pudendal nerve block)
- Operative services, including inspections around site, intra-amniotic injections, examination for cervical dilation, delivery of fetus and secundines, and hemostasis
- Appropriate post-op E/M visit(s)

Additional Notes

- For the outpatient medical treatment of an induced abortion (medication abortion), report the appropriate E/M code
- If D&C or D&E is required, report 59851 instead
- If hysterotomy is required, report 59852 instead
- If placement of vaginal prostaglandins or cervical osmotic dilators is performed, report 59855 instead

SURGERY

CPT® CODE 59851

Induced abortion, by 1 or more intra-amniotic injections (amniocentesis-injections), including hospital admission and visits, delivery of fetus and secundines; with dilation and curettage and/or evacuation

POLICY INDICATORS

Global Period
90 day post-op period

Assistants at Surgery
Submit reason for assistant

Co-Surgeons Allowed
No co-surgeon

Reduction for Multiple Procedures
Subject to 50% reduction

Bilateral Surgery Payment
N/A

Applicable Medicare Policies
Inpatient-only list

Relative Value Units (RVUs)

Work RVUs	5.92
Non-Facility Total	Only valued for facility
Facility Total	12.99

Coding Assistance

59851 includes:

- Positioning and prepping patient
- Examination of site after anesthesia
- Hospital admission and visits
- Uncomplicated bladder catheterization or catheter insertion
- Injection of anesthetic nerve block (eg, paracervical, pudendal nerve block)
- Operative services, including inspections around site, intra-amniotic injections, examination for cervical dilation, delivery of fetus and secundines, and hemostasis
- Appropriate post-op E/M visit(s)

Additional Notes

- For the outpatient medical treatment of an induced abortion (medication abortion), report the appropriate E/M code
- If placement of vaginal prostaglandins or cervical osmotic dilators is performed, report 59856 instead

CPT® CODE 59852

Induced abortion, by 1 or more intra-amniotic injections (amniocentesis-injections), including hospital admission and visits, delivery of fetus and secundines; with hysterotomy (failed intra-amniotic injection)

POLICY INDICATORS

Global Period
90 day post-op period

Assistants at Surgery
Submit reason for assistant

Co-Surgeons Allowed
No co-surgeon

Reduction for Multiple Procedures
Subject to 50% reduction

Bilateral Surgery Payment
N/A

Applicable Medicare Policies
Inpatient-only list

Relative Value Units (RVUs)

Work RVUs	8.23
Non-Facility Total	Only valued for facility
Facility Total	17.80

Coding Assistance

59852 includes:

- Positioning and prepping patient
- Examination of site after anesthesia
- Hospital admission and visits
- Uncomplicated bladder catheterization or catheter insertion
- Injection of anesthetic nerve block (eg, paracervical, pudendal nerve block)
- Operative services, including inspections around site, intra-amniotic injections, examination for cervical dilation, exploratory laparotomy, delivery of fetus and secundines via hysterotomy, hemostasis and closure
- Appropriate post-op E/M visit(s)

Additional Notes

- For the outpatient medical treatment of an induced abortion (medication abortion), report the appropriate E/M code
- If placement of vaginal prostaglandins or cervical osmotic dilators is performed, report 59857 instead

CPT® CODE 59855

Induced abortion, by 1 or more vaginal suppositories (eg, prostaglandin) with or without cervical dilation (eg, laminaria), including hospital admission and visits, delivery of fetus and secundines

POLICY INDICATORS

Global Period
90 day post-op period

Assistants at Surgery
Submit reason for assistant

Co-Surgeons Allowed
No co-surgeon

Reduction for Multiple Procedures
Subject to 50% reduction

Bilateral Surgery Payment
N/A

Applicable Medicare Policies
Inpatient-only list

Relative Value Units (RVUs)

Work RVUs	6.43
Non-Facility Total	Only valued for facility
Facility Total	12.87

Coding Assistance

59855 includes:

- Positioning and prepping patient
- Examination of site after anesthesia
- Hospital admission and visits
- Uncomplicated bladder catheterization or catheter insertion
- Injection of anesthetic nerve block (eg, paracervical, pudendal nerve block)
- Operative services, including inspections around site, placement of vaginal suppositories and/or cervical osmotic dilators, examination for cervical dilation, delivery of fetus and secundines, and hemostasis
- Appropriate post-op E/M visit(s)

Additional Notes

- For the outpatient medical treatment of an induced abortion (medication abortion), report the appropriate E/M code
- If D&C or D&E is required, report 59856 instead
- If hysterotomy is required, report 59857 instead

CPT® CODE 59856

Induced abortion, by 1 or more vaginal suppositories (eg, prostaglandin) with or without cervical dilation (eg, laminaria), including hospital admission and visits, delivery of fetus and secundines; with dilation and curettage and/or evacuation

POLICY INDICATORS

Global Period
90 day post-op period

Assistants at Surgery
Submit reason for assistant

Co-Surgeons Allowed
No co-surgeon

Reduction for Multiple Procedures
Subject to 50% reduction

Bilateral Surgery Payment
N/A

Applicable Medicare Policies
Inpatient-only list

Relative Value Units (RVUs)

Work RVUs	7.79
Non-Facility Total	Only valued for facility
Facility Total	15.07

Coding Assistance

59856 includes:

- Positioning and prepping patient
- Examination of site after anesthesia
- Hospital admission and visits
- Uncomplicated bladder catheterization or catheter insertion
- Injection of anesthetic nerve block (eg, paracervical, pudendal nerve block)
- Operative services, including inspections around site, placement of vaginal suppositories and/or cervical osmotic dilators, examination for cervical dilation, delivery of fetus and secundines, dilation and curettage and/or evacuation, and hemostasis
- Appropriate post-op E/M visit(s)

Additional Notes

- For the outpatient medical treatment of an induced abortion (medication abortion), report the appropriate E/M code

CPT® CODE 59857

Induced abortion, by 1 or more vaginal suppositories (eg, prostaglandin) with or without cervical dilation (eg, laminaria), including hospital admission and visits, delivery of fetus and secundines; with hysterotomy (failed medical evacuation)

POLICY INDICATORS

Global Period
90 day post-op period

Assistants at Surgery
Submit reason for assistant

Co-Surgeons Allowed
No co-surgeon

Reduction for Multiple Procedures
Subject to 50% reduction

Bilateral Surgery Payment
N/A

Applicable Medicare Policies
Inpatient-only list

Relative Value Units (RVUs)

Work RVUs	9.33
Non-Facility Total	Only valued for facility
Facility Total	17.55

Coding Assistance

59857 includes:

- Positioning and prepping patient
- Examination of site after anesthesia
- Hospital admission and visits
- Uncomplicated bladder catheterization or catheter insertion
- Injection of anesthetic nerve block (eg, paracervical, pudendal nerve block)
- Operative services, including inspections around site, placement of vaginal suppositories and/or cervical osmotic dilators, examination for cervical dilation, exploratory laparotomy, delivery of fetus and secundines via hysterotomy, hemostasis and closure
- Appropriate post-op E/M visit(s)

Additional Notes

- For the outpatient medical treatment of an induced abortion (medication abortion), report the appropriate E/M code

CPT® CODE 59866

Multifetal pregnancy reduction(s) (MPR)

POLICY INDICATORS

Global Period
0 day post-op period

Assistants at Surgery
Assistant allowed

Co-Surgeons Allowed
Submit reason for co-surgeon

Reduction for Multiple Procedures
Subject to 50% reduction

Bilateral Surgery Payment
N/A

Applicable Medicare Policies

Relative Value Units (RVUs)

Work RVUs	3.99
Non-Facility Total	Only valued for facility
Facility Total	7.17

Coding Assistance

59866 includes:

- Positioning and prepping patient
- Examination of site after anesthesia
- Uncomplicated bladder catheterization or catheter insertion
- Injection of anesthetic nerve block (eg, paracervical, pudendal nerve block)
- Operative services, including inspections around site, intra-amniotic and/or intrafetal injections, repetition as needed for number of fetuses to be reduced, and hemostasis

Additional Notes

- For the inpatient medical treatment of an induced abortion with hospital admission, by 1 or more intra-amniotic injections, report 59850, 59851, or 59852 as appropriate

CPT® CODE 59870

Uterine evacuation and curettage for hydatidiform mole

POLICY INDICATORS

Global Period
90 day post-op period

Assistants at Surgery
Assistant allowed

Co-Surgeons Allowed
No co-surgeon

Reduction for Multiple Procedures
Subject to 50% reduction

Bilateral Surgery Payment
N/A

Applicable Medicare Policies

Relative Value Units (RVUs)

Work RVUs	6.57
Non-Facility Total	Only valued for facility
Facility Total	16.19

Coding Assistance

59870 includes:

- Positioning and prepping patient
- Examination of site after anesthesia
- Uncomplicated bladder catheterization or catheter insertion
- Injection of anesthetic nerve block (eg, paracervical, pudendal nerve block)
- Operative services, including inspections around site, injection of vasopressors or other medications, dilation and curettage or evacuation, and hemostasis
- Appropriate post-op E/M visit(s)

CPT® CODE 59871

Removal of cerclage suture under anesthesia (other than local)

POLICY INDICATORS

Global Period
0 day post-op period

Assistants at Surgery
Submit reason for assistant

Co-Surgeons Allowed
No co-surgeon

Reduction for Multiple Procedures
Subject to 50% reduction

Bilateral Surgery Payment
N/A

Applicable Medicare Policies

Relative Value Units (RVUs)

Work RVUs	2.13
Non-Facility Total	Only valued for facility
Facility Total	4.01

Coding Assistance

59871 includes:

- Positioning and prepping patient
- Examination of site after anesthesia
- Uncomplicated bladder catheterization or catheter insertion
- Injection of anesthetic nerve block (eg, paracervical, pudendal nerve block)
- Operative services, including inspections around site, application of traction device, cutting and removal of cerclage suture, hemostasis and closure

Additional Notes

- If cerclage removal is performed with local anesthesia, report an appropriate E/M code instead

CPT® CODE 64425

Injection(s), anesthetic agent(s) and/or steroid; ilioinguinal, iliohypogastric nerves

POLICY INDICATORS

Global Period
0 day post-op period

Assistants at Surgery
No assistant

Co-Surgeons Allowed
No co-surgeon

Reduction for Multiple Procedures
Subject to 50% reduction

Bilateral Surgery Payment
150% paid if bilateral

Applicable Medicare Policies

Relative Value Units (RVUs)

Work RVUs	1.00
Non-Facility Total	3.28
Facility Total	1.63

Coding Assistance

64425 includes:

- Positioning and prepping patient
- Examination of site after anesthesia
- Operative services, including inspections around site, injection(s) of anesthetic agent(s) and/or steroid, and hemostasis

Additional Notes

- Report once per nerve plexus, nerve, or branch as described by the code regardless of the number of injections performed along the nerve plexus, nerve, or branch

CPT® CODE 64430

Injection(s), anesthetic agent(s) and/or steroid; pudendal nerve

POLICY INDICATORS

Global Period
0 day post-op period

Assistants at Surgery
No assistant

Co-Surgeons Allowed
No co-surgeon

Reduction for Multiple Procedures
Subject to 50% reduction

Bilateral Surgery Payment
150% paid if bilateral

Applicable Medicare Policies

Relative Value Units (RVUs)

Work RVUs	1.00
Non-Facility Total	2.93
Facility Total	1.65

Coding Assistance

64430 includes:

- Positioning and prepping patient
- Examination of site after anesthesia
- Operative services, including inspections around site, injection(s) of anesthetic agent(s) and/or steroid, and hemostasis

Additional Notes

- Report once per nerve plexus, nerve, or branch as described by the code regardless of the number of injections performed along the nerve plexus, nerve, or branch

CPT® CODE 64435

Injection(s), anesthetic agent(s) and/or steroid; paracervical (uterine) nerve

POLICY INDICATORS

Global Period
0 day post-op period

Assistants at Surgery
No assistant

Co-Surgeons Allowed
No co-surgeon

Reduction for Multiple Procedures
Subject to 50% reduction

Bilateral Surgery Payment
150% paid if bilateral

Applicable Medicare Policies

Relative Value Units (RVUs)

Work RVUs	0.75
Non-Facility Total	2.38
Facility Total	1.31

Coding Assistance

64435 includes:

- Positioning and prepping patient
- Examination of site after anesthesia
- Operative services, including inspections around site, injection(s) of anesthetic agent(s) and/or steroid, and hemostasis

Additional Notes

- Report once per nerve plexus, nerve, or branch as described by the code regardless of the number of injections performed along the nerve plexus, nerve, or branch

CPT® CODE 64450

Injection(s), anesthetic agent(s) and/or steroid; other peripheral nerve or branch

POLICY INDICATORS

Global Period
0 day post-op period

Assistants at Surgery
No assistant

Co-Surgeons Allowed
No co-surgeon

Reduction for Multiple Procedures
Subject to 50% reduction

Bilateral Surgery Payment
150% paid if bilateral

Applicable Medicare Policies

Relative Value Units (RVUs)

Work RVUs	0.75
Non-Facility Total	2.22
Facility Total	1.24

Coding Assistance

64450 includes:

- Positioning and prepping patient
- Examination of site after anesthesia
- Operative services, including inspections around site, injection(s) of anesthetic agent(s) and/or steroid, and hemostasis

Additional Notes

- Report once per nerve plexus, nerve, or branch as described by the code regardless of the number of injections performed along the nerve plexus, nerve, or branch

CPT® CODE 64561

Percutaneous implantation of neurostimulator electrode array; sacral nerve (transforaminal placement) including image guidance, if performed

POLICY INDICATORS

Global Period
10 day post-op period

Assistants at Surgery
No assistant

Co-Surgeons Allowed
No co-surgeon

Reduction for Multiple Procedures
Subject to 50% reduction

Bilateral Surgery Payment
150% paid if bilateral

Applicable Medicare Policies

Relative Value Units (RVUs)

Work RVUs	5.44
Non-Facility Total	21.41
Facility Total	9.09

Coding Assistance

64561 includes:

- Positioning and prepping patient
- Examination of site after anesthesia
- Operative services, including inspections around site, placement of foramen needle, imaging guidance if used, placement of electrode, test stimulation, hemostasis and closure
- Electronic analysis and programming of implanted neurostimulator at the time of implantation
- Appropriate post-op E/M visit(s)

Additional Notes

- Used for both temporary and permanent placement of percutaneous electrode arrays
- For percutaneous electrical neuromuscular stimulation or neuromodulation using needle(s) or needle electrode(s) (eg, PENS, PNT), use 64999

SURGERY

CPT® CODE 64566

Posterior tibial neurostimulation, percutaneous needle electrode, single treatment, includes programming

POLICY INDICATORS

Global Period
0 day post-op period

Assistants at Surgery
Submit reason for assistant

Co-Surgeons Allowed
No co-surgeon

Reduction for Multiple Procedures
Subject to 50% reduction

Bilateral Surgery Payment
N/A

Applicable Medicare Policies

Relative Value Units (RVUs)

Work RVUs	0.60
Non-Facility Total	3.39
Facility Total	0.89

Coding Assistance

64566 includes:

- Positioning and prepping patient
- Examination of site after anesthesia
- Operative services, including inspections around site, placement of PTNS needle, activation of stimulator, hemostasis and closure
- Electronic analysis and programming of implanted neurostimulator at the time of implantation

Additional Notes

- Do not report in conjunction with 64555, 95970-95972

CPT® CODE 64575

Open implantation of neurostimulator electrode array; peripheral nerve (excludes sacral nerve)

POLICY INDICATORS

Global Period
90 day post-op period

Assistants at Surgery
No assistant

Co-Surgeons Allowed
No co-surgeon

Reduction for Multiple Procedures
Subject to 50% reduction

Bilateral Surgery Payment
N/A

Applicable Medicare Policies

Relative Value Units (RVUs)

Work RVUs	4.42
Non-Facility Total	Only valued for facility
Facility Total	9.53

Coding Assistance

64575 includes:

- Positioning and prepping patient
- Examination of site after anesthesia
- Injection of local anesthesia
- Operative services, including inspections around site, hemostasis and closure
- Appropriate post-op E/M visit(s)

CPT® CODE 64580

Open implantation of neurostimulator electrode array; neuromuscular

POLICY INDICATORS

Global Period
90 day post-op period

Assistants at Surgery
Assistant allowed

Co-Surgeons Allowed
No co-surgeon

Reduction for Multiple Procedures
Subject to 50% reduction

Bilateral Surgery Payment
N/A

Applicable Medicare Policies

Relative Value Units (RVUs)

Work RVUs	4.19
Non-Facility Total	Only valued for facility
Facility Total	9.60

Coding Assistance

64580 includes:

- Positioning and prepping patient
- Examination of site after anesthesia
- Injection of local anesthesia
- Operative services, including inspections around site, hemostasis and closure
- Appropriate post-op E/M visit(s)

CPT® CODE 64581

Open implantation of neurostimulator electrode array; sacral nerve (transforaminal placement)

POLICY INDICATORS

Global Period
90 day post-op period

Assistants at Surgery
No assistant

Co-Surgeons Allowed
No co-surgeon

Reduction for Multiple Procedures
Subject to 50% reduction

Bilateral Surgery Payment
N/A

Applicable Medicare Policies

Relative Value Units (RVUs)

Work RVUs	12.20
Non-Facility Total	Only valued for facility
Facility Total	19.72

Coding Assistance

64581 includes:

- Positioning and prepping patient
- Examination of site after anesthesia
- Injection of local anesthesia
- Operative services, including inspections around site, placement of foramen needle, imaging guidance if used, placement of electrode, tunneling the lead subcutaneously, test stimulation, hemostasis and closure
- Electronic analysis and programming of implanted neurostimulator at the time of implantation
- Appropriate post-op E/M visit(s)

CPT® CODE 64585

Revision or removal of peripheral neurostimulator electrode array

POLICY INDICATORS

Global Period
10 day post-op period

Assistants at Surgery
No assistant

Co-Surgeons Allowed
No co-surgeon

Reduction for Multiple Procedures
Subject to 50% reduction

Bilateral Surgery Payment
N/A

Applicable Medicare Policies

Relative Value Units (RVUs)

Work RVUs	2.11
Non-Facility Total	7.18
Facility Total	4.35

Coding Assistance

64585 includes:

- Positioning and prepping patient
- Examination of site after anesthesia
- Injection of local anesthesia
- Operative services, including inspections around site, revision or removal of electrode lead, hemostasis and closure
- Appropriate post-op E/M visit(s)

CPT® CODE 64590

Insertion or replacement of peripheral, sacral, or gastric neurostimulator pulse generator or receiver, requiring pocket creation and connection between electrode array and pulse generator or receiver

POLICY INDICATORS

Global Period
10 day post-op period

Assistants at Surgery
Submit reason for assistant

Co-Surgeons Allowed
Submit reason for co-surgeon

Reduction for Multiple Procedures
Subject to 50% reduction

Bilateral Surgery Payment
N/A

Applicable Medicare Policies

Relative Value Units (RVUs)

Work RVUs	5.10
Non-Facility Total	12.43
Facility Total	8.87

Coding Assistance

64590 includes:

- Positioning and prepping patient
- Examination of site after anesthesia
- Injection of local anesthesia
- Operative services, including inspections around site, incising and dissection to create or access a pocket site, insertion of pulse generator into the pocket, connecting the previously tunneled electrode lead, pulse generator testing, hemostasis and closure
- Appropriate post-op E/M visit(s)

CPT® CODE 64595

Revision or removal of peripheral, sacral, or gastric neurostimulator pulse generator or receiver, with detachable connection to electrode array

POLICY INDICATORS

Global Period
10 day post-op period

Assistants at Surgery
Submit reason for assistant

Co-Surgeons Allowed
No co-surgeon

Reduction for Multiple Procedures
Subject to 50% reduction

Bilateral Surgery Payment
N/A

Applicable Medicare Policies

Relative Value Units (RVUs)

Work RVUs	3.79
Non-Facility Total	10.11
Facility Total	6.94

Coding Assistance

64595 includes:

- Positioning and prepping patient
- Examination of site after anesthesia
- Injection of local anesthesia
- Operative services, including inspections around site, incising and dissection to access the pulse generator, removal of the pulse generator, hemostasis and closure
- Appropriate post-op E/M visit(s)

CPT® CODE 64630

Destruction by neurolytic agent; pudendal nerve

POLICY INDICATORS

Global Period
10 day post-op period

Assistants at Surgery
Submit reason for assistant

Co-Surgeons Allowed
No co-surgeon

Reduction for Multiple Procedures
Subject to 50% reduction

Bilateral Surgery Payment
N/A

Applicable Medicare Policies

Relative Value Units (RVUs)

Work RVUs	3.05
Non-Facility Total	7.75
Facility Total	5.82

Coding Assistance

64630 includes:

- Positioning and prepping patient
- Examination of site after anesthesia
- Injection of local anesthesia
- Operative services, including inspections around site, injection(s) of neurolytic agent(s), and hemostasis
- Appropriate post-op E/M visit(s)

Additional Notes

- Includes the injection of other therapeutic agents (eg, corticosteroids). Do not report diagnostic or therapeutic injections separately
- For therapies that are not destructive of the target nerve (eg, pulsed radiofrequency), use 64999

CPT® CODE 64640

Destruction by neurolytic agent; other peripheral nerve or branch

POLICY INDICATORS

Global Period
10 day post-op period

Assistants at Surgery
No assistant

Co-Surgeons Allowed
No co-surgeon

Reduction for Multiple Procedures
Subject to 50% reduction

Bilateral Surgery Payment
150% paid if bilateral

Applicable Medicare Policies

Relative Value Units (RVUs)

Work RVUs	1.98
Non-Facility Total	7.45
Facility Total	3.62

Coding Assistance

64640 includes:

- Positioning and prepping patient
- Examination of site after anesthesia
- Injection of local anesthesia
- Operative services, including inspections around site, injection(s) of neurolytic agent(s), and hemostasis
- Appropriate post-op E/M visit(s)

Additional Notes

- Includes the injection of other therapeutic agents (eg, corticosteroids). Do not report diagnostic or therapeutic injections separately.
- For therapies that are not destructive of the target nerve (eg, pulsed radiofrequency), use 64999

CPT® CODE 64642

Chemodenervation of one extremity; 1-4 muscle(s)

POLICY INDICATORS

Global Period
0 day post-op period

Assistants at Surgery
No assistant

Co-Surgeons Allowed
No co-surgeon

Reduction for Multiple Procedures
Subject to 50% reduction

Bilateral Surgery Payment
N/A

Applicable Medicare Policies

Relative Value Units (RVUs)

Work RVUs	1.65
Non-Facility Total	4.63
Facility Total	3.23

Coding Assistance

64642 includes:

- Positioning and prepping patient
- Examination of site after anesthesia
- Injection of local anesthesia
- Operative services, including inspections around site, injection(s) of neurolytic agent(s), and hemostasis

Additional Notes

- Includes the injection of other therapeutic agents (eg, corticosteroids). Do not report diagnostic or therapeutic injections separately.
- For therapies that are not destructive of the target nerve (eg, pulsed radiofrequency), use 64999.
- Report separately the supply of the chemodenervation agent (eg, botulinum toxin).
- Report 64642 once per extremity.
- Do not report modifier -50 in conjunction with 64642

CPT® CODE 64646

Chemodenervation of trunk muscle(s); 1-5 muscle(s)

POLICY INDICATORS

Global Period
0 day post-op period

Assistants at Surgery
No assistant

Co-Surgeons Allowed
No co-surgeon

Reduction for Multiple Procedures
Subject to 50% reduction

Bilateral Surgery Payment
N/A

Applicable Medicare Policies

Relative Value Units (RVUs)

Work RVUs	1.80
Non-Facility Total	4.87
Facility Total	3.52

Coding Assistance

64646 includes:

- Positioning and prepping patient
- Examination of site after anesthesia
- Injection of local anesthesia
- Operative services, including inspections around site, injection(s) of neurolytic agent(s), and hemostasis

Additional Notes

- Includes the injection of other therapeutic agents (eg, corticosteroids). Do not report diagnostic or therapeutic injections separately.
- For therapies that are not destructive of the target nerve (eg, pulsed radiofrequency), use 64999.
- Report separately the supply of the chemodenervation agent (eg, botulinum toxin).
- Report 64646 or 64647 for chemodenervation for muscles of the trunk. Trunk muscles include the erector spinae and paraspinal muscles, rectus abdominus and obliques. All other somatic muscles are extremity muscles, head muscles, or neck muscles.
- Do not report modifier -50 in conjunction with 64646.

CPT® CODE 64647

Chemodenervation of trunk muscle(s); 6 or more muscles

POLICY INDICATORS

Global Period
0 day post-op period

Assistants at Surgery
No assistant

Co-Surgeons Allowed
No co-surgeon

Reduction for Multiple Procedures
Subject to 50% reduction

Bilateral Surgery Payment
N/A

Applicable Medicare Policies

Relative Value Units (RVUs)

Work RVUs	2.11
Non-Facility Total	5.48
Facility Total	3.99

Coding Assistance

64647 includes:

- Positioning and prepping patient
- Examination of site after anesthesia
- Injection of local anesthesia
- Operative services, including inspections around site, injection(s) of neurolytic agent(s), and hemostasis

Additional Notes

- Includes the injection of other therapeutic agents (eg, corticosteroids). Do not report diagnostic or therapeutic injections separately.
- For therapies that are not destructive of the target nerve (eg, pulsed radiofrequency), use 64999.
- Report separately the supply of the chemodenervation agent (eg, botulinum toxin).
- Report 64646 or 64647 for chemodenervation for muscles of the trunk. Trunk muscles include the erector spinae and paraspinal muscles, rectus abdominus and obliques. All other somatic muscles are extremity muscles, head muscles, or neck muscles.
- Do not report modifier -50 in conjunction with 64647

CPT® CODE 96547

Intraoperative hyperthermic intraperitoneal chemotherapy (HIPEC) procedure, including separate incision(s) and closure, when performed; first 60 minutes (List separately in addition to code for primary procedure.)

POLICY INDICATORS

Global Period
Global for primary procedure applies

Assistants at Surgery
N/A

Co-Surgeons Allowed
N/A

Reduction for Multiple Procedures
N/A

Bilateral Surgery Payment
N/A

Applicable Medicare Policies
Carrier Priced

Relative Value Units (RVUs)

Work RVUs	6.53
Non-Facility Total	Only valued for facility
Facility Total	10.85

Coding Assistance

96547 includes:

- Positioning and prepping patient
- Examination of site after anesthesia
- Operative services, including inspections around site and closure
- Appropriate post-op E/M visit(s)
- Chemotherapy

Add-On Code:

- Follow Primary Code Policies

CPT® CODE 96548

Intraoperative hyperthermic intraperitoneal chemotherapy (HIPEC) procedure, including separate incision(s) and closure, when performed; each additional 30 minutes (List separately in addition to code for primary procedure.)

POLICY INDICATORS

Global Period
Global for primary procedure applies

Assistants at Surgery
N/A

Co-Surgeons Allowed
N/A

Reduction for Multiple Procedures
N/A

Bilateral Surgery Payment
N/A

Applicable Medicare Policies
Carrier Priced

Relative Value Units (RVUs)

Work RVUs	3.00
Non-Facility Total	Only valued for facility
Facility Total	4.97

Coding Assistance

96548 includes:

- Positioning and prepping patient
- Examination of site after anesthesia
- Operative services, including inspections around site and closure
- Appropriate post-op E/M visit(s)
- Chemotherapy

Add-On Code:

- Follow Primary Code Policies

Maternity Codes

CPT® CODE 59400

Routine obstetric care including antepartum care, vaginal delivery (with or without episiotomy, and/or forceps) and postpartum care

POLICY INDICATORS

Global Period
Visit after confirmation of pregnancy – 6 weeks postpartum

Assistants at Delivery
No assistant

Co-Surgeons Allowed
No co-surgeon

Reduction for Multiple Procedures
Subject to 100/50 reduction

Bilateral Surgery Payment
N/A

Applicable Medicare Policies

Relative Value Units (RVUs)

Work RVUs	37.00
Non-Facility Total	Only valued for delivery in a facility
Facility Total	72.82

Coding Assistance

59400 includes:

- All prenatal visits, including weight, blood pressure, fetal heart tones and routine chemical urinalysis. This does not include the "confirmation of pregnancy" visit.
- E/M visit(s) performed the day before or day of delivery
- Admission to L&D, update of history and physical
- Management of labor including fetal monitoring
- Catheterization
- Vaginal delivery, with or without forceps or vacuum extraction
- Delivery of placenta, any method
- Episiotomy and repair. This does not include the repair of 3rd or 4th degree lacerations (use CPT 12041-12047 or 13131-13133)
- Local anesthesia
- Administration of oxytocin
- Exploration of uterus
- Placement of hemostatic pack or agent
- Simple removal of cerclage (not under anesthesia)
- Recovery room visit(s)
- Postpartum visits, including uncomplicated inpatient and outpatient visits, for up to 6 weeks postpartum. This includes any discussion of contraception. Traditionally, this includes 2 inpatient postpartum days and 1 routine outpatient postpartum visit.

Additional Notes

- If multiples are delivered vaginally, report 59409-59 for the subsequent delivery(ies)
- For a patient seen for more than 13 visits due to a complication related to the pregnancy, report each visit separately at the time of delivery
- Visits unrelated to the pregnancy should be reported separately at the time of the service, independent of the prenatal visits

CPT® CODE 59409

Vaginal delivery only (with or without episiotomy and/or forceps)

POLICY INDICATORS

Global Period
Day before or day of admission – delivery

Assistants at Delivery
Submit reason for assistant

Co-Surgeons Allowed
No co-surgeon

Reduction for Multiple Procedures
Subject to 100/50 reduction

Bilateral Surgery Payment
N/A

Applicable Medicare Policies

Relative Value Units (RVUs)

Work RVUs	14.37
Non-Facility Total	Only valued for delivery in a facility
Facility Total	23.99

Coding Assistance

59409 includes:

- E/M visit(s) performed the day before or day of delivery
- Admission to L&D, update of history and physical
- Management of labor including fetal monitoring
- Catheterization
- Vaginal delivery, with or without forceps or vacuum extraction
- Delivery of placenta, any method
- Episiotomy and repair. This does not include the repair of 3rd or 4th degree lacerations (use CPT 12041-12047 or 13131-13133)
- Local anesthesia
- Administration of oxytocin
- Exploration of uterus
- Placement of hemostatic pack or agent
- Simple removal of cerclage (not under anesthesia)
- Recovery room visit(s)

Additional Notes

- If inpatient postpartum care is performed and outpatient E/M services are not being reported, report those services separately with the appropriate inpatient E/M code(s)
- If multiples are delivered vaginally, report 59409-59 for the subsequent delivery(ies)
- Use 59410 if all postpartum care also performed

MATERNITY

CPT® CODE 59410

Vaginal delivery only (with or without episiotomy and/or forceps); including postpartum care

POLICY INDICATORS

Global Period
Day before or day of admission – 6 weeks after delivery

Assistants at Delivery
No assistant

Co-Surgeons Allowed
No co-surgeon

Reduction for Multiple Procedures
Subject to 100/50 reduction

Bilateral Surgery Payment
N/A

Applicable Medicare Policies

Relative Value Units (RVUs)

Work RVUs	18.76
Non-Facility Total	Only valued for delivery in a facility
Facility Total	32.49

Coding Assistance

59410 includes:

- E/M visit(s) performed the day before or day of delivery
- Admission to L&D, update of history and physical
- Management of labor including fetal monitoring
- Catheterization
- Vaginal delivery, with or without forceps or vacuum extraction
- Delivery of placenta, any method
- Episiotomy and repair. This does not include the repair of 3rd or 4th degree lacerations (use CPT 12041-12047 or 13131-13133)
- Local anesthesia
- Administration of oxytocin
- Exploration of uterus
- Placement of hemostatic pack or agent
- Simple removal of cerclage (not under anesthesia)
- Recovery room visit(s)
- Postpartum visits, including uncomplicated inpatient and outpatient visits, for up to 6 weeks postpartum. This includes any discussion of contraception. Traditionally, this includes 2 inpatient postpartum days and 1 routine outpatient postpartum visit.

Additional Notes

- If inpatient postpartum care is performed and outpatient E/M services are not being reported, report those services separately with the appropriate inpatient E/M code(s)
- If multiples are delivered vaginally, report 59409-59 for the subsequent delivery(ies)
- Use 59400 if prenatal care is also performed

CPT® CODE 59412

External cephalic version, with or without tocolysis

POLICY INDICATORS

Global Period
Day of procedure

Assistants at Delivery
Submit reason for assistant

Co-Surgeons Allowed
No co-surgeon

Reduction for Multiple Procedures
Not subject to multiple surgery reduction

Bilateral Surgery Payment
N/A

Applicable Medicare Policies

Relative Value Units (RVUs)

Work RVUs	1.71
Non-Facility Total	Only valued for delivery in a facility
Facility Total	3.09

Coding Assistance

59412 includes:

- Procedure includes proper positioning and administration of intravenous tocolysis, if performed
- E/M visit on the day of the procedure that are related to the procedure. Unrelated E/M visits are separately reportable on the day of the procedure, if a 25 modifier is attached
- Fetal monitoring
- Completion of patient record
- Patient evaluation and stabilization
- Dictation of procedure report
- Patient instructions
- Consultation with family

CPT® CODE 59414

Delivery of placenta (separate procedure)

POLICY INDICATORS

Global Period
Day of procedure

Assistants at Delivery
Submit reason for assistant

Co-Surgeons Allowed
No co-surgeon

Reduction for Multiple Procedures
Subject to 100/50 reduction

Bilateral Surgery Payment
N/A

Applicable Medicare Policies

Relative Value Units (RVUs)

Work RVUs	1.61
Non-Facility Total	Only valued for delivery in a facility
Facility Total	2.73

Coding Assistance

59414 includes:

- Delivery of placenta, any method
- Catheterization
- Repair of episiotomy/suturing of laceration(s)
- Local anesthesia
- Administration of oxytocin
- Exploration of uterus
- Placement of hemostatic pack or agent

Additional Notes

- If a delivery is also performed, do not report 59414. It is considered an integral part of the delivery and should generally not be reported separately unless it is unrelated to the delivery. A -59 modifier should be used, along with a distinct ICD-10-CM code.

CPT® CODE 59425

Antepartum care only; 4-6 visits

POLICY INDICATORS

Global Period
Visit after confirmation of pregnancy – 6 visits

Assistants at Delivery
Submit reason for assistant

Co-Surgeons Allowed
No co-surgeon

Reduction for Multiple Procedures
Not subject to multiple surgery reduction

Bilateral Surgery Payment
N/A

Applicable Medicare Policies

Relative Value Units (RVUs)

Work RVUs	7.80
Non-Facility Total	16.96
Facility Total	13.02

Coding Assistance

59425 includes:

- 4-6 antepartum visits, including a visit for initial history and physical examination and subsequent weight, blood pressure, fetal heart tones and routine chemical urinalysis

Additional Notes

- If the patient is seen only 1-3 times, report each visit separately using the appropriate Evaluation and Management code
- If the patient is seen more than 6 times for prenatal care only, report 59426

CPT® CODE 59426

Antepartum care only; 7 or more visits

POLICY INDICATORS

Global Period
Visit after confirmation of pregnancy - day of delivery

Assistants at Delivery
Submit reason for assistant

Co-Surgeons Allowed
No co-surgeon

Reduction for Multiple Procedures
Not subject to multiple surgery reduction

Bilateral Surgery Payment
N/A

Applicable Medicare Policies

Relative Value Units (RVUs)

Work RVUs	14.30
Non-Facility Total	31.05
Facility Total	23.91

Coding Assistance

59426 includes:

- 4-6 antepartum visits, including a visit for initial history and physical examination and subsequent weight, blood pressure, fetal heart tones and routine chemical urinalysis

Additional Notes

- If the patient is seen only 1-3 times, report each visit separately using the appropriate Evaluation and Management code
- If the patient is seen 4-6 times for prenatal care only, report 59425

CPT® CODE 59430

Postpartum care only (separate procedure)

POLICY INDICATORS

Global Period
After discharge for 6 weeks

Assistants at Delivery
No assistant

Co-Surgeons Allowed
No co-surgeon

Reduction for Multiple Procedures
Subject to 100/50 reduction

Bilateral Surgery Payment
N/A

Applicable Medicare Policies

Relative Value Units (RVUs)

Work RVUs	3.22
Non-Facility Total	7.90
Facility Total	5.36

Coding Assistance

59430 includes:

- Routine outpatient postpartum visits, for up to 6 weeks postpartum. This includes any discussion of contraception. Traditionally, this includes 1 routine outpatient postpartum visit for a vaginal delivery and 2 routine outpatient postpartum visits for a cesarean delivery.

Additional Notes

- If a vaginal delivery is also performed, report 59410 or 59614
- If a cesarean delivery is also performed, report 59515 or 59622
- 59430 is considered an integral part of the delivery and should generally not be reported separately unless it is unrelated to the delivery. A -59 modifier should be used, along with a distinct ICD-10-CM code

CPT® CODE 59510

Routine obstetric care including antepartum care, cesarean delivery, and postpartum care

POLICY INDICATORS

Global Period
Visit after confirmation of pregnancy – 6 weeks postpartum

Assistants at Delivery
No assistant

Co-Surgeons Allowed
No co-surgeon

Reduction for Multiple Procedures
Subject to 100/50 reduction

Bilateral Surgery Payment
N/A

Applicable Medicare Policies

Relative Value Units (RVUs)

Work RVUs	41.05
Non-Facility Total	Only valued for delivery in a facility
Facility Total	80.89

Coding Assistance

59510 includes:

- All prenatal visits, including weight, blood pressure, fetal heart tones and routine chemical urinalysis. This does not include the "confirmation of pregnancy" visit.
- E/M visit(s) performed the day before or day of delivery
- Admission to L&D, update of history and physical
- Management of labor including fetal monitoring
- Catheterization and anesthesia
- Preparation of abdomen and abdominal incision
- Incision into uterus with delivery of fetus, placenta, and fetal membranes
- Uterine repair and closure
- Hemostasis
- Administration of oxytocin
- Simple removal of cerclage
- Recovery room visit(s)
- Removal of sutures or staples
- Postpartum visits, including uncomplicated inpatient and outpatient visits, for up to 6 weeks postpartum. This includes any discussion of contraception. Traditionally, this includes 2 inpatient postpartum days and 1 routine outpatient postpartum visit.

Additional Notes

- If one twin is delivered vaginally and one by cesarean, report 59510 and 59409-51. If both are delivered by cesarean only, report 59510
- For a patient seen for more than 13 visits due to a complication related to the pregnancy, report each visit separately at the time of delivery
- Visits unrelated to the pregnancy should be reported separately at the time of the service, independent of the prenatal visits

MATERNITY

CPT® CODE 59514

Cesarean delivery only

POLICY INDICATORS

Global Period
Day before or day of admission – delivery

Assistants at Delivery
Assistant allowed

Co-Surgeons Allowed
Submit reason for co-surgeon

Reduction for Multiple Procedures
Subject to 100/50 reduction

Bilateral Surgery Payment
N/A

Applicable Medicare Policies
Inpatient-only list

Relative Value Units (RVUs)

Work RVUs	16.13
Non-Facility Total	Only valued for delivery in a facility
Facility Total	27.21

Coding Assistance

59514 includes:

- E/M visit(s) performed the day before or day of delivery
- Admission to L&D, update of history and physical
- Management of labor including fetal monitoring
- Catheterization and anesthesia
- Preparation of abdomen and abdominal incision
- Incision into uterus with delivery of fetus, placenta, and fetal membranes
- Uterine repair and closure
- Hemostasis
- Administration of oxytocin
- Simple removal of cerclage
- Recovery room visit(s)
- Removal of sutures or staples

Additional Notes

- If one twin is delivered vaginally and one by cesarean, report 59514 and 59409-51. If both are delivered by cesarean only, report 59514
- If inpatient and outpatient postpartum care is also performed, report 59515 instead of 59514
- If inpatient postpartum care is performed without outpatient postpartum care, report the appropriate subsequent inpatient Evaluation and Management code(s)

CPT® CODE 59515

Cesarean delivery only; including postpartum care

POLICY INDICATORS

Global Period
Day before or day of admission – 6 weeks after delivery

Assistants at Delivery
No assistant

Co-Surgeons Allowed
No co-surgeon

Reduction for Multiple Procedures
Subject to 100/50 reduction

Bilateral Surgery Payment
N/A

Applicable Medicare Policies

Relative Value Units (RVUs)

Work RVUs	22.79
Non-Facility Total	Only valued for delivery in a facility
Facility Total	40.30

Coding Assistance

59515 includes:

- E/M visit(s) performed the day before or day of delivery
- Admission to L&D, update of history and physical
- Management of labor including fetal monitoring
- Catheterization and anesthesia
- Preparation of abdomen and abdominal incision
- Incision into uterus with delivery of fetus, placenta, and fetal membranes
- Uterine repair and closure
- Hemostasis
- Administration of oxytocin
- Simple removal of cerclage
- Recovery room visit(s)
- Removal of sutures or staples
- Postpartum visits, including uncomplicated inpatient and outpatient visits, for up to 6 weeks postpartum. This includes any discussion of contraception. Traditionally, this includes 2 inpatient postpartum days and 1 routine outpatient postpartum visit.

Additional Notes

- If antepartum services are provided, report 59510 instead

CPT® CODE 59525

Subtotal or total hysterectomy after cesarean delivery
(List separately in addition to code for primary procedure)

POLICY INDICATORS

Global Period
Global for primary procedure applies

Assistants at Surgery
Assistant allowed

Co-Surgeons Allowed
Submit reason for co-surgeon

Reduction for Multiple Procedures
Not subject to multiple surgery reduction

Bilateral Surgery Payment
N/A

Applicable Medicare Policies
Inpatient-only list

Relative Value Units (RVUs)

Work RVUs	8.53
Non-Facility Total	Only valued for delivery in a facility
Facility Total	14.41

Coding Assistance

59525 includes:

- Hysterectomy after cesarean delivery (an indwelling catheter is usually in place)
- Removal of the uterine fundus and possibly the uterine cervix
- Exploratory laparotomy
- Removal of tubes and ovaries
- Placement of pelvic drains
- Pelvic examination under anesthesia
- Hemostasis
- Wound closure

Add-On Code:

- Follow Primary Code Policies

Additional Notes

- This is an add-on code that can only be reported when a cesarean delivery code is also reported. No modifier is necessary.

CPT® CODE 59610

Routine obstetric care including antepartum care, vaginal delivery (with or without episiotomy, and/or forceps) and postpartum care, after previous cesarean delivery

POLICY INDICATORS

Global Period
Visit after confirmation of pregnancy – 6 weeks postpartum

Assistants at Delivery
Submit reason for assistant

Co-Surgeons Allowed
No co-surgeon

Reduction for Multiple Procedures
Subject to 100/50 reduction

Bilateral Surgery Payment
N/A

Applicable Medicare Policies

Relative Value Units (RVUs)

Work RVUs	38.71
Non-Facility Total	Only valued for delivery in a facility
Facility Total	76.28

Coding Assistance

59610 includes:

- All prenatal visits, including weight, blood pressure, fetal heart tones and routine chemical urinalysis. This does not include the "confirmation of pregnancy" visit.
- E/M visit(s) performed the day before or day of delivery
- Admission to L&D, update of history and physical
- Management of labor including fetal monitoring
- Catheterization
- Vaginal delivery, with or without forceps or vacuum extraction
- Delivery of placenta, any method
- Episiotomy and repair. This does not include the repair of 3rd or 4th degree lacerations (use CPT 12041-12047 or 13131-13133)
- Local anesthesia
- Administration of oxytocin
- Exploration of uterus
- Placement of hemostatic pack or agent
- Simple removal of cerclage (not under anesthesia)
- Recovery room visit(s)
- Postpartum visits, including uncomplicated inpatient and outpatient visits, for up to 6 weeks postpartum. This includes any discussion of contraception. Traditionally, this includes 2 inpatient postpartum days and 1 routine outpatient postpartum visit.

Additional Notes

- If vaginal delivery of twins is performed, report 59612-59 for the subsequent delivery(ies)
- For a patient seen for more than 13 visits due to a complication related to the pregnancy, report each visit separately at the time of delivery
- Visits unrelated to the pregnancy should be reported separately at the time of the service, independent of the prenatal visits

CPT® CODE 59612

Vaginal delivery only, after previous cesarean delivery (with or without episiotomy and/or forceps)

POLICY INDICATORS

Global Period
Day before or day of admission – delivery

Assistants at Delivery
Submit reason for assistant

Co-Surgeons Allowed
No co-surgeon

Reduction for Multiple Procedures
Subject to 100/50 reduction

Bilateral Surgery Payment
N/A

Applicable Medicare Policies

Relative Value Units (RVUs)

Work RVUs	16.09
Non-Facility Total	Only valued for delivery in a facility
Facility Total	27.19

Coding Assistance

59612 includes:

- E/M visit(s) performed the day before or day of delivery
- Admission to L&D, update of history and physical
- Management of labor including fetal monitoring
- Catheterization
- Vaginal delivery, with or without forceps or vacuum extraction
- Delivery of placenta, any method
- Episiotomy and repair. This does not include the repair of 3rd or 4th degree lacerations (use CPT 12041-12047 or 13131-13133)
- Local anesthesia
- Administration of oxytocin
- Exploration of uterus
- Placement of hemostatic pack or agent
- Simple removal of cerclage (not under anesthesia)
- Recovery room visit(s)

Additional Notes

- If inpatient postpartum care is performed and outpatient E/M services are not being reported, report those services separately with the appropriate inpatient E/M code(s).
- If multiples are delivered vaginally, report 59612-59 for the subsequent delivery(ies)
- Use 59614 if all postpartum care also performed

CPT® CODE 59614

Vaginal delivery only, after previous cesarean delivery (with or without episiotomy and/or forceps); including postpartum care

POLICY INDICATORS

Global Period
Day before or day of admission – 6 weeks after delivery

Assistants at Delivery
Submit reason for assistant

Co-Surgeons Allowed
No co-surgeon

Reduction for Multiple Procedures
Subject to 100/50 reduction

Bilateral Surgery Payment
N/A

Applicable Medicare Policies

Relative Value Units (RVUs)

Work RVUs	20.48
Non-Facility Total	Only valued for delivery in a facility
Facility Total	35.14

Coding Assistance

59614 includes:

- E/M visit(s) performed the day before or day of delivery
- Admission to L&D, update of history and physical
- Management of labor including fetal monitoring
- Catheterization
- Vaginal delivery, with or without forceps or vacuum extraction
- Delivery of placenta, any method
- Episiotomy and repair. This does not include the repair of 3rd or 4th degree lacerations (use CPT 12041-12047 or 13131-13133)
- Local anesthesia
- Administration of oxytocin
- Exploration of uterus
- Placement of hemostatic pack or agent
- Simple removal of cerclage (not under anesthesia)
- Recovery room visit(s)
- Postpartum visits, including uncomplicated inpatient and outpatient visits, for up to 6 weeks postpartum. This includes any discussion of contraception. Traditionally, this includes 2 inpatient postpartum days and 1 routine outpatient postpartum visit.

Additional Notes

- If inpatient postpartum care is performed and outpatient E/M services are not being reported, report those services separately with the appropriate inpatient E/M code(s).
- Use 59610 if prenatal care is also performed

CPT® CODE 59618

Routine obstetric care including antepartum care, cesarean delivery, and postpartum care, following attempted vaginal delivery after previous cesarean delivery

POLICY INDICATORS

Global Period
Visit after confirmation of pregnancy – 6 weeks postpartum

Assistants at Delivery
Submit reason for assistant

Co-Surgeons Allowed
No co-surgeon

Reduction for Multiple Procedures
Subject to 100/50 reduction

Bilateral Surgery Payment
N/A

Applicable Medicare Policies

Relative Value Units (RVUs)

Work RVUs	41.57
Non-Facility Total	Only valued for delivery in a facility
Facility Total	81.75

Coding Assistance

59618 includes:

- All prenatal visits, including weight, blood pressure, fetal heart tones and routine chemical urinalysis. This does not include the "confirmation of pregnancy" visit.
- E/M visit(s) performed the day before or day of delivery
- Admission to L&D, update of history and physical
- Management of labor including fetal monitoring
- Catheterization and anesthesia
- Preparation of abdomen and abdominal incision
- Incision into uterus with delivery of fetus, placenta, and fetal membranes
- Uterine repair and closure
- Hemostasis
- Administration of oxytocin
- Simple removal of cerclage
- Recovery room visit(s)
- Removal of sutures or staples
- Postpartum visits, including uncomplicated inpatient and outpatient visits, for up to 6 weeks postpartum. This includes any discussion of contraception. Traditionally, this includes 2 inpatient postpartum days and 1 routine outpatient postpartum visit.

Additional Notes

- If one twin is delivered vaginally and one by cesarean, report 59618 and 59612-51. If both are delivered by cesarean only, report 59618-22
- For a patient seen for more than 13 visits due to a complication related to the pregnancy, report each visit separately at the time of delivery
- Visits unrelated to the pregnancy should be reported separately at the time of the service, independent of the prenatal visits

CPT® CODE 59620

Cesarean delivery only, following attempted vaginal delivery after previous cesarean delivery

POLICY INDICATORS

Global Period
Day before or day of admission – delivery

Assistants at Delivery
Assistant allowed

Co-Surgeons Allowed
No co-surgeon

Reduction for Multiple Procedures
Subject to 100/50 reduction

Bilateral Surgery Payment
N/A

Applicable Medicare Policies
Inpatient-only list

Relative Value Units (RVUs)

Work RVUs	16.66
Non-Facility Total	Only valued for delivery in a facility
Facility Total	28.15

Coding Assistance

59620 includes:

- E/M visit(s) performed the day before or day of delivery
- Admission to L&D, update of history and physical
- Management of labor including fetal monitoring
- Catheterization and anesthesia
- Preparation of abdomen and abdominal incision
- Incision into uterus with delivery of fetus, placenta, and fetal membranes
- Uterine repair and closure
- Hemostasis
- Administration of oxytocin
- Simple removal of cerclage
- Recovery room visit(s)
- Removal of sutures or staples

Additional Notes

- If inpatient and outpatient postpartum care is also performed, report 59622 instead of 59620
- If inpatient postpartum care is performed without outpatient postpartum care, report the appropriate subsequent inpatient Evaluation and Management code(s)

CPT® CODE 59622

Cesarean delivery only, following attempted vaginal delivery after previous cesarean delivery; including postpartum care

POLICY INDICATORS

Global Period
Day before or day of admission – 6 weeks after delivery

Assistants at Delivery
Submit reason for assistant

Co-Surgeons Allowed
No co-surgeon

Reduction for Multiple Procedures
Subject to 100/50 reduction

Bilateral Surgery Payment
N/A

Applicable Medicare Policies

Relative Value Units (RVUs)

Work RVUs	23.32
Non-Facility Total	Only valued for delivery in a facility
Facility Total	41.70

Coding Assistance

59622 includes:

- E/M visit(s) performed the day before or day of delivery
- Admission to L&D, update of history and physical
- Management of labor including fetal monitoring
- Catheterization and anesthesia
- Preparation of abdomen and abdominal incision
- Incision into uterus with delivery of fetus, placenta, and fetal membranes
- Uterine repair and closure
- Hemostasis
- Administration of oxytocin
- Simple removal of cerclage
- Recovery room visit(s)
- Removal of sutures or staples
- Postpartum visits, including uncomplicated inpatient and outpatient visits, for up to 6 weeks postpartum. This includes any discussion of contraception. Traditionally, this includes 2 inpatient postpartum days and 1 routine outpatient postpartum visit.

Additional Notes

- If antepartum services are provided, report 59618 instead.

Imaging Codes

CPT® CODE 76000

Fluoroscopy (separate procedure), up to 1 hour physician or other qualified health care professional time

Relative Value Units (RVUs)

Work RVUs	0.30
Non-Facility Total	1.29
Facility Total	Only valued for non-facility

CPT® CODE 76376

3D rendering with interpretation and reporting of computed tomography, magnetic resonance imaging, ultrasound, or other tomographic modality with image postprocessing under concurrent supervision; not requiring image postprocessing on an independent workstation

Relative Value Units (RVUs)

Work RVUs	0.20
Non-Facility Total	0.77
Facility Total	Only valued for non-facility

CPT® CODE 76377

3D rendering with interpretation and reporting of computed tomography, magnetic resonance imaging, ultrasound, or other tomographic modality with image postprocessing under concurrent supervision; requiring image postprocessing on an independent workstation

Relative Value Units (RVUs)

Work RVUs	0.79
Non-Facility Total	2.38
Facility Total	Only valued for non-facility

CPT® CODE 76380

Computed tomography, limited or localized follow-up study

Relative Value Units (RVUs)

Work RVUs	0.98
Non-Facility Total	3.98
Facility Total	Only valued for non-facility

CPT® CODE 76641

Ultrasound, breast, unilateral, real time with image documentation, including axilla when performed; complete

Relative Value Units (RVUs)

Work RVUs	0.73
Non-Facility Total	3.06
Facility Total	Only valued for non-facility

CPT® CODE 76642

Ultrasound, breast, unilateral, real time with image documentation, including axilla when performed; limited

Relative Value Units (RVUs)

Work RVUs	0.68
Non-Facility Total	2.54
Facility Total	Only valued for non-facility

CPT® CODE 76700

Ultrasound, abdominal, real time with image documentation; complete

Relative Value Units (RVUs)

Work RVUs	0.81
Non-Facility Total	3.46
Facility Total	Only valued for non-facility

CPT® CODE 76705

Ultrasound, abdominal, real time with image documentation; limited (eg, single organ, quadrant, follow-up)

Relative Value Units (RVUs)

Work RVUs	0.59
Non-Facility Total	2.60
Facility Total	Only valued for non-facility

CPT® CODE 76706

Ultrasound, abdominal aorta, real time with image documentation, screening study for abdominal aortic aneurysm (AAA)

Relative Value Units (RVUs)

Work RVUs	0.55
Non-Facility Total	3.20
Facility Total	Only valued for non-facility

CPT® CODE 76770

Ultrasound, retroperitoneal (eg, renal, aorta, nodes), real time with image documentation; complete

Relative Value Units (RVUs)

Work RVUs	0.74
Non-Facility Total	3.23
Facility Total	Only valued for non-facility

CPT® CODE 76775

Ultrasound, retroperitoneal (eg, renal, aorta, nodes), real time with image documentation; limited

Relative Value Units (RVUs)

Work RVUs	0.58
Non-Facility Total	1.82
Facility Total	Only valued for non-facility

CPT® CODE 76801

Ultrasound, pregnant uterus, real time with image documentation, fetal and maternal evaluation, first trimester (< 14 weeks 0 days), transabdominal approach; single or first gestation

Relative Value Units (RVUs)

Work RVUs	0.99
Non-Facility Total	3.49
Facility Total	Only valued for non-facility

INCLUDED IN THIS PROCEDURE

- Determination of number of gestational sacs and fetuses
- Gestational sac/fetal measurements
- Survey of visible fetal and placental anatomic structures
- Qualitative assessment of amniotic fluid volume and gestational sac shape
- Examination of maternal uterus and adnexae
- Limited ultrasound (76815)

Additional Notes

- In cases of multiple gestation, report 76802 in addition to this code
- The highest valued ultrasound procedure should be listed first on the claim form. No modifier -51 is necessary
- Follow-up care is not included in the ultrasound procedure
- ACOG clinical policy recognizes the need for multiple ultrasounds in the first trimester of pregnancy for certain clinical conditions. Clinical conditions include—but are not limited to:
  - First trimester bleeding
  - Suspected or known ectopic pregnancy
  - Pelvic pain
  - Ovarian cycts
  - Uncertain dating
  - Gestational trophoblastic disease
  - Mullerian anomalies
  - Risk of multiple gestation
  - History of recurrent pregnancy loss
  - Suspected or known early pregnancy loss

CPT® CODE 76802

Ultrasound, pregnant uterus, real time with image documentation, fetal and maternal evaluation, first trimester (< 14 weeks 0 days), transabdominal approach; each additional gestation (List separately in addition to code for primary procedure)

Relative Value Units (RVUs)

Work RVUs	0.83
Non-Facility Total	1.79
Facility Total	Only valued for non-facility

CPT® CODE 76805

Ultrasound, pregnant uterus, real time with image documentation, fetal and maternal evaluation, after first trimester (> or = 14 weeks 0 days), transabdominal approach; single or first gestation

INCLUDED IN THIS PROCEDURE

- Determination of number of gestational sacs and fetuses
- Gestational sac/fetal measurements
- Survey of intracranial, spinal and abdominal anatomy
- Evaluation of four-chambered heart
- Assessment of umbilical cord insertion site
- Survey of placenta location and amniotic fluid assessment
- When visible, examination of maternal adnexa
- Limited ultrasound (76815)

Relative Value Units (RVUs)

Work RVUs	0.99
Non-Facility Total	4.02
Facility Total	Only valued for non-facility

Additional Notes

- In cases of multiple gestation, report 76810 in addition to this code
- For first trimester fetal and maternal evaluation, report 76801 instead of this code
- When there are multiple evaluations for medical reasons, and all elements this code are documented, report this code
- The highest valued ultrasound procedure should be listed first on the claim form. No modifier -51 is necessary
- Follow-up care is not included in the ultrasound procedure

CPT® CODE 76810

Ultrasound, pregnant uterus, real time with image documentation, fetal and maternal evaluation, after first trimester (> or = 14 weeks 0 days), transabdominal approach; each additional gestation
(List separately in addition to code for primary procedure)

Relative Value Units (RVUs)

Work RVUs	0.98
Non-Facility Total	2.59
Facility Total	Only valued for non-facility

CPT® CODE 76811

Ultrasound, pregnant uterus, real time with image documentation, fetal and maternal evaluation plus detailed fetal anatomic examination, transabdominal approach; single or first gestation

INCLUDED IN THIS PROCEDURE

- All components of 76805 and 76810
- Detailed anatomic evaluation of fetal brain, ventricles, face, heart, outflow tracts, chest anatomy, abdominal organ specific anatomy, and the number, length and architecture of limbs
- Detailed evaluation of umbilical cord, placenta and other fetal anatomy as indicated
- Limited ultrasound (76815)

Relative Value Units (RVUs)

Work RVUs	1.90
Non-Facility Total	5.32
Facility Total	Only valued for non-facility

Additional Notes

- Codes 76811 and 76812 are reported when performed for a suspected or known fetal anomaly, not for routine screening.
- In cases of multiple gestation, report 76812 in addition to this code
- When there are multiple evaluations for medical reasons, and all elements this code are documented, report this code
- The highest valued ultrasound procedure should be listed first on the claim form. No modifier -51 is necessary
- Follow-up care is not included in the ultrasound procedure

CPT® CODE 76812

Ultrasound, pregnant uterus, real time with image documentation, fetal and maternal evaluation plus detailed fetal anatomic examination, transabdominal approach; each additional gestation (List separately in addition to code for primary procedure)

Relative Value Units (RVUs)

Work RVUs	1.78
Non-Facility Total	5.67
Facility Total	Only valued for non-facility

CPT® CODE 76813

Ultrasound, pregnant uterus, real time with image documentation, first trimester fetal nuchal translucency measurement, transabdominal or transvaginal approach; single or first gestation

INCLUDED IN THIS PROCEDURE

- Mid-sagittal view of embryo
- Crown-rump measurement
- Embryonic neck in neutral position
- Observation of spontaneous embryonic movement that allows differentiation between outer edge of nuchal skin and the amnion
- At least 3 measurements between the inner edges of nuchal translucency
- Comparison of crown-rump length and gestational age
- Calculation of Down's risk
- Limited ultrasound (76815)

Relative Value Units (RVUs)

Work RVUs	1.18
Non-Facility Total	3.40
Facility Total	Only valued for non-facility

Additional Notes

- In cases of multiple gestation, report 76812 in addition to this code
- When there are multiple evaluations for medical reasons, and all elements this code are documented, report this code
- The highest valued ultrasound procedure should be listed first on the claim form. No modifier -51 is necessary
- Follow-up care is not included in the ultrasound procedure

CPT® CODE 76814

Ultrasound, pregnant uterus, real time with image documentation, first trimester fetal nuchal translucency measurement, transabdominal or transvaginal approach; each additional gestation
(List separately in addition to code for primary procedure)

Relative Value Units (RVUs)

Work RVUs	0.99
Non-Facility Total	2.20
Facility Total	Only valued for non-facility

CPT® CODE 76815

Ultrasound, pregnant uterus, real time with image documentation, limited (eg, fetal heart beat, placental location, fetal position and/or qualitative amniotic fluid volume), 1 or more fetuses

INCLUDED IN THIS PROCEDURE

This examination is a general assessment of one or more of the following:

- Fetal position
- Fetal heart beat
- Placental location
- Qualitative amniotic fluid volume

Relative Value Units (RVUs)

Work RVUs	0.65
Non-Facility Total	2.42
Facility Total	Only valued for non-facility

Additional Notes

- When a comprehensive maternal and fetal evaluation is performed, report 76801-76810
- This code is reported once regardless of the gestation number
- This code is reported once per examination, not per element
- The highest valued ultrasound procedure should be listed first on the claim form. No modifier -51 is necessary
- Follow-up care is not included in the ultrasound procedure
- ACOG clinical policy recognizes the need for multiple ultrasounds in the first trimester of pregnancy for certain clinical conditions. Clinical conditions include—but are not limited to:
  - First trimester bleeding
  - Suspected or known ectopic pregnancy
  - Pelvic pain
  - Ovarian cycts
  - Uncertain dating
  - Gestational trophoblastic disease
  - Mullerian anomalies
  - Risk of multiple gestation
  - History of recurrent pregnancy loss
  - Suspected or known early pregnancy loss

CPT® CODE 76816

Ultrasound, pregnant uterus, real time with image documentation, follow-up (eg, re-evaluation of fetal size by measuring standard growth parameters and amniotic fluid volume, re-evaluation of organ system(s) suspected or confirmed to be abnormal on a previous scan), transabdominal approaoch, per fetus

INCLUDED IN THIS PROCEDURE

- Transabdominal evaluation of either of the following:
  - Re-evaluation of fetal size by measuring growth and amniotic fluid
  - Re-evaluation of organ
- Limited ultrasound (76815)

Relative Value Units (RVUs)

Work RVUs	0.85
Non-Facility Total	3.25
Facility Total	Only valued for non-facility

Additional Notes

- Consider 76805 or 76810 based on the elements documented for the second trimester evaluation
- Report this code separately for each gestation using the modifier -59 to the additional codes
- The highest valued ultrasound procedure should be listed first on the claim form. No modifier -51 is necessary
- Follow-up care is not included in the ultrasound procedure
- ACOG clinical policy recognizes the need for multiple ultrasounds in the first trimester of pregnancy for certain clinical conditions. Clinical conditions include – but are not limited to:
  - First trimester bleeding
  - Suspected or known ectopic pregnancy
  - Pelvic pain
  - Ovarian cycts
  - Uncertain dating
  - Gestational trophoblastic disease
  - Mullerian anomalies
  - Risk of multiple gestation
  - History of recurrent pregnancy loss
- Suspected or known early pregnancy loss

IMAGING

CPT® CODE 76817

Ultrasound, pregnant uterus, real time with image documentation, transvaginal

INCLUDED IN THIS PROCEDURE

Transvaginal evaluation of either of the following:

- Evaluation of the embryo(s) and gestational sac(s)
- Evaluation of maternal uterus, adnexa and/or cervix

Relative Value Units (RVUs)

Work RVUs	0.75
Non-Facility Total	2.75
Facility Total	Only valued for non-facility

Additional Notes

- When a comprehensive maternal and fetal evaluation is performed, report 76801-76810
- This code is reported once regardless of the gestation number
- This code is reported once per examination, not per element
- The highest valued ultrasound procedure should be listed first on the claim form. No modifier -51 is necessary
- Follow-up care is not included in the ultrasound procedure
- ACOG clinical policy recognizes the need for multiple ultrasounds in the first trimester of pregnancy for certain clinical conditions. Clinical conditions include but are not limited to:
  - First trimester bleeding
  - Suspected or known ectopic pregnancy
  - Pelvic pain
  - Ovarian cycts
  - Uncertain dating
  - Gestational trophoblastic disease
  - Mullerian anomalies
  - Risk of multiple gestation
  - History of recurrent pregnancy loss
- Suspected or known early pregnancy loss

CPT® CODE 76818

- Fetal biophysical profile; with non-stress testing

INCLUDED IN THIS PROCEDURE

- Fetal breathing movements
  - 1 or more episodes of rhythmic fetal breathing movement of 30 seconds or more within 30 minutes
- Fetal movements
  - 3 or more discrete body or limb movements within 30 minutes
- Fetal tone
  - 1 or more episodes of fetal extremity extension with return to flexion
- Quanitification of amniotic fluid

Relative Value Units (RVUs)

Work RVUs	1.05
Non-Facility Total	3.56
Facility Total	Only valued for non-facility

Additional Notes

- Report this code separately for each gestation using the modifier -59 to the additional codes
- The highest valued ultrasound procedure should be listed first on the claim form. No modifier -51 is necessary
- Follow-up care is not included in the ultrasound procedure

CPT® CODE 76819

- Fetal biophysical profile; without non-stress testing

INCLUDED IN THIS PROCEDURE

- Fetal breathing movements
  - 1 or more episodes of rhythmic fetal breathing movement of 30 seconds or more within 30 minutes
- Fetal movements
  - 3 or more discrete body or limb movements within 30 minutes
- Fetal tone
  - 1 or more episodes of fetal extremity extension with return to flexion
- Quantification of amniotic fluid

Relative Value Units (RVUs)

Work RVUs	0.77
Non-Facility Total	2.57
Facility Total	Only valued for non-facility

Additional Notes

- If an obstetrician performs a non-stress test and a radiologist performs the biophysical profile, the obstetrician should report 59025 and the radiologist should report 76819
- If a fetal non-stress test is performed, report 76818 instead of this code
- If an amniotic fluid index test is also performed, report 76818 instead of this code
- Report this code separately for each gestation using the modifier -59 to the additional codes
- The highest valued ultrasound procedure should be listed first on the claim form. No modifier -51 is necessary
- Follow-up care is not included in the ultrasound procedure

CPT® CODE 76820

Doppler velocimetry, fetal; umbilical artery

INCLUDED IN THIS PROCEDURE

- Visualization of a segment of the umbilical cord and umbilical artery
- Recording 2-4 waveforms during fetal inactivity
- Measurement of peak systolic and end diastolic frequency shift
- Comparing the average of 2-4 waveforms with normative values for gestational age

Relative Value Units (RVUs)

Work RVUs	0.50
Non-Facility Total	1.32
Facility Total	Only valued for non-facility

Additional Notes

- Report this code separately for each gestation using the modifier -59 to the additional codes
- The highest valued ultrasound procedure should be listed first on the claim form. No modifier -51 is necessary
- Follow-up care is not included in the ultrasound procedure

CPT® CODE 76821

Doppler velocimetry, fetal; middle cerebral artery

INCLUDED IN THIS PROCEDURE

- Location of the fetal head and anterior wing of the sphenoid bone
- Visualization of the middle cerebral artery near the origin from the circle of Willis
- Recording the highest velocity
- Comparing 2-4 measurements with normative values for gestational age

Relative Value Units (RVUs)

Work RVUs	0.70
Non-Facility Total	2.63
Facility Total	Only valued for non-facility

Additional Notes

- Report this code separately for each gestation using the modifier -59 to the additional codes
- The highest valued ultrasound procedure should be listed first on the claim form. No modifier -51 is necessary
- Follow-up care is not included in the ultrasound procedure

CPT® CODE 76825

Echocardiography, fetal, cardiovascular system, real time with image documentation (2D), with or without M-mode recording

INCLUDED IN THIS PROCEDURE

- Fetal orientation, fetal cephalic and caudal ends, extremities, and spine
- Determination of fetal situs
- Evaluation of the heart, including venous connections, chambers, competence, great arterial connections and movement of valves
- Evaluation of cardiac function

Relative Value Units (RVUs)

Work RVUs	1.67
Non-Facility Total	7.67
Facility Total	Only valued for non-facility

Additional Notes

- Report this code separately for each gestation using the modifier -59 to the additional codes
- The highest valued ultrasound procedure should be listed first on the claim form. No modifier -51 is necessary
- Follow-up care is not included in the ultrasound procedure

CPT® CODE 76826

Echocardiography, fetal, cardiovascular system, real time with image documentation (2D), with or without M-mode recording; follow-up or repeat study

INCLUDED IN THIS PROCEDURE

Evaluation of cardiac function

Relative Value Units (RVUs)

Work RVUs	0.83
Non-Facility Total	4.61
Facility Total	Only valued for non-facility

Additional Notes

- If all of the elements of 76825 are documented, it is appropriate to report 76825

CPT® CODE 76827

Doppler echocardiography, fetal, pulsed wave and/or continuous wave with spectral display; complete

INCLUDED IN THIS PROCEDURE

- Identification of vessels studied
- Quantification of results
- Assessment of amniotic fluid volume

Relative Value Units (RVUs)

Work RVUs	0.58
Non-Facility Total	2.06
Facility Total	Only valued for non-facility

Additional Notes

- Report 76820 or 76821 or velocimetry of umbilical or middle cerebral arteries
- Report this code separately for each gestation using the modifier -59 to the additional codes
- The highest valued ultrasound procedure should be listed first on the claim form. No modifier -51 is necessary
- Follow-up care is not included in the ultrasound procedure

CPT® CODE 76830

Ultrasound, transvaginal

INCLUDED IN THIS PROCEDURE

Imaging of uterus, tubes, ovaries, and pelvic structures as indicated

Relative Value Units (RVUs)

Work RVUs	0.69
Non-Facility Total	3.53
Facility Total	Only valued for non-facility

Additional Notes

- If the patient is pregnant, report 76817 instead of this code
- It is appropriate to bill both transvaginal and transabdominal approaches when medically necessary to view all structures
- The highest valued ultrasound procedure should be listed first on the claim form. No modifier -51 is necessary
- Follow-up care is not included in the ultrasound procedure

CPT® CODE 76831

Saline infusion sonohysterography (SIS), including color flow Doppler, when performed

INCLUDED IN THIS PROCEDURE

- Imaging of uterus, tubes, ovaries and pelvic structures as indicated
- Transvaginal ultrasound (76830)

Relative Value Units (RVUs)

Work RVUs	0.72
Non-Facility Total	3.42
Facility Total	Only valued for non-facility

Additional Notes

- The highest valued ultrasound procedure should be listed first on the claim form. No modifier -51 is necessary
- Follow-up care is not included in the ultrasound procedure

CPT® CODE 76856

Ultrasound, pelvic (nonobstetric), real time with image documentation; complete

INCLUDED IN THIS PROCEDURE

- Complete evaluation of pelvic anatomy
- Measurements of:
  - Uterus
  - Adnexal structures
  - Endometrium
  - Bladder (when indicated)
- Description of pelvic pathology

Relative Value Units (RVUs)

Work RVUs	0.69
Non-Facility Total	3.14
Facility Total	Only valued for non-facility

Additional Notes

- The highest valued ultrasound procedure should be listed first on the claim form. No modifier -51 is necessary
- Follow-up care is not included in the ultrasound procedure

CPT® CODE 76857

Ultrasound, pelvic (nonobstetric), real time with image documentation; limited or follow-up (eg, for follicles)

INCLUDED IN THIS PROCEDURE

At least one element from 76856 and/or re-evaluation of pelvic abnormalities

Relative Value Units (RVUs)

Work RVUs	0.50
Non-Facility Total	1.50
Facility Total	Only valued for non-facility

Additional Notes

- For complete pelvic echography, report 76856 instead
- If kidneys are assessed, report 76770 instead of this code
- For bladder volume without imaging, report 51798
- The highest valued ultrasound procedure should be listed first on the claim form. No modifier -51 is necessary
- Follow-up care is not included in the ultrasound procedure

CPT® CODE 76941

Ultrasonic guidance for intrauterine fetal transfusion or cordocentesis, imaging supervision and interpretation

INCLUDED IN THIS PROCEDURE

Real-time visualization of placental and umbilical cord anatomy for the percutaneous placement of a needle for fetal transfusion or cordocentesis

Relative Value Units (RVUs)

Work RVUs	0.00
Non-Facility Total	0.00
Facility Total	Only valued for non-facility

Additional Notes

- The highest valued ultrasound procedure should be listed first on the claim form. No modifier -51 is necessary
- Follow-up care is not included in the ultrasound procedure

CPT® CODE 76942

Ultrasonic guidance for needle placement (eg, biopsy, aspiration, injection, localization device), imaging supervision and interpretation

INCLUDED IN THIS PROCEDURE

Real-time visualization for separately reportable intervention which necessitates the needle placement.

Relative Value Units (RVUs)

Work RVUs	0.67
Non-Facility Total	1.77
Facility Total	Only valued for non-facility

Additional Notes

- The highest valued ultrasound procedure should be listed first on the claim form. No modifier -51 is necessary
- Follow-up care is not included in the ultrasound procedure

CPT® CODE 76945

Ultrasonic guidance for chorionic villus sampling, imaging supervision and interpretation

INCLUDED IN THIS PROCEDURE

Real-time visualization of intrauterine gestation and placenta for percutaneous placement of the CVS catheter

Relative Value Units (RVUs)

Work RVUs	0.00
Non-Facility Total	0.00
Facility Total	Only valued for non-facility

Additional Notes

- The highest valued ultrasound procedure should be listed first on the claim form. No modifier -51 is necessary
- Follow-up care is not included in the ultrasound procedure

CPT® CODE 76946

Ultrasonic guidance for amniocentesis, imaging supervision and interpretation

INCLUDED IN THIS PROCEDURE

Real-time visualization of intrauterine gestation for percutaneous placement into the amniotic sac

Relative Value Units (RVUs)

Work RVUs	0.38
Non-Facility Total	1.00
Facility Total	Only valued for non-facility

Additional Notes

- The highest valued ultrasound procedure should be listed first on the claim form. No modifier -51 is necessary
- Follow-up care is not included in the ultrasound procedure

CPT® CODE 76948

Ultrasonic guidance for aspiration of ova, imaging supervision and interpretation

INCLUDED IN THIS PROCEDURE

Real-time visualization of intrauterine gestation for percutaneous placement into the amniotic sac

Relative Value Units (RVUs)

Work RVUs	0.67
Non-Facility Total	2.39
Facility Total	Only valued for non-facility

Additional Notes

- The highest valued ultrasound procedure should be listed first on the claim form. No modifier -51 is necessary
- Follow-up care is not included in the ultrasound procedure

CPT® CODE 76977

Ultrasound bone density measurement and interpretation, peripheral site(s), any method

INCLUDED IN THIS PROCEDURE

- Measurement of one or more peripheral sites like the wrist or knee
- This code includes both measurement and interpretation

Relative Value Units (RVUs)

Work RVUs	0.05
Non-Facility Total	0.22
Facility Total	Only valued for non-facility

Additional Notes

- The highest valued ultrasound procedure should be listed first on the claim form. No modifier -51 is necessary
- Follow-up care is not included in the ultrasound procedure

CPT® CODE 76998

Ultrasonic guidance, intraoperative

INCLUDED IN THIS PROCEDURE

Examination of organs and other tissues for abnormalities during surgical procedure

Relative Value Units (RVUs)

Work RVUs	0.00
Non-Facility Total	0.00
Facility Total	Only valued for non-facility

Additional Notes

- Report second to the surgical procedure

CPT® CODE 77002

Fluoroscopic guidance for needle placement (eg, biopsy, aspiration, injection, localization device) (List separately in addition to code for primary procedure)

INCLUDED IN THIS PROCEDURE

Real-time visualization for separately reportable procedure

Relative Value Units (RVUs)

Work RVUs	0.54
Non-Facility Total	3.41
Facility Total	Only valued for non-facility

Coding Assistance

Add-On Code:

- Follow Primary Code Policies

CPT® CODE 77014

Computed tomography guidance for placement of radiation therapy fields

INCLUDED IN THIS PROCEDURE

Real-time visualization for separately reportable procedure

Relative Value Units (RVUs)

Work RVUs	0.85
Non-Facility Total	3.58
Facility Total	Only valued for non-facility

Reproductive Medicine Codes

CPT® CODE 89250

Culture of oocyte(s)/embryo(s), less than 4 days

INCLUDED PROCEDURES

Culture of oocyte(s) or embryo(s) for less than 4 days, including the day of insemination

Additional Notes

- Report for culturing fresh or cryopreserved oocyte(s) or embryo(s)
- If co-culture is performed, report 89251 instead of this code
- If culture is extended beyond 3 days, report 89272 in addition to this code

CPT® CODE 89251

Culture of oocyte(s)/embryo(s), less than 4 days; with co-culture of oocyte(s)/embryos

INCLUDED PROCEDURES

- Culture of oocyte(s) or embryo(s) for less than 4 days, including the day of insemination
- Co-culture with feeder cells

Additional Notes

- Report for culturing fresh or cryopreserved oocyte(s) or embryo(s)
- If culture is extended beyond 3 days, report 89272 in addition to this code

CPT® CODE 89253

Assisted embryo hatching, microtechniques (any method)

INCLUDED PROCEDURES

Micromanipulation technique to assist hatching of the embryo from the zona

Additional Notes

- Report for culturing fresh or cryopreserved oocyte(s) or embryo(s)

CPT® CODE 89254

Oocyte identification from follicular fluid

INCLUDED PROCEDURES

Identification of oocytes contained in the fluid aspirated at oocyte retrieval

Additional Notes

- Report this code once per IVF cycle regardless of the number of oocytes identified

CPT® CODE 89255

Preparation of embryo for transfer (any method)

INCLUDED PROCEDURES

- Embryo removal, preparation, transportation
- Examination of catheter after embryo(s) transfer

Additional Notes

- Report for culturing fresh or cryopreserved embryo(s)

CPT® CODE 89257

Sperm identification from aspiration (other than seminal fluid)

INCLUDED PROCEDURES

Identification of sperm from the vas deferens or epididymis

Additional Notes

- Report 89300-89322, 89260-89261 if sperm identification is from seminal fluid
- Report 89264 if sperm identification is from testis tissue

CPT® CODE 89258

Cryopreservation; embryo(s)

INCLUDED PROCEDURES

Cryopreservation at any stage of development

Additional Notes

- Report this code once for each day of cryopreservation during the IVF cycle
- Report 89335 for cryopreservation of testicular tissue
- Report 89398 for cryopreservation of ovarian tissue
- Report 89337 for cryopreservation of oocytes
- This code does not include equipment or supplies for long-term storage

CPT® CODE 89259

Cryopreservation; sperm

INCLUDED PROCEDURES

Cryopreservation; sperm

Additional Notes

- Report 89335 for cryopreservation of testicular tissue
- Report 89398 for cryopreservation of ovarian tissue
- Report 89337 for cryopreservation of oocytes
- This code does not include equipment or supplies for long-term storage

CPT® CODE 89260

Sperm isolation; simple prep (eg, sperm wash and swim-up) for insemination or diagnosis with semen analysis

INCLUDED PROCEDURES

- Performance of sperm wash or swim-up
- 89300-89320

Additional Notes

- Report 89261 for complex prep instead of this code
- Report 58323 for sperm washing without semen analysis instead of this code
- Report 89320 for semen analysis without sperm wash or swim-up instead of this code

CPT® CODE 89261

Sperm isolation; complex prep (eg, Percoll gradient, albumin gradient) for insemination or diagnosis with semen analysis

INCLUDED PROCEDURES

- Performance of sperm isolation from complex prep
- 89300-89320

Additional Notes

- Report 89260 for simple prep instead of this code
- Report 58323 for sperm washing without semen analysis instead of this code
- Report 89320 for semen analysis without sperm wash or swim-up instead of this code

CPT® CODE 89264

Sperm identification from testis tissue, fresh or cryopreserved

INCLUDED PROCEDURES

Identification and isolation of sperm

Additional Notes

- Report 54500-54505 for biopsy of testis

CPT® CODE 89268

Insemination of oocytes

INCLUDED PROCEDURES

In vitro insemination

Additional Notes

- Report for inseminating fresh or cryopreserved oocyte(s) or embryo(s)

CPT® CODE 89272

Extended culture of oocyte(s)/ embryo(s), 4-7 days

INCLUDED PROCEDURES

- Culture of oocyte(s) or embryo(s) on days 4-7
- Co-culture with feeder cells

Additional Notes

- Report in addition to 89250 or 89251 for cultures that extend 4-7 days
- Report for culturing fresh or cryopreserved oocyte(s) or embryo(s)

CPT® CODE 89280

Assisted oocyte fertilization, microtechnique; less than or equal to 10 oocytes

INCLUDED PROCEDURES

Any micromanipulation technique to assist fertilization of the oocyte

Additional Notes

- Report 89281 for fertilization of 10 or more oocytes instead of this code
- Report 89268 along with this code if conventional insemination is performed for diagnostic purposes

CPT® CODE 89281

Assisted oocyte fertilization, microtechnique; greater than 10 oocytes

INCLUDED PROCEDURES

Any micromanipulation technique to assist fertilization of the oocyte

Additional Notes

- Report 89280 for fertilization of less than 10 oocytes instead of this code
- Report 89268 in addition to this code if conventional insemination is performed for diagnostic purposes

CPT® CODE 89290

Biopsy, oocyte polar body or embryo blastomere, microtechnique (for pre-implantation genetic diagnosis); less than or equal to 5 embryos

INCLUDED PROCEDURES

Biopsy of oocyte polar body or embryo blastomere

Additional Notes

- Report 89291 in addition to this code for more than 5 biopsies
- Report for biopsies for fresh or cryopreserved oocyte(s) or embryo(s)

CPT® CODE 89291

Biopsy, oocyte polar body or embryo blastomere, microtechnique (for pre-implantation genetic diagnosis); greater than 5 embryos

INCLUDED PROCEDURES

Biopsy of oocyte polar body or embryo blastomere

Additional Notes

- Report 89290 instead of this code for less than 5 biopsies
- Report for biopsies for fresh or cryopreserved oocyte(s) or embryo(s)

CPT® CODE 89300

Semen analysis; presence and/or motility of sperm including Huhner test (postcoital)

INCLUDED PROCEDURES

Semen analysis including Huhner test

Additional Notes

- Report 89310-89322 for semen analysis that does not include a Huhner test

CPT® CODE 89310

Semen analysis; motility and count (not including Huhner test)

INCLUDED PROCEDURES

Motility and count

Additional Notes

- Report 89321 for analysis that does not include sperm count instead of this code
- Report 89320 for complete semen analysis instead of this code
- Report 89331 and appropriate semen analysis code for retrograde ejaculation

CPT® CODE 89320

Semen analysis; volume, count, motility, and differential

INCLUDED PROCEDURES

Volume, count, and differential

Additional Notes

- Report 89260 or 89261 if sperm isolation is also performed instead of this code
- Report 89322 for semen analysis that includes differential using strict morphologic criteria instead of this code
- Report 89331 and appropriate semen analysis code for retrograde ejaculation

CPT® CODE 89321

Semen analysis; sperm presence and motility of sperm, if performed

INCLUDED PROCEDURES

Presence and/or motility

Additional Notes

- Report 89300 if analysis includes Huhner test instead of this code
- Report 89310 if analysis includes sperm count instead of this code
- Report 89320 if analysis includes sperm count, volume and differential instead of this code
- Report 89331 and appropriate semen analysis code for retrograde ejaculation

CPT® CODE 89322

Semen analysis; volume, count, motility, and differential using strict morphologic criteria (eg, Kruger)

INCLUDED PROCEDURES

- Volume, count and differential
- Manual, complicated differential analysis including the assessment of several hundred sperm
- 89310
- 89320

Additional Notes

- Report 89320 if the analysis does not include strict morphologic criteria, instead of this code

CPT® CODE 89325

Sperm antibodies

INCLUDED PROCEDURES

Test for antibodies in cervical mucus, seminal plasma, sperm, or serum

CPT® CODE 89329

Sperm evaluation; hamster penetration test

INCLUDED PROCEDURES

Evaluation using hamster penetration test

Additional Notes

- Report 89330 for cervical mucus penetration test instead of this code

REPRODUCTIVE MEDICINE

CPT® CODE 89330

Sperm evaluation; cervical mucus penetration test, with or without spinnbarkeit test

INCLUDED PROCEDURES

Cervical mucus penetration test

Additional Notes

- Report 89329 if the hamster penetration test is performed

CPT® CODE 89331

Sperm evaluation, for retrograde ejaculation, urine (sperm concentration, motility, and morphology, as indicated)

INCLUDED PROCEDURES

- Sperm concentration, motility and morphology
- 81015

CPT® CODE 89335

Cryopreservation, reproductive tissue, testicular

INCLUDED PROCEDURES

Cryopreservation of testicular tissue

Additional Notes

- Report 89258 for cryopreservation of embryos instead of this code
- Report 89259 for cryopreservation of sperm instead of this code
- Report 89337 for cryopreservation of oocytes instead of this code
- Report 89398 for cryopreservation of ovarian reproductive tissue instead of this code
- This code does not include equipment or supplies for long-term storage

CPT® CODE 89337

Cryopreservation, mature oocyte(s)

INCLUDED PROCEDURES

Cryopreservation of oocytes

Additional Notes

- Report 89258 for cryopreservation of embryos instead of this code
- Report 89259 for cryopreservation of sperm instead of this code
- Report 89335 for cryopreservation of testicular reproductive tissue instead of this code
- Report 89398 for cryopreservation of ovarian reproductive tissue instead of this code
- This code does not include equipment or supplies for long-term storage

CPT® CODE 89342

Storage (per year); embryo(s)

INCLUDED PROCEDURES

Annual storage

Additional Notes

- This code does not include equipment or supplies for long-term storage

CPT® CODE 89343

Storage (per year); sperm/semen

INCLUDED PROCEDURES

Annual storage

Additional Notes

- This code does not include equipment or supplies for long-term storage

CPT® CODE 89344

Storage (per year); reproductive tissue, testicular/ovarian

INCLUDED PROCEDURES

Annual storage

Additional Notes

- This code does not include equipment or supplies for long-term storage

CPT® CODE 89346

Storage (per year); oocyte(s)

INCLUDED PROCEDURES

Annual storage

Additional Notes

- This code does not include equipment or supplies for long-term storage

CPT® CODE 89352

Thawing of cryopreserved; embryo(s)

INCLUDED PROCEDURES

- Thawing
- Culture if performed on same date

Additional Notes

- Report 89250, 89251, or 89272 if thawed embryo(s) are cultured beyond the date of the thaw
- This code does not include equipment or supplies for long-term storage

CPT® CODE 89353

Thawing of cryopreserved; sperm/semen, each aliquot

INCLUDED PROCEDURES

Thawing

Additional Notes

- This code does not include equipment or supplies for long-term storage

CPT® CODE 89354

Thawing of cryopreserved; reproductive tissue, testicular/ovarian

INCLUDED PROCEDURES

- Culture of oocyte(s) or embryo(s) for less than 4 days, including the day of insemination
- Co-culture with feeder cells

Additional Notes

- This code does not include equipment or supplies for long-term storage

CPT® CODE 89356

Thawing of cryopreserved; oocytes, each aliquot

INCLUDED PROCEDURES

Thawing

Additional Notes

- This code does not include equipment or supplies for long-term storage

Diagnostic Codes

CPT® CODE 51725

Simple cystometrogram (CMG) (eg, spinal manometer)

Relative Value Units (RVUs)

Work RVUs	1.51
Non-Facility Total	6.21
Facility Total	Only valued for non-facility

CPT® CODE 51726

Complex cystometrogram (ie, calibrated electronic equipment)

Relative Value Units (RVUs)

Work RVUs	1.71
Non-Facility Total	8.32
Facility Total	Only valued for non-facility

CPT® CODE 51727

Complex cystometrogram (ie, calibrated electronic equipment); with urethral pressure profile studies (ie, urethral closure pressure profile), any technique

Relative Value Units (RVUs)

Work RVUs	2.11
Non-Facility Total	10.21
Facility Total	Only valued for non-facility

CPT® CODE 51728

Complex cystometrogram (ie, calibrated electronic equipment); with voiding pressure studies (ie, bladder voiding pressure), any technique

Relative Value Units (RVUs)

Work RVUs	2.11
Non-Facility Total	10.16
Facility Total	Only valued for non-facility

CPT® CODE 51729

Complex cystometrogram (ie, calibrated electronic equipment); with voiding pressure studies (ie, bladder voiding pressure) and urethral pressure profile studies (ie, urethral closure pressure profile), any technique

Relative Value Units (RVUs)

Work RVUs	2.51
Non-Facility Total	10.76
Facility Total	Only valued for non-facility

CPT® CODE 51736

Simple uroflowmetry (UFR) (eg, stop-watch flow rate, mechanical uroflowmeter)

Relative Value Units (RVUs)

Work RVUs	0.17
Non-Facility Total	0.41
Facility Total	Only valued for non-facility

CPT® CODE 51741

Complex uroflowmetry (eg, calibrated electronic equipment)

Relative Value Units (RVUs)

Work RVUs	0.17
Non-Facility Total	0.43
Facility Total	Only valued for non-facility

CPT® CODE 51784

Electromyography studies (EMG) of anal or urethral sphincter, other than needle, any technique

Relative Value Units (RVUs)

Work RVUs	0.75
Non-Facility Total	1.92
Facility Total	Only valued for non-facility

CPT® CODE 51785

Needle electromyography studies (EMG) of anal or urethral sphincter, any technique

Relative Value Units (RVUs)

Work RVUs	1.53
Non-Facility Total	11.82
Facility Total	Only valued for non-facility

CPT® CODE 51792

Stimulus evoked response (eg, measurement of bulbocavernosus reflex latency time)

Relative Value Units (RVUs)

Work RVUs	1.10
Non-Facility Total	7.57
Facility Total	Only valued for non-facility

CPT® CODE 51797

Voiding pressure studies, intra-abdominal (ie, rectal, gastric, intraperitoneal)
(List separately in addition to code for primary procedure)

Relative Value Units (RVUs)

Work RVUs	0.80
Non-Facility Total	4.98
Facility Total	Only valued for non-facility

CPT® CODE 51798

Measurement of post-voiding residual urine and/or bladder capacity by ultrasound, non-imaging

Relative Value Units (RVUs)

Work RVUs	0.00
Non-Facility Total	0.35
Facility Total	Only valued for non-facility

CPT® CODE 59050

Fetal monitoring during labor by consulting physician (ie, non-attending physician) with written report; supervision and interpretation

Relative Value Units (RVUs)

Work RVUs	0.89
Non-Facility Total	Only valued for Facility
Facility Total	1.50

POLICY INDICATORS

Global Period
N/A

Assistants at Surgery
Submit reason for assistant

Co-Surgeons Allowed
No co-surgeon

Reduction for Multiple Procedures
Not subject to multiple surgery reduction

Bilateral Surgery Payment
N/A

Applicable Medicare Policies

CPT® CODE 95970

Electronic analysis of implanted neurostimulator pulse generator/transmitter (eg, contact group[s], interleaving, amplitude, pulse width, frequency [Hz], on/off cycling, burst, magnet mode, dose lockout, patient selectable parameters, responsive neurostimulation, detection algorithms, closed loop parameters, and passive parameters) by physician or other qualified health care professional; with brain, cranial nerve, spinal cord, peripheral nerve, or sacral nerve, neurostimulator pulse generator/transmitter, without programming

Relative Value Units (RVUs)

Work RVUs	0.35
Non-Facility Total	0.56
Facility Total	0.55

CPT® CODE 95971

Electronic analysis of implanted neurostimulator pulse generator/transmitter (eg, contact group[s], interleaving, amplitude, pulse width, frequency [Hz], on/off cycling, burst, magnet mode, dose lockout, patient selectable parameters, responsive neurostimulation, with simple spinal cord or peripheral nerve (eg, sacral nerve) neurostimulator pulse generator/transmitter programming by physician or other qualified health care professional

Relative Value Units (RVUs)

Work RVUs	0.78
Non-Facility Total	1.43
Facility Total	1.15

On telehealth list

CPT® CODE 95972

Electronic analysis of implanted neurostimulator pulse generator/transmitter (eg, contact group[s], interleaving, amplitude, pulse width, frequency [Hz], on/off cycling, burst, magnet mode, dose lockout, patient selectable parameters, responsive neurostimulation, with complex spinal cord or peripheral nerve (eg, sacral nerve) neurostimulator pulse generator/transmitter programming by physician or other qualified health care professional

On telehealth list

Relative Value Units (RVUs)

Work RVUs	0.80
Non-Facility Total	1.70
Facility Total	1.18

CPT® CODE 99091

Collection and interpretation of physiologic data (eg, ECG, blood pressure, glucose monitoring) digitally stored and/or transmitted by the patient and/or caregiver to the physician or other qualified health care professional, qualified by education, training, licensure/regulation (when applicable) requiring a minimum of 30 minutes of time, each 30 days

Relative Value Units (RVUs)

Work RVUs	1.10
Non-Facility Total	1.60
Facility Total	1.60

Telemedicine Codes

CPT® CODE 98000 SYNCHRONOUS AUDIO-VIDEO VISIT: NEW PATIENT

Synchronous audio-video visits for the evaluation and management of a new patient, which requires a medically appropriate history and/or examination and straightforward medical decision making. When using total time on the date of the encounter for code selection, 15 minutes must be met or exceeded.

Relative Value Units (RVUs)

Work RVUs	0.93
Non-Facility Total	1.54
Facility Total	1.35

CPT® CODE 98001

Synchronous audio-video visit for the evaluation and management of a new patient, which requires a medically appropriate history and/or examination and low medical decision making. When using total time on the date of the encounter for code selection, 30 minutes must be met or exceeded.

Relative Value Units (RVUs)

Work RVUs	1.60
Non-Facility Total	2.54
Facility Total	2.33

CPT® CODE 98002

Synchronous audio-video visit for the evaluation and management of a new patient, which requires a medically appropriate history and/or examination and moderate medical decision making. When using total time on the date of the encounter for code selection, 45 minutes must be met or exceeded.

Relative Value Units (RVUs)

Work RVUs	2.60
Non-Facility Total	4.05
Facility Total	3.78

CPT® CODE 98003

Synchronous audio-video visit for the evaluation and management of a new patient, which requires a medically appropriate history and/or examination and high medical decision making. When using total time on the date of the encounter for code selection, 60 minutes must be met or exceeded. (For services 75 minutes or longer, use prolonged services code 99417)

Relative Value Units (RVUs)

Work RVUs	3.50
Non-Facility Total	5.37
Facility Total	5.08

CPT® CODE 98004 SYNCHRONOUS AUDIO-VIDEO VISIT: ESTABLISHED PATIENT

Synchronous audio-video visit for the evaluation and management of an established patient, which requires a medically appropriate history and/or examination and straightforward medical decision making. When using total time on the date of the encounter for code selection, 10 minutes must be met or exceeded.

Relative Value Units (RVUs)

Work RVUs	0.70
Non-Facility Total	1.54
Facility Total	1.01

CPT® CODE 98005

Synchronous audio-video visit for the evaluation and management of an established patient, which requires a medically appropriate history and/or examination and low medical decision making. When using total time on the date of the encounter for code selection, 20 minutes must be met or exceeded.

Relative Value Units (RVUs)

Work RVUs	1.30
Non-Facility Total	2.08
Facility Total	1.88

CPT® CODE 98006

Synchronous audio-video visit for the evaluation and management of an established patient, which requires a medically appropriate history and/or examination and moderate medical decision making. When using total time on the date of the encounter for code selection, 30 minutes must be met or exceeded.

Relative Value Units (RVUs)

Work RVUs	1.92
Non-Facility Total	3.07
Facility Total	2.80

CPT® CODE 98007

Synchronous audio-video visit for the evaluation and management of an established patient, which requires a medically appropriate history and/or examination and high medical decision making. When using total time on the date of the encounter for code selection, 40 minutes must be met or exceeded.

Relative Value Units (RVUs)

Work RVUs	2.60
Non-Facility Total	4.07
Facility Total	3.78

CPT® CODE 98008 SYNCHRONOUS AUDIO-ONLY VISIT: NEW PATIENT

Synchronous audio-only visit for the evaluation and management of a new patient, which requires a medically appropriate history and/or examination, straightforward medical decision making, and more than 10 minutes of medical discussion. When using total time on the date of the encounter for code selection, 15 minutes must be met or exceeded.

Relative Value Units (RVUs)

Work RVUs	0.90
Non-Facility Total	1.46
Facility Total	1.29

CPT® CODE 98009

Synchronous audio-only visit for the evaluation and management of a new patient, which requires a medically appropriate history and/or examination, low medical decision making, and more than 10 minutes of medical discussion. When using total time on the date of the encounter for code selection, 30 minutes must be met or exceeded.

Relative Value Units (RVUs)

Work RVUs	1.55
Non-Facility Total	2.42
Facility Total	2.24

CPT® CODE 98010

Synchronous audio-only visit for the evaluation and management of a new patient, which requires a medically appropriate history and/or examination, moderate medical decision making, and more than 10 minutes of medical discussion. When using total time on the date of the encounter for code selection, 45 minutes must be met or exceeded.

Relative Value Units (RVUs)

Work RVUs	2.42
Non-Facility Total	3.77
Facility Total	3.53

CPT® CODE 98011

Synchronous audio-only visit for the evaluation and management of a new patient, which requires a medically appropriate history and/or examination, high medical decision making, and more than 10 minutes of medical discussion. When using total time on the date of the encounter for code selection, 60 minutes must be met or exceeded. (For services 75 minutes or longer, use prolonged services code 99417)

Relative Value Units (RVUs)

Work RVUs	3.20
Non-Facility Total	4.90
Facility Total	4.64

CPT® CODE 98012 SYNCHRONOUS AUDIO-ONLY VISIT: ESTABLISHED PATIENT

Synchronous audio-only visit for the evaluation and management of an established patient, which requires a medically appropriate history and/or examination, straightforward medical decision making, and more than 10 minutes of medical discussion. When using total time on the date of the encounter for code selection, 10 minutes must be exceeded.

Relative Value Units (RVUs)

Work RVUs	0.65
Non-Facility Total	1.09
Facility Total	0.95

CPT® CODE 98013

Synchronous audio-only visit for the evaluation and management of an established patient, which requires a medically appropriate history and/or examination, low medical decision making, and more than 10 minutes of medical discussion. When using total time on the date of the encounter for code selection, 20 minutes must be met or exceeded.

Relative Value Units (RVUs)

Work RVUs	1.20
Non-Facility Total	1.90
Facility Total	1.73

CPT® CODE 98014

Synchronous audio-only visit for the evaluation and management of an established patient, which requires a medically appropriate history and/or examination, moderate medical decision making, and more than 10 minutes of medical discussion. When using total time on the date of the encounter for code selection, 30 minutes must be met or exceeded.

Relative Value Units (RVUs)

Work RVUs	1.75
Non-Facility Total	2.78
Facility Total	2.56

CPT® CODE 98015

Synchronous audio-only visit for the evaluation and management of an established patient, which requires a medically appropriate history and/or examination, high medical decision making, and more than 10 minutes of medical discussion. When using total time on the date of the encounter for code selection, 40 minutes must be met or exceeded. (For services 55 minutes or longer, use prolonged services code 99417)

Relative Value Units (RVUs)

Work RVUs	2.60
Non-Facility Total	4.04
Facility Total	3.78

CPT® CODE 98016 BRIEF SYNCHRONOUS COMMUNICATION TECHNOLOGY (VIRTUAL CHECK-IN)

Brief communication technology-based service (e.g., virtual check-in) by a physician or other qualified health care professional who can report evaluation and management services provided to an established patient, not originating from a related evaluation and management service provided within the previous 7 days nor leading to an evaluation and management service or procedure within the next 24 hours or the soonest available appointment, 5-10 minutes of medical discussion

Relative Value Units (RVUs)

Work RVUs	0.30
Non-Facility Total	0.49
Facility Total	0.45

Evaluation and Management Codes

CPT® CODE 99202 NEW PATIENT: OUTPATIENT

Office or other outpatient visit for the evaluation and management of a new patient, which requires a medically appropriate history and/or examination and straightforward medical decision making. When using total time on the date of the encounter for code selection, 15 minutes must be met or exceeded.

Relative Value Units (RVUs)

Work RVUs	0.93
Non-Facility Total	2.16
Facility Total	1.40

CPT® CODE 99203

Office or other outpatient visit for the evaluation and management of a new patient, which requires a medically appropriate history and/or examination and low level of medical decision making. When using total time on the date of the encounter for code selection, 30 minutes must be met or exceeded.

Relative Value Units (RVUs)

Work RVUs	1.60
Non-Facility Total	3.37
Facility Total	2.45

CPT® CODE 99204

Office or other outpatient visit for the evaluation and management of a new patient, which requires a medically appropriate history and/or examination and moderate level of medical decision making. When using total time on the date of the encounter for code selection, 45 minutes must be met or exceeded.

Relative Value Units (RVUs)

Work RVUs	2.60
Non-Facility Total	5.05
Facility Total	3.99

CPT® CODE 99205

Office or other outpatient visit for the evaluation and management of a new patient, which requires a medically appropriate history and/or examination and high level of medical decision making. When using total time on the date of the encounter for code selection, 60 minutes must be met or exceeded.

Relative Value Units (RVUs)

Work RVUs	3.50
Non-Facility Total	6.67
Facility Total	5.43

EVALUATION AND MANAGEMENT

CPT® CODE 99211 ESTABLISHED PATIENT: OUTPATIENT

Office or other outpatient visit for the evaluation and management of an established patient that may not require the presence of a physician or other qualified health care professional

Relative Value Units (RVUs)

Work RVUs	0.18
Non-Facility Total	0.70
Facility Total	0.26

CPT® CODE 99212

Office or other outpatient visit for the evaluation and management of an established patient, which requires a medically appropriate history and/or examination and straightforward medical decision making. When using total time on the date of the encounter for code selection, 10 minutes must be met or exceeded.

Relative Value Units (RVUs)

Work RVUs	0.70
Non-Facility Total	1.70
Facility Total	1.05

CPT® CODE 99213

Office or other outpatient visit for the evaluation and management of an established patient, which requires a medically appropriate history and/or examination and low level of medical decision making. When using total time on the date of the encounter for code selection, 20 minutes must be met or exceeded.

Relative Value Units (RVUs)

Work RVUs	1.30
Non-Facility Total	2.75
Facility Total	1.97

CPT® CODE 99214

Office or other outpatient visit for the evaluation and management of an established patient, which requires a medically appropriate history and/or examination and moderate level of medical decision making. When using total time on the date of the encounter for code selection, 30 minutes must be met or exceeded.

Relative Value Units (RVUs)

Work RVUs	1.92
Non-Facility Total	3.87
Facility Total	2.90

CPT® CODE 99215

Office or other outpatient visit for the evaluation and management of an established patient, which requires a medically appropriate history and/or examination and high level of medical decision making. When using total time on the date of the encounter for code selection, 40 minutes must be met or exceeded.

Relative Value Units (RVUs)

Work RVUs	2.80
Non-Facility Total	5.43
Facility Total	4.29

CPT® CODE 99221 INPATIENT OR OBSERVATION: INITIAL

Initial hospital inpatient or observation care, per day, for the evaluation and management of a patient, which requires a medically appropriate history and/or examination and straightforward or low-level medical decision making. When using total time on the date of the encounter for code selection, 40 minutes must be met or exceeded.

Relative Value Units (RVUs),

Work RVUs	1.63
Non-Facility Total	Only valued for facility
Facility Total	2.46

CPT® CODE 99222

Initial hospital inpatient or observation care, per day, for the evaluation and management of a patient, which requires a medically appropriate history and/or examination and moderate level of medical decision making. When using total time on the date of the encounter for code selection, 55 minutes must be met or exceeded.

Relative Value Units (RVUs)

Work RVUs	2.60
Non-Facility Total	Only valued for facility
Facility Total	3.88

CPT® CODE 99223

Initial hospital inpatient or observation care, per day, for the evaluation and management of a patient, which requires a medically appropriate history and/or examination and high level of medical decision making. When using total time on the date of the encounter for code selection, 75 minutes must be met or exceeded.

Relative Value Units (RVUs)

Work RVUs	3.50
Non-Facility Total	Only valued for facility
Facility Total	5.17

CPT® CODE 99231 INPATIENT OR OBSERVATION: SUBSEQUENT

Subsequent hospital inpatient or observation care, per day, for the evaluation and management of a patient, which requires a medically appropriate history and/or examination and straightforward or low level of medical decision making. When using total time on the date of the encounter for code selection, 25 minutes must be met or exceeded.

Relative Value Units (RVUs)

Work RVUs	1.00
Non-Facility Total	Only valued for facility
Facility Total	1.46

CPT® CODE 99232

Subsequent hospital inpatient or observation care, per day, for the evaluation and management of a patient, which requires a medically appropriate history and/or examination and moderate level of medical decision making. When using total time on the date of the encounter for code selection, 35 minutes must be met or exceeded.

Relative Value Units (RVUs)

Work RVUs	1.59
Non-Facility Total	Only valued for facility
Facility Total	2.36

CPT® CODE 99233

Subsequent hospital inpatient or observation care, per day, for the evaluation and management of a patient, which requires a medically appropriate history and/or examination and high level of medical decision making. When using total time on the date of the encounter for code selection, 50 minutes must be met or exceeded.

Relative Value Units (RVUs)

Work RVUs	2.40
Non-Facility Total	Only valued for facility
Facility Total	3.52

CPT® CODE 99234

INPATIENT OR OBSERVATION: SAME-DAY ADMISSION AND DISCHARGE

Hospital inpatient or observation care, for the evaluation and management of a patient including admission and discharge on the same date, which requires a medically appropriate history and/or examination and straightforward or low level of medical decision making. When using total time on the date of the encounter for code selection, 45 minutes must be met or exceeded.

Relative Value Units (RVUs)

Work RVUs	2.00
Non-Facility Total	Only valued for facility
Facility Total	2.90

CPT® CODE 99235

Hospital inpatient or observation care, for the evaluation and management of a patient including admission and discharge on the same date, which requires a medically appropriate history and/or examination and moderate level of medical decision making. When using total time on the date of the encounter for code selection, 70 minutes must be met or exceeded.

Relative Value Units (RVUs)

Work RVUs	3.24
Non-Facility Total	Only valued for facility
Facility Total	4.72

CPT® CODE 99236

Hospital inpatient or observation care, for the evaluation and management of a patient including admission and discharge on the same date, which requires a medically appropriate history and/or examination and high level of medical decision making. When using total time on the date of the encounter for code selection, 85 minutes must be met or exceeded.

Relative Value Units (RVUs)

Work RVUs	4.30
Non-Facility Total	Only valued for facility
Facility Total	6.17

CPT® CODE 99238 INPATIENT OR OBSERVATION: DISCHARGE ONLY

Hospital inpatient or observation discharge day management; 30 minutes or less on the date of the encounter.

Relative Value Units (RVUs)

Work RVUs	1.50
Non-Facility Total	Only valued for facility
Facility Total	2.42

CPT® CODE 99239

Hospital inpatient or observation discharge day management more than 30 minutes on the date of the encounter.

Relative Value Units (RVUs)

Work RVUs	2.15
Non-Facility Total	Only valued for facility
Facility Total	3.42

EVALUATION AND MANAGEMENT

CPT® CODE 99242 OUTPATIENT CONSULTATION

Office or other outpatient consultation for a new or established patient, which requires a medically appropriate history and/or examination and straightforward medical decision making. When using total time on the date of the encounter for code selection, 20 minutes must be met or exceeded.

Relative Value Units (RVUs)

Work RVUs	1.08
Non-Facility Total	2.24
Facility Total	1.65

CPT® CODE 99243

Office or other outpatient consultation for a new or established patient, which requires a medically appropriate history and/or examination and low level of medical decision making. When using total time on the date of the encounter for code selection, 30 minutes must be met or exceeded.

Relative Value Units (RVUs)

Work RVUs	1.80
Non-Facility Total	3.38
Facility Total	2.63

CPT® CODE 99244

Office or other outpatient consultation for a new or established patient, which requires a medically appropriate history and/or examination and moderate level of medical decision making. When using total time on the date of the encounter for code selection, 40 minutes must be met or exceeded.

Relative Value Units (RVUs)

Work RVUs	2.69
Non-Facility Total	4.81
Facility Total	3.99

CPT® CODE 99245

Office or other outpatient consultation for a new or established patient, which requires a medically appropriate history and/or examination and high level of medical decision making. When using total time on the date of the encounter for code selection, 55 minutes must be met or exceeded.

Relative Value Units (RVUs)

Work RVUs	3.75
Non-Facility Total	6.27
Facility Total	5.36

CPT® CODE 99252 INPATIENT OR OBSERVATION CONSULTATION

Inpatient or observation consultation for a new or established patient, which requires a medically appropriate history and/or examination and straightforward medical decision making. When using total time on the date of the encounter for code selection, 35 minutes must be met or exceeded.

Relative Value Units (RVUs)

Work RVUs	1.50
Non-Facility Total	Only valued for facility
Facility Total	2.10

CPT® CODE 99253

Inpatient or observation consultation for a new or established patient, which requires a medically appropriate history and/or examination and low level of medical decision making. When using total time on the date of the encounter for code selection, 45 minutes must be met or exceeded.

Relative Value Units (RVUs)

Work RVUs	2.00
Non-Facility Total	Only valued for facility
Facility Total	2.97

CPT® CODE 99254

Inpatient or observation consultation for a new or established patient, which requires a medically appropriate history and/or examination and moderate level of medical decision making. When using total time on the date of the encounter for code selection, 60 minutes must be met or exceeded.

Relative Value Units (RVUs)

Work RVUs	2.72
Non-Facility Total	Only valued for facility
Facility Total	4.11

CPT® CODE 99255

Inpatient or observation consultation for a new or established patient, which requires a medically appropriate history and/or examination and high level of medical decision making. When using total time on the date of the encounter for code selection, 80 minutes must be met or exceeded.

Relative Value Units (RVUs)

Work RVUs	3.86
Non-Facility Total	Only valued for facility
Facility Total	5.52

CPT® CODE 99281

EMERGENCY DEPARTMENT

Emergency department visit for the evaluation and management of a patient that may not require the presence of a physician or other qualified health care professional.

Relative Value Units (RVUs)

Work RVUs	0.25
Non-Facility Total	Only valued for facility
Facility Total	0.34

CPT® CODE 99282

Emergency department visit for the evaluation and management of a patient, which requires a medically appropriate history and/or examination and straightforward medical decision making.

Relative Value Units (RVUs)

Work RVUs	0.93
Non-Facility Total	Only valued for facility
Facility Total	1.25

CPT® CODE 99283

Emergency department visit for the evaluation and management of a patient, which requires a medically appropriate history and/or examination and low level of medical decision making.

Relative Value Units (RVUs)

Work RVUs	1.60
Non-Facility Total	Only valued for facility
Facility Total	2.11

CPT® CODE 99284

Emergency department visit for the evaluation and management of a patient, which requires a medically appropriate history and/or examination and moderate level of medical decision making.

Relative Value Units (RVUs)

Work RVUs	2.74
Non-Facility Total	Only valued for facility
Facility Total	3.60

CPT® CODE 99285

Emergency department visit for the evaluation and management of a patient, which requires a medically appropriate history and/or examination and high level of medical decision making.

Relative Value Units (RVUs)

Work RVUs	4.00
Non-Facility Total	Only valued for facility
Facility Total	5.22

CPT® CODE 99358 PROLONGED SERVICES: NON-FACE-TO-FACE TIME

Prolonged evaluation and management service before and/or after direct patient care; first hour.

Relative Value Units (RVUs)

Work RVUs	1.80
Non-Facility Total	2.67
Facility Total	2.63

CPT® CODE 99359

Prolonged evaluation and management service before and/or after direct patient care each additional 30 minutes.
(List separately in addition to code for prolonged service.) (Use 99359 in conjunction with 99358.)

Relative Value Units (RVUs)

Work RVUs	0.75
Non-Facility Total	1.13
Facility Total	1.08

Additional Notes

- Codes 99358 and 99359 are used when a prolonged service is provided on a date other than the date of a face-to-face evaluation and management encounter with the patient and/or family/caregiver. Codes 99358 and 99359 may be reported for prolonged services in relation to any evaluation and management service on a date other than the face-to-face service, whether or not time was used to select the level of the face-to-face service.
- If the non-face-to-face work was less than 30 minutes, do not report.
- Report 99358 for 30-74 minutes.
- Add 99359 for additional 30 minutes after 74 minutes, and 2 units after 104 minutes.

CPT® CODE 99360 STANDBY SERVICE

Standby service, requiring prolonged attendance, each 30 minutes (eg, operative standby, standby for frozen section, for cesarean/high risk delivery, for monitoring EEG)

Relative Value Units (RVUs)

Work RVUs	1.20
Non-Facility Total	Only valued for facility
Facility Total	1.73

CPT® CODE 99366 MEDICAL TEAM CONFERENCE

Medical team conference with interdisciplinary team of health care professionals, face-to-face with patient and/or family, 30 minutes or more, participation by nonphysician qualified health care professional

Relative Value Units (RVUs)

Work RVUs	0.82
Non-Facility Total	1.21
Facility Total	1.18

CPT® CODE 99367

Medical team conference with interdisciplinary team of health care professionals, patient and/or family not present, 30 minutes or more; participation by physician

Relative Value Units (RVUs)

Work RVUs	1.10
Non-Facility Total	Only valued for facility
Facility Total	1.59

CPT® CODE 99368

Medical team conference with interdisciplinary team of health care professionals, patient and/or family not present, 30 minutes or more; participation by nonphysician qualified health care professional

Relative Value Units (RVUs)

Work RVUs	0.72
Non-Facility Total	Only valued for facility
Facility Total	1.04

CPT® CODE 99383 INITIAL PREVENTIVE VISIT

Initial comprehensive preventive medicine evaluation and management of an individual including an age and gender appropriate history, examination, counseling/anticipatory guidance/risk factor reduction interventions, and the ordering of laboratory/diagnostic tests; late childhood (age 5 through 11 years)

Relative Value Units (RVUs)

Work RVUs	1.70
Non-Facility Total	3.57
Facility Total	2.47

CPT® CODE 99384

Initial comprehensive preventive medicine evaluation and management of an individual including an age and gender appropriate history, examination, counseling/anticipatory guidance/risk factor reduction interventions, and the ordering of laboratory/diagnostic tests; adolescent (age 12 through 17 years)

Relative Value Units (RVUs)

Work RVUs	2.00
Non-Facility Total	4.01
Facility Total	2.92

CPT® CODE 99385

Initial comprehensive preventive medicine evaluation and management of an individual including an age and gender appropriate history, examination, counseling/anticipatory guidance/risk factor reduction interventions, and the ordering of laboratory/diagnostic tests; 18-39 years

Relative Value Units (RVUs)

Work RVUs	1.92
Non-Facility Total	3.90
Facility Total	2.80

CPT® CODE 99386

Initial comprehensive preventive medicine evaluation and management of an individual including an age and gender appropriate history, examination, counseling/anticipatory guidance/risk factor reduction interventions, and the ordering of laboratory/diagnostic tests; 40-64 years

Relative Value Units (RVUs)

Work RVUs	2.33
Non-Facility Total	4.49
Facility Total	3.39

CPT® CODE 99387

Initial comprehensive preventive medicine evaluation and management of an individual including an age and gender appropriate history, examination, counseling/anticipatory guidance/risk factor reduction interventions, and the ordering of laboratory/diagnostic tests; 65 years and older

Relative Value Units (RVUs)

Work RVUs	2.50
Non-Facility Total	4.88
Facility Total	3.64

CPT® CODE 99393 PERIODIC PREVENTIVE VISIT

Periodic comprehensive preventive medicine reevaluation and management of an individual including an age and gender appropriate history, examination, counseling/anticipatory guidance/risk factor reduction interventions, and the ordering of laboratory/diagnotic tests; late childhood (age 5 through 11 years)

Relative Value Units (RVUs)

Work RVUs	1.50
Non-Facility Total	3.13
Facility Total	2.17

CPT® CODE 99394

Periodic comprehensive preventive medicine reevaluation and management of an individual including an age and gender appropriate history, examination, counseling/anticipatory guidance/risk factor reduction interventions, and the ordering of laboratory/diagnotic tests; adolescent (age 12 through 17 years)

Relative Value Units (RVUs)

Work RVUs	1.70
Non-Facility Total	3.42
Facility Total	2.47

CPT® CODE 99395

Periodic comprehensive preventive medicine reevaluation and management of an individual including an age and gender appropriate history, examination, counseling/anticipatory guidance/risk factor reduction interventions, and the ordering of laboratory/diagnostic tests; 18-39 years

Relative Value Units (RVUs)

Work RVUs	1.75
Non-Facility Total	3.52
Facility Total	2.56

CPT® CODE 99396

Periodic comprehensive preventive medicine reevaluation and management of an individual including an age and gender appropriate history, examination, counseling/anticipatory guidance/risk factor reduction interventions, and the ordering of laboratory/diagnostic tests; 40-64 years

Relative Value Units (RVUs)

Work RVUs	1.90
Non-Facility Total	3.74
Facility Total	2.78

CPT® CODE 99397

Periodic comprehensive preventive medicine reevaluation and management of an individual including an age and gender appropriate history, examination, counseling/anticipatory guidance/risk factor reduction interventions, and the ordering of laboratory/diagnostic tests; 65 years and older

Relative Value Units (RVUs)

Work RVUs	2.00
Non-Facility Total	4.03
Facility Total	2.92

CPT® CODE 99401 PREVENTIVE MEDICINE COUNSELING

Preventive medicine counseling and/or risk factor reduction intervention(s) provided to an individual (separate procedure); approximately 15 minutes

Relative Value Units (RVUs)

Work RVUs	0.48
Non-Facility Total	1.15
Facility Total	0.70

CPT® CODE 99402

Preventive medicine counseling and/or risk factor reduction intervention(s) provided to an individual (separate procedure); approximately 30 minutes

Relative Value Units (RVUs)

Work RVUs	0.98
Non-Facility Total	1.87
Facility Total	1.41

CPT® CODE 99403

Preventive medicine counseling and/or risk factor reduction intervention(s) provided to an individual (separate procedure); approximately 45 minutes

Relative Value Units (RVUs)

Work RVUs	1.46
Non-Facility Total	2.56
Facility Total	2.11

CPT® CODE 99404

Preventive medicine counseling and/or risk factor reduction intervention(s) provided to an individual (separate procedure); approximately 60 minutes

Relative Value Units (RVUs)

Work RVUs	1.95
Non-Facility Total	3.30
Facility Total	2.85

CPT® CODE 99406 SMOKING AND TOBACCO COUNSELING

Smoking and tobacco use cessation counseling visit; intermediate, greater than 3 minutes up to 10 minutes

Relative Value Units (RVUs)

Work RVUs	0.24
Non-Facility Total	0.43
Facility Total	0.35

CPT® CODE 99407

Smoking and tobacco use cessation counseling visit; intensive, greater than 10 minutes

Relative Value Units (RVUs)

Work RVUs	0.50
Non-Facility Total	0.82
Facility Total	0.74

CPT® CODE 99408 ALCOHOL/SUBSTANCE ABUSE COUNSELING

Alcohol and/or substance (other than tobacco) abuse structured screening (eg, AUDIT, DAST), and brief intervention (SBI) services; 15 to 30 minutes

Relative Value Units (RVUs)

Work RVUs	0.65
Non-Facility Total	1.02
Facility Total	0.95

CPT® CODE 99409

Alcohol and/or substance (other than tobacco) abuse structured screening (eg, AUDIT, DAST), and brief intervention (SBI) services; greater than 30 minutes

Relative Value Units (RVUs)

Work RVUs	1.30
Non-Facility Total	1.96
Facility Total	1.88

CPT® CODE 99411 GROUP COUNSELING

Preventive medicine counseling and/or risk factor reduction intervention(s) provided to individuals in a group setting (separate procedure); approximately 30 minutes

Relative Value Units (RVUs)

Work RVUs	0.15
Non-Facility Total	0.59
Facility Total	0.22

CPT® CODE 99412

Preventive medicine counseling and/or risk factor reduction intervention(s) provided to individuals in a group setting (separate procedure); approximately 60 minutes

Relative Value Units (RVUs)

Work RVUs	0.25
Non-Facility Total	0.74
Facility Total	0.37

CPT® CODE 99415 PROLONGED SERVICES: CLINICAL STAFF

Prolonged clinical staff service (the service beyond the highest time in the range of total time of the service) during an evaluation and management service in the office or outpatient setting, direct patient contact with physician supervision; first hour. (List separately in addition to code for outpatient Evaluation and Management service.)

Relative Value Units (RVUs)

Work RVUs	0.00
Non-Facility Total	0.62
Facility Total	Only valued for non-facility

CPT® CODE 99416

Each additional 30 minutes. (List separately in addition to code for prolonged service.) (Use 99416 in conjunction with 99415.)

Relative Value Units (RVUs)

Work RVUs	0.00
Non-Facility Total	0.29
Facility Total	Only valued for non-facility

CPT® CODE 99417 PROLONGED SERVICE: SAME DAY AS E/M

Prolonged outpatient evaluation and management service(s) time with or without direct patient contact beyond the required time of the primary service when the primary service level has been selected using total time, each 15 minutes of total time. (List separately in addition to the code of the outpatient Evaluation and Management service.)

(Use 99417 in conjunction with 99205, 99215, 99245, 99345, 99350, 99483.) (Do not report 99417 for any time unit less than 15 minutes.)

Relative Value Units (RVUs)

Work RVUs	0.61
Non-Facility Total	0.92
Facility Total	0.89

EVALUATION AND MANAGEMENT

CPT® CODE 99421 ONLINE VISIT: ESTABLISHED PATIENT

Online digital evaluation and management service, for an established patient, for up to 7 days, cumulative time during the 7 days; 5-10 minutes

Relative Value Units (RVUs)

Work RVUs	0.25
Non-Facility Total	0.45
Facility Total	0.38

CPT® CODE 99422

Online digital evaluation and management service, for an established patient, for up to 7 days, cumulative time during the 7 days; 11-20 minutes

Relative Value Units (RVUs)

Work RVUs	0.50
Non-Facility Total	0.88
Facility Total	0.76

CPT® CODE 99423

Online digital evaluation and management service, for an established patient, for up to 7 days, cumulative time during the 7 days; 21 or more minutes

Relative Value Units (RVUs)

Work RVUs	0.80
Non-Facility Total	1.39
Facility Total	1.18

CPT® CODE 99446 TELEPHONE/INTERNET/EHR CONSULTATION

Interprofessional telephone/Internet/electronic health record assessment and management service provided by a consultative physician, including a verbal and written report to the patient's treating/requesting physician or other qualified health care professional; 5-10 minutes of medical consultative discussion and review

Relative Value Units (RVUs)

Work RVUs	0.35
Non-Facility Total	0.53
Facility Total	0.53

CPT® CODE 99447

Interprofessional telephone/Internet/electronic health record assessment and management service provided by a consultative physician, including a verbal and written report to the patient's treating/requesting physician or other qualified health care professional; 11-21 minutes of medical consultative discussion and review

Relative Value Units (RVUs)

Work RVUs	0.70
Non-Facility Total	1.07
Facility Total	1.07

CPT® CODE 99448

Interprofessional telephone/Internet/electronic health record assessment and management service provided by a consultative physician, including a verbal and written report to the patient's treating/requesting physician or other qualified health care professional; 21-30 minutes of medical consultative discussion and review

Relative Value Units (RVUs)

Work RVUs	1.05
Non-Facility Total	1.59
Facility Total	1.59

CPT® CODE 99449

Interprofessional telephone/Internet/electronic health record assessment and management service provided by a consultative physician, including a verbal and written report to the patient's treating/requesting physician or other qualified health care professional; 31 minutes or more of medical consultative discussion and review

Relative Value Units (RVUs)

Work RVUs	1.40
Non-Facility Total	2.15
Facility Total	2.15

CPT® CODE 99451

Interprofessional telephone/Internet/electronic health record assessment and management service provided by a consultative physician, including a verbal and written report to the patient's treating/requesting physician or other qualified health care professional; 5 minutes or more of medical consultative discussion and review

Relative Value Units (RVUs)

Work RVUs	0.70
Non-Facility Total	1.02
Facility Total	1.02

CPT® CODE 99452

Interprofessional telephone/Internet/electronic health record referral service(s) provided by a treating/requesting physician or other qualified health care professional, 30 minutes

Relative Value Units (RVUs)

Work RVUs	0.70
Non-Facility Total	1.04
Facility Total	1.04

CPT® CODE 99453 REMOTE PHYSIOLOGIC MONITORING

Remote monitoring of physiologic parameter(s) (eg, weight, blood pressure, pulse oximetry, respiratory flow rate), initial; set-up and patient education on use of equipment

Relative Value Units (RVUs)

Work RVUs	0.00
Non-Facility Total	0.61
Facility Total	Only valued for non-facility

CPT® CODE 99454

Remote monitoring of physiologic parameter(s) (eg, weight, blood pressure, pulse oximetry, respiratory flow rate), initial; device(s) supply with daily recording(s) or programmed alert(s) transmission, each 30 days

Relative Value Units (RVUs)

Work RVUs	0.00
Non-Facility Total	1.33
Facility Total	Only valued for non-facility

CPT® CODE 99457

Remote physiologic monitoring treatment management services, clinical staff/physician/other qualified health care professional time in a calendar month requiring interactive communication with the patient/caregiver during the month; first 20 minutes

Relative Value Units (RVUs)

Work RVUs	0.61
Non-Facility Total	1.48
Facility Total	0.89

CPT® CODE 99458

Remote physiologic monitoring treatment management services, clinical staff/physician/other qualified health care professional time in a calendar month requiring interactive communication with the patient/caregiver during the month; each additional 20 minutes
(List separately in addition to code for primary procedure)

Relative Value Units (RVUs)

Work RVUs	0.61
Non-Facility Total	1.19
Facility Total	0.89

CPT® CODE 99459

Pelvic examination
(List separately in addition to code for primary procedure.)

Relative Value Units (RVUs)

Work RVUs	0.00
Non-Facility Total	0.64
Facility Total	0.00

CPT® CODE 99473 PATIENT EDUCATION FOR SELF-MONITORING

Self-measured blood pressure using a device validated for clinical accuracy; patient education/training and device calibration

Relative Value Units (RVUs)

Work RVUs	0.00
Non-Facility Total	0.43
Facility Total	Only valued for non-facility

CPT® CODE 99474 SELF-MONITORING: DATA COLLECTION

Self-measured blood pressure using a device validated for clinical accuracy; separate self-measurements of two readings one minute apart, twice daily over a 30-day period (minimum of 12 readings), collection of data reported by the patient and/or caregiver to the physician or other qualified health care professional, with report of average systolic and diastolic pressures and subsequent communication of a treatment plan to the patient

Relative Value Units (RVUs)

Work RVUs	0.18
Non-Facility Total	0.51
Facility Total	0.26

CPT® CODE 99484 CARE MANAGEMENT SERVICES

Care management services for behavioral health conditions, at least 20 minutes of clinical staff time, directed by a physician or other qualified health care professional, per calendar month, with the following required elements: initial assessment or follow-up monitoring, including the use of applicable validated rating scales; behavioral health care planning in relation to behavioral/psychiatric health problems, including revision for patients who are not progressing or whose status changes; facilitating and coordinating treatment such as psychotherapy, pharmacotherapy, counseling and/or psychiatric consultation; and continuity of care with a designated member of the care team.

Relative Value Units (RVUs)

Work RVUs	0.93
Non-Facility Total	1.64
Facility Total	1.28

CPT® CODE 99497 ADVANCED CARE PLANNING

Advance care planning including the explanation and discussion of advance directives such as standard forms (with completion of such forms, when performed), by the physician or other qualified health care professional; first 30 minutes, face-to-face with the patient, family member(s), and/or surrogate

Relative Value Units (RVUs)

Work RVUs	1.50
Non-Facility Total	2.46
Facility Total	2.24

CPT® CODE 99498

Advance care planning including the explanation and discussion of advance directives such as standard forms (with completion of such forms, when performed), by the physician or other qualified health care professional; each additional 30 minutes
(List separately in addition to code for primary procedure)

Relative Value Units (RVUs)

Work RVUs	1.40
Non-Facility Total	2.13
Facility Total	2.12

PART III
Appendices

Appendix A

OFFICE/OUTPATIENT E/M: NEW PATIENT VISITS

CPT CODE	CODE DESCRIPTION	MEDICAL DECISION MAKING	TOTAL TIME (MINUTES)
99202	Office or other outpatient visit for the evaluation and management of a new patient, which requires a medically appropriate history and/or examination and straightforward medical decision making. When using total time on the date of the encounter for code selection, 15 minutes must be met or exceeded.	Straightforward	15 or more
99203	Office or other outpatient visit for the evaluation and management of a new patient, which requires a medically appropriate history and/or examination and low level of medical decision making. When using total time on the date of the encounter for code selection, 30 minutes must be met or exceeded.	Low	30 or more
99204	Office or other outpatient visit for the evaluation and management of a new patient, which requires a medically appropriate history and/or examination and moderate level of medical decision making. When using total time on the date of the encounter for code selection, 45 minutes must be met or exceeded.	Moderate	45 or more
99205	Office or other outpatient visit for the evaluation and management of a new patient, which requires a medically appropriate history and/or examination and high level of medical decision making. When using total time on the date of the encounter for code selection, 60 minutes must be met or exceeded. (For services 75 minutes or longer, see Prolonged Services 99417)	High	60 or more

Appendix B

OFFICE/OUTPATIENT E/M: ESTABLISHED PATIENT VISITS

CPT CODE	CODE DESCRIPTION	MEDICAL DECISION MAKING	TOTAL TIME (MINUTES)
99211	Office or other outpatient visit for the evaluation and management of an established patient that may not require the presence of a physician or other qualified health care professional. Usually, the presenting problem(s) are minimal.	N/A	N/A
99212	Office or other outpatient visit for the evaluation and management of an established patient that requires a medically appropriate history and/or examination and straightforward medical decision making. When using total time on the date of the encounter for code selection, 10 minutes must be met or exceeded.	Straightforward	10 or more
99213	Office or other outpatient visit for the evaluation and management of an established patient that requires a medically appropriate history and/or examination and low level of medical decision making. When using total time on the date of the encounter for code selection, 20 minutes must be met or exceeded.	Low	20 or more
99214	Office or other outpatient visit for the evaluation and management of an established patient that requires a medically appropriate history and/or examination and moderate level of medical decision making. When using total time on the date of the encounter for code selection, 30 minutes must be met or exceeded.	Moderate	30 or more
99215	Office or other outpatient visit for the evaluation and management of an established patient that requires a medically appropriate history and/or examination and high level of medical decision making. When using total time on the date of the encounter for code selection, 40 minutes must be met or exceeded. (For services 55 minutes or longer, see Prolonged Services 99417)	High	40 or more

Appendix C

DOCUMENTING OFFICE E/M SERVICES: MEDICAL DECISION MAKING

LEVEL OF MDM (BASED ON 2 OUT OF 3 ELEMENTS OF MDM)	NUMBER AND COMPLEXITY OF PROBLEMS ADDRESSED AT THE ENCOUNTER	AMOUNT AND/OR COMPLEXITY OF DATA TO BE REVIEWED AND ANALYZED	RISK OF COMPLICATIONS AND/OR MORBIDITY OR MORTALITY OF PATIENT MANAGEMENT
Straightforward	Minimal 1 self-limited* or minor problem	Minimal or none	Minimal risk of morbidity from additional diagnostic testing or treatment
Low Complexity	Limited Stable†, uncomplicated, single problem or 2 or more self-limited/minor problems	Limited 2 tests/documents from Category I‡ **or** an assessment requiring an independent historian(s)	Low risk of morbidity from additional diagnostic testing or treatment
Moderate Complexity	Multiple problems Unstable illness with exacerbation, progression, side effects of treatment, uncertain prognosis, systemic symptoms or complicated injury; or 2 or more stable chronic illnesses	Moderate (1 out of the following): 3 tests/documents from Category I‡ **or** Category II‡, independent interpretation of tests (not separately reported) **or** Category III‡, discussion of management or test interpretation (not separately reported)	Moderate risk of morbidity from additional diagnostic testing or treatment Examples: ▪ Prescription drug management ▪ Minor surgery with patient or procedure risk factors ▪ Major surgery ▪ Limitations due to social determinants of health
High Complexity	Very ill Illnesses with severe exacerbation, progression, side effects of treatment, or pose a threat to life or bodily function	Extensive (2 out of the following): 3 tests/documents from Category I‡ **or** Category II‡, independent interpretation of tests (not separately reported); **or** Category III‡, discussion of management or test interpretation (not separately reported)	High risk of morbidity from additional diagnostic testing or treatment Examples: ▪ Drug therapy requiring intensive monitoring for toxicity ▪ Major surgery with identified patient or procedure risk factors ▪ Emergency major surgery ▪ Hospitalization ▪ Decision not to resuscitate or to de-escalate care because of poor prognosis

*Self-limited or minor problem: A problem that runs a definite and prescribed course, is transient in nature, and is not likely to permanently alter health status.

†Stable in the context of specific treatment goals for an individual patient.

‡Category I: Tests, documents, orders, or independent historian(s)—each unique test, order, or document is counted. Category II: Independent interpretation of tests not reported separately. Category III: Discussion of management or test interpretation with external physician/other QHP/appropriate source

Appendix D

INITIAL HOSPITAL INPATIENT/OBSERVATION CARE: NEW OR ESTABLISHED PATIENT

CPT CODE	CODE DESCRIPTION	MEDICAL DECISION MAKING	TOTAL TIME (minutes)
99221	Initial hospital inpatient or observation care, per day, for the evaluation and management of a patient, which requires a medically appropriate history and/or examination and straightforward or low-level medical decision making. When using total time on the date of encounter for code selection, 40 minutes must be met or exceeded.	Straightforward/ low	40 or more
99222	Initial hospital inpatient or observation care, per day, for the evaluation and management of a patient, which requires a medically appropriate history and/or examination and moderate-level medical decision making. When using total time on the date of encounter for code selection, 55 minutes must be met or exceeded.	Moderate	55 or more
99223	Initial hospital inpatient or observation care, per day, for the evaluation and management of a patient, which requires a medically appropriate history and/or examination and high-level medical decision making. When using total time on the date of encounter for code selection, 75 minutes must be met or exceeded.	High	75 or more
Note: For services of 90 minutes or longer, use prolonged service code 993X0.			

SUBSEQUENT HOSPITAL INPATIENT/OBSERVATION CARE

CPT CODE	CODE DESCRIPTION	MEDICAL DECISION MAKING	TOTAL TIME (minutes)
99231	Subsequent hospital inpatient or observation care, per day, for the evaluation and management of a patient, which requires a medically appropriate history and/or examination and straightforward or low level of medical decision making. When using total time on the date of the encounter for code selection, 25 minutes must be met or exceeded.	Straightforward/ low	25 or more
99232	Subsequent hospital inpatient or observation care, per day, for the evaluation and management of a patient, which requires a medically appropriate history and/or examination and moderate level of medical decision making. When using total time on the date of the encounter for code selection, 35 minutes must be met or exceeded.	Moderate	35 or more
99233	Subsequent hospital inpatient or observation care, per day, for the evaluation and management of a patient, which requires a medically appropriate history and/or examination and high level of medical decision making. When using total time on the date of the encounter for code selection, 50 minutes must be met or exceeded.	High	50 or more
Note: For services of 65 minutes or longer, use prolonged service code 993X0.			

Appendix E

HOSPITAL INPATIENT/OBSERVATION CARE SERVICES: INCLUDING ADMISSION AND DISCHARGE SERVICES

CPT CODE	CODE DESCRIPTION	MEDICAL DECISION MAKING	TOTAL TIME (minutes)
99234	Hospital inpatient or observation care, for the evaluation and management of a patient including admission and discharge on the same date, which requires a medically appropriate history and/or examination and straightforward or low level of medical decision making. When using total time on the date of the encounter for code selection, 45 minutes must be met or exceeded.	Straightforward/ low	45 or more
99235	Hospital inpatient or observation care, for the evaluation and management of a patient including admission and discharge on the same date, which requires a medically appropriate history and/or examination and moderate level of medical decision making. When using total time on the date of the encounter for code selection, 70 minutes must be met or exceeded.	Moderate	70 or more
99236	Hospital inpatient or observation care, for the evaluation and management of a patient including admission and discharge on the same date, which requires a medically appropriate history and/or examination and high level of medical decision making. When using total time on the date of the encounter for code selection, 85 minutes must be met or exceeded.	High	85 or more

HOSPITAL INPATIENT/OBSERVATION DISCHARGE SERVICES

99238	Hospital inpatient or observation discharge day management; 30 minutes or less on the date of the encounter.		30 or less
99239	Hospital inpatient or observation discharge day management; more than 30 minutes on the date of the encounter.		30 or more

Appendix F

OFFICE/OTHER OUTPATIENT CONSULTATIONS: NEW/ESTABLISHED PATIENT

CPT CODE	CODE DESCRIPTION	MEDICAL DECISION MAKING	TOTAL TIME (minutes)
99242	Office or other outpatient consultation for a new or established patient, which requires a medically appropriate history and/or examination and straightforward medical decision making. When using total time on the date of the encounter for code selection, 20 minutes must be met or exceeded.	Straightforward	20 or more
99243	Office or other outpatient consultation for a new or established patient, which requires a medically appropriate history and/or examination and low level of medical decision making. When using total time on the date of the encounter for code selection, 30 minutes must be met or exceeded.	Low	30 or more
99244	Office or other outpatient consultation for a new or established patient, which requires a medically appropriate history and/or examination and moderate level of medical decision making. When using total time on the date of the encounter for code selection, 40 minutes must be met or exceeded.	Moderate	40 or more
99245	Office or other outpatient consultation for a new or established patient, which requires a medically appropriate history and/or examination and high level of medical decision making. When using total time on the date of the encounter for code selection, 55 minutes must be met or exceeded.	High	55 or more
Note: For services of 70 minutes or longer, use prolonged service code 99417.			

INPATIENT/OBSERVATION CONSULTATIONS: NEW/ESTABLISHED PATIENT

CPT CODE	CODE DESCRIPTION	MEDICAL DECISION MAKING	TOTAL TIME (minutes)
99252	Inpatient or observation consultation for a new or established patient, which requires a medically appropriate history and/or examination and straightforward medical decision making. When using total time on the date of the encounter for code selection, 35 minutes must be met or exceeded.	Straightforward	35 or more
99253	Inpatient or observation consultation for a new or established patient, which requires a medically appropriate history and/or examination and low level of medical decision making. When using total time on the date of the encounter for code selection, 45 minutes must be met or exceeded.	Low	45 or more

(continued)

Appendix F: Inpatient/Observation Consultations: New/Established Patient (continued)

CPT CODE	CODE DESCRIPTION	MEDICAL DECISION MAKING	TOTAL TIME (minutes)
99254	Inpatient or observation consultation for a new or established patient, which requires a medically appropriate history and/or examination and moderate level of medical decision making. When using total time on the date of the encounter for code selection, 60 minutes must be met or exceeded.	Moderate	60 or more
99255	Inpatient or observation consultation for a new or established patient, which requires a medically appropriate history and/or examination and high level of medical decision making. When using total time on the date of the encounter for code selection, 80 minutes must be met or exceeded.	High	80 or more
Note: For services of 95 minutes or longer, use prolonged services code 993X0.			

Appendix G

EMERGENCY DEPARTMENT SERVICES: NEW/ESTABLISHED PATIENT

CPT CODE	CODE DESCRIPTION	MEDICAL DECISION MAKING
99281	Emergency department visit for the evaluation and management of a patient that may not require the presence of a physician or other qualified health care professional.	N/A
99282	Emergency department visit for the evaluation and management of a patient, which requires a medically appropriate history and/or examination and straightforward medical decision making.	Straightforward
99283	Emergency department visit for the evaluation and management of a patient, which requires a medically appropriate history and/or examination and low level of medical decision making.	Low
99284	Emergency department visit for the evaluation and management of a patient, which requires a medically appropriate history and/or examination and moderate level of medical decision making.	Moderate
99285	Emergency department visit for the evaluation and management of a patient, which requires a medically appropriate history and/or examination and high level of medical decision making.	High
Note: Time is not a descriptive component for the emergency department levels of E/M services, as emergency department services are typically provided based on a variable intensity, involving multiple encounters with several patients over an extended period of time.		

OTHER EMERGENCY SERVICES

99288	Physician or other qualified health care professional direction of emergency medical systems (EMS) emergency care, advanced life support.	

Appendix H

EXAMPLES OF LEVELS OF RISK IN MEDICAL DECISION MAKING

E/M NOT Inclusive of Outpatient E/M Codes (See Appendix C)

LEVEL OF RISK	PRESENTING PROBLEM(S)	DIAGNOSTIC PROCEDURE(S) ORDERED	MANAGEMENT OPTIONS SELECTED
Minimal	*1 self-limited/minor problem* (eg, cold, insect bite, tinea corporis)	*Imaging studies* – ultrasound, EKG	Rest Elastic bandages
Low	*2 or more self-limited/ minor problems* *1 or more chronic illness* – stable, eg, non-insulin dependent diabetes Acute illness or injury – uncomplicated	*Imaging studies with contrast* – non-cardiovascular, eg, barium enema *Biopsies* – skin or superficial needle	*Minor surgery* – no identified risk factors *Drugs* – over the counter
Moderate	*Undiagnosed new problem* with uncertain prognosis – eg, breast lump *1 or more chronic illnesses* – with mild exacerbation/progression, or side effects of treatment *Acute illness* with systemic symptoms *Acute injury* – complicated	*Imaging studies with contrast* – No identified risk factors *Diagnostic endoscopies* with no identifiable risk factors *Biopsies* – deep needle or incisional	*Minor surgery* – identifiable risk factors *Major surgery* – elective with no identifiable risk factors *Drugs* – management of prescription drugs
High	*1 or more chronic illnesses* – severe exacerbation/progression/ side effects of treatment *Acute illnesses or injuries* posing threat to life/bodily function Abrupt change in neurologic status	*Imaging studies with contrast* – identified risk factors *Diagnostic endoscopies* with identified risk factors	*Major surgery* – elective with identifiable risk factors OR emergency surgery *Drugs* – therapy requiring intensive monitoring for toxicity

Appendix I

E/M SERVICES MODIFIERS

MODIFIER	DESCRIPTION	COMMENTS
24	Unrelated E/M service. E/M service provided by the surgeon during a global surgical period.	A postoperative service was provided during the global surgical period. Diagnosis code indicates the service is unrelated to the original surgical procedure.
25	Significant, Separately Identifiable E/M Service. E/M service provided on the same day as a procedure or other service	*E/M service and a procedure on same day* – The E/M service may have led to the decision to perform the procedure or may have involved the evaluation of a problem unrelated to the procedure. Medicare states that this modifier is used when the decision to perform minor surgery is made on the day of or day before the surgery. For major surgery, see modifier 57. *Two E/M services on the same day* – Each service must be significant and separately identifiable. Primarily used when a preventive visit and problem-oriented visit are provided on the same day. See chapter 3.
32	Mandated Services. A consultation and/or related services required by a private payer, governmental, legislative or regulatory entity.	E/M service was required by insurer; eg, a second opinion.
57	Decision for Surgery. An E/M Service resulted in the initial decision to perform a surgical procedure.	The decision to perform the surgery was made during this E/M service. Medicare states that this modifier is used when the decision is made to perform *major* surgery on the day of or day before the surgery. For minor surgery, see modifier 25.

Appendix J

PREVENTIVE MEDICINE CPT CODES

CODE	DESCRIPTOR
99381	**Initial comprehensive preventive medicine** evaluation and management of an individual including an age and gender appropriate history, examination, counseling/anticipatory guidance/ risk factor reduction interventions, and the ordering of laboratory/diagnostic procedures, new patient; infant (age younger than 1 year)
99382	... early childhood (age 1 through 4 years)
99383	... late childhood (age 5 through 11 years)
99384	... adolescent (age 12 through 17 years)
99385	... 18-39 years
99386	... 40-64 years
99387	... 65 years and older
99391	**Periodic comprehensive preventive medicine** reevaluation and management of an individual including an age and gender appropriate history, examination, counseling/anticipatory guidance/ risk factor reduction interventions, and the ordering of laboratory/diagnostic procedures, established patient; infant (age younger than 1 year)
99392	... early childhood (age 1 through 4 years)
99393	... late childhood (age 5 through 11 years)
99394	... adolescent (age 12 through 17 years)
99395	... 18-39 years
99396	... 40-64 years
99397	... 65 years and older

Appendix K

INITIAL PREVENTIVE PHYSICAL EXAMINATION AND ANNUAL WELLNESS VISIT*

Code	Description
G0402	**Initial preventive physical examination**; face to face visit, services limited to new beneficiary during first (12) months of Medicare enrollment
G0403	Electrocardiogram, routine ECG with at least 12 leads; performed as a screening for the **initial preventive physical examination** with interpretation and report
G0404	Tracing only, without interpretation and report, performed as a component of the **initial preventive physical examination**
G0405	Interpretation and report only, performed as a component of the **initial preventive physical examination**
G0468	Federally qualified health center: a FQHC visit that includes an **initial preventive physical examination** (IPPE) or **annual wellness visit** (AWV) and includes a typical bundle of Medicare covered services that would be furnished per diem to a patient receiving an IPPE or AWV.
G0438	**Annual wellness visit**; includes a personalized prevention plan of service (PPPS), initial visit
G0439	**Annual wellness visit**; includes a personalized prevention plan of service (PPPS), subsequent visit
99497	**Advance care planning** including the explanation and discussion of advance directives such as standard forms (with completion of such forms, when performed), by the physician or other qualified health professional; first 30 minutes, face to face with the patient, family member(s) and/or surrogate
99498	**Advance care planning** including the explanation and discussion of advance directives such as standard forms (with completion of such forms, when performed), by the physician or other qualified health care professional; each additional 30 minutes (List separately in addition to code for primary procedure)

*https://www.cms.gov/Medicare/Prevention/PrevntionGenInfo/medicare-preventive-services/MPS-QuickReferenceChart-1.html

Appendix L

MEDICARE SCREENING SERVICES: PELVIC EXAMINATION AND CYTOPATHOLOGY (PAP)

SCREENING	HIGH-RISK	FREQUENCY	LOW RISK	FREQUENCY
G0101: Pelvic examination (including breast exam)	Z72.51, Z72.52, Z72.53, Z77.29, Z77.9, Z91.89, and Z92.89	Annually	Z01.411, Z01.419, Z12.4, Z12.72, Z12.79, and Z12.89	Every 2 years
G0123: Screening cytopathology, cervical or vaginal (any reporting system), collected in preservative fluid, automated thin layer preparation, screening by cytotechnologist under physician supervision				
G0124: Screening cytopathology, cervical or vaginal (any reporting system), collected in preservative fluid, automated thin layer preparation, requiring interpretation by physician				
G0141: Screening cytopathology smears, cervical or vaginal, performed by automated system, with manual rescreening, requiring interpretation by physician				
G0143: Screening cytopathology, cervical or vaginal (any reporting system), collected in preservative fluid, automated thin layer preparation, with manual screening and rescreening by cytotechnologist under physician supervision				
G0144: Screening cytopathology, cervical or vaginal (any reporting system), collected in preservative fluid, automated thin layer preparation, with screening by automated system, under physician supervision				
G0145: Screening cytopathology, cervical or vaginal (any reporting system), collected in preservative fluid, automated thin layer preparation, with screening by automated system and manual rescreening under physician supervision				
G0147: Screening cytopathology smears, cervical or vaginal, performed by automated system under physician supervision				
G0148: Screening cytopathology smears, cervical or vaginal, performed by automated system with manual rescreening				
P3000: Screening papanicolaou smear, cervical or vaginal, up to three smears, by technician under physician supervision				
P3001: Screening papanicolaou smear, cervical or vaginal, up to three smears, requiring interpretation by physician				
Q0091: Screening papanicolaou smear; obtaining, preparing and conveyance of cervical or vaginal smear to laboratory				

Appendix M

MEDICARE SCREENING SERVICES: MAMMOGRAM AND BONE MASS

SCREENING	ICD-10	INDICATIONS	FREQUENCY
77067: Screening mammography, bilateral (2-view study of each breast), including computer-aided detection (CAD) when performed ▪ Use 77063 as an add-on code to 77067 when tomosynthesis is used in addition to 2-D mammography	N63.15, N63.25, Z12.31	Age	Aged 35 through 39: One baseline Aged 40 and older: Annually
0554T: Bone strength and fracture risk using finite element analysis of functional data, and bone-mineral density, utilizing data from a computed tomography scan; retrieval and transmission of the scan data, assessment of bone strength and fracture risk and bone mineral density, interpretation and report **0555T:** Retrieval and transmission of the scan data **0556T:** Assessment of bone strength and fracture risk and bone mineral density **0557T:** Interpretation and report **0558T:** Computed tomography scan taken for the purpose of biomechanical computed tomography analysis **76977:** Ultrasound bone density measurement and interpretation, peripheral site(s), any method **77078:** Computed tomography, bone mineral density study, 1 or more sites; axial skeleton (eg, hips, pelvis, spine) **77080:** Dual-energy X-ray absorptiometry (DXA), bone density study, 1 or more sites; axial skeleton (eg, hips, pelvis, spine) **77081:** Dual-energy X-ray absorptiometry (DXA), bone density study, 1 or more sites; appendicular skeleton (peripheral) (eg, radius, wrist, heel) **77085:** Dual-energy X-ray absorptiometry (DXA), bone density study, 1 or more sites; axial skeleton (eg, hips, pelvis, spine), including vertebral fracture assessment **G0130:** Single energy X-ray absorptiometry (SEXA) bone density study, 1 or more sites, appendicular skeleton (peripheral) (eg, radius, wrist, heel)	E21.0, E21.3, E23.0, E34.2, E89.40, E89.41, M80.08xA, M80.88xA, M84.58xA, M84.68xA, N95.8, N95.9, Q78.0, S34.3xxA, Z78.0, Z79.3, Z79.51, Z79.52, Z79.811, Z79.818, Z79.83, Z87.310	▪ Women determined to be estrogen deficient and at clinical risk for osteoporosis ▪ Individuals with vertebral abnormalities ▪ Individuals getting glucocorticoid therapy > 3 months ▪ Individuals with hyperparathyroidism ▪ Individuals being monitored for FDA-approved osteoporosis drug therapy	Every 2 years

Appendix N

MEDICARE SCREENING SERVICES: HEPATITIS B AND C

SCREENING	HIGH-RISK	FREQUENCY	LOW-RISK	FREQUENCY
G0499: Hepatitis B screening in non-pregnant, high risk individual includes hepatitis B surface antigen (HBSAG) followed by a neutralizing confirmatory test for initially reactive results, and antibodies to HBSAG (anti-HBS) and hepatitis B core antigen (anti-HBC)	Z11.59 **and** Z72.89	Annually only for those who have continued high risk who do not get hepatitis B vaccination	**Subsequent visits:** Z11.59 **and one of:** F11.10–F11.99, F13.10–F13.99, F14.10–F14.99, F15.10–F15.99, Z20.2, Z20.5, Z72.52, Z72.53	
FOR PREGNANT WOMEN: **86704:** Hepatitis B core antibody (HBcAb); total **86706:** Hepatitis B surface antibody (HBsAb) **87340:** Infectious agent antigen detection by immunoassay technique, (eg, enzyme immunoassay [EIA], enzyme-linked immunosorbent assay [ELISA], immunochemiluminometric assay [IMCA]) qualitative or semiquantitative, multiple-step method; hepatitis B surface antigen (HBsAg) **87341:** Infectious agent antigen detection by immunoassay technique, (eg, enzyme immunoassay [EIA], enzyme-linked immunosorbent assay [ELISA], immunochemiluminometric assay [IMCA]) qualitative or semiquantitative, multiple-step method; hepatitis B surface antigen (HBsAg) neutralization	Z11.59 **and** Z72.89 **and one of the following:** Z34.00, Z34.01, Z34.02, Z34.03, Z34.80, Z34.81, Z34.82, Z34.83, Z34.90, Z34.91, Z34.92, Z34.93, O09.90, O09.91, O09.92, O09.93	One screening for pregnant women at the first prenatal visit for each pregnancy and rescreening at the time of delivery for those with new or continued risk factors	Z11.59 **and one of the following:** Z34.00, Z34.80, Z34.90, O09.90	One screening for pregnant women at the first prenatal visit for each pregnancy
G0472: Hepatitis C antibody screening, for individual at high risk and other covered indication(s)	Z72.89 and F19.20	Initial screening: blood transfusion before 1992, current or past history of injection drug use Annually for injection drug use	Z11.59	Once for patients born from 1945–1965 who are not high risk

Appendix O

MEDICARE SCREENING SERVICES: HUMAN PAPILLOMAVIRUS (HPV), HUMAN IMMUNODEFICIENCY VIRUS (HIV), AND SEXUALLY TRANSMITTED DISEASE

SCREENING	HIGH-RISK	FREQUENCY	LOW-RISK	FREQUENCY
G0476: Infectious agent detection by nucleic acid (DNA or RNA); human papillomavirus (HPV), high-risk types (eg, 16, 18, 31, 33, 35, 39, 45, 51, 52, 56, 58, 59, 68) for cervical cancer screening, must be performed in addition to Papanicolaou test	Z11.51 **and either** Z01.411 **or** Z01.419	Every 5 years	N/A	N/A
HIV NON-OBSTETRIC **G0432:** Infectious agent antibody detection by enzyme immunoassay (EIA) technique, HIV-1 and/or HIV-2, screening **G0433:** Infectious agent antibody detection by enzyme-linked immunosorbent assay (ELISA) technique, HIV-1 and/or HIV-2, screening **G0435:** Infectious agent antibody detection by rapid antibody test, HIV-1 and/or HIV-2, screening **G0475:** HIV antigen/antibody, combination assay, screening	Z11.4 and Z72.51, Z72.52, Z72.53, or Z72.89	Annually for ages younger than 15 and older than 65	Z11.4	Annually for ages 15–65
HIV OBSTETRIC	**ALL PREGNANCIES:** Z11.4 and Z34.00, Z34.01, Z34.02, Z34.03, Z34.80, Z34.81, Z34.82, Z34.83, Z34.90, Z34.91, Z34.92, Z34.93, O09.90, O09.91, O09.92, or O09.93			1. Initial pregnancy test 2. 3rd trimester 3. At labor
Chlamydia (86631, 86632, 87110, 87270, 87320, 87490, 87491, 87810, 87800) **Gonorrhea** (87590, 87591, 87850, 87800) **Syphilis** (86592, 86593, 86780) **Hepatitis B** (87340, 87341) **HIBC** (G0445)	**SEXUALLY ACTIVE:** Z11.3, Z11.59, Z34.00, Z34.01, Z34.02, Z34.03, Z34.80, Z34.81, Z34.82, Z34.83, Z34.90, Z34.91, Z34.92, Z34.93, Z72.51, Z72.52, Z72.53, Z72.89, O09.90, O09.91, O09.92, and O09.93			As indicated

Appendix P

MEDICARE SCREENING SERVICES: TESTS AND COUNSELING*

SCREENING	ICD-10	INDICATIONS	FREQUENCY
Alcohol Misuse **G0442:** Annual alcohol misuse screening, 15 minutes **G0443:** Brief face-to-face behavioral counseling for alcohol misuse, 15 minutes	N/A	No indications	Annually for testing; 4x/year for counseling
Cardiovascular (80061, 82465, 83718, 84478)	Z13.6	No indications	Every 5 years
Colorectal (81528, 82270, G0104, G0105, G0106, G0120, G0121, G0328, 00812)	Z86.004	Age 50 and older	Dependent on test type: range every 1–10 years
Depression **G0444:** Annual depression screening, 15 minutes	N/A	No indications	Annually
Diabetes (82947, 82950, 82951)	Z13.1	No indications	Annually for normal results; every 6 months for abnormal
Obesity **G0447:** Face-to-face behavioral counseling for obesity, 15 minutes **G0473:** Face-to-face behavioral counseling for obesity, group (2–10), 30 minutes	Z68.30, Z68.31, Z68.32, Z68.33, Z68.34, Z68.35, Z68.36, Z68.37, Z68.38, Z68.39, Z68.41, Z68.42, Z68.43, Z68.44, or Z68.45	Body Mass Index (BMI) ≥30 kilograms (kg) per meter squared	Up to 22 visits in 12 months
Tobacco Cessation **99406:** Smoking and tobacco use cessation counseling visit; intermediate, greater than 3 minutes up to 10 minutes **99407:** Smoking and tobacco use cessation counseling visit; intensive, greater than 10 minutes	F17.210, F17.211, F17.213, F17.218, F17.219, F17.220, F17.221, F17.223, F17.228, F17.229, F17.290, F17.291, F17.293, F17.298, F17.299, T65.211A, T65.212A, T65.213A, T65.214A, T65.221A, T65.222A, T65.223A, T65.224A, T65.291A, T65.292A, T65.293A, T65.294A, and Z87.891	Use of tobacco	8 sessions per year

*https://www.cms.gov/Medicare/Prevention/PrevntionGenInfo/medicare-preventive-services/MPS-QuickReferenceChart-1.html

Appendix Q

MEDICARE SCREENING SERVICES: IMMUNIZATIONS

ICD-10 for Immunizations: Z23

Hepatitis B: As recommended by the Centers for Disease Control and Prevention (https://www.cdc.gov/hepatitis/hbv/)
90739: Hepatitis B vaccine (HepB), adult dosage, 2 dose schedule, for intramuscular use **90740:** Hepatitis B vaccine (HepB), dialysis or immunosuppressed patient dosage, 3 dose schedule, for intramuscular use **90743:** Hepatitis B vaccine (HepB), adolescent, 2 dose schedule, for intramuscular use **90744:** Hepatitis B vaccine (HepB), pediatric/adolescent dosage, 3 dose schedule, for intramuscular use **90746:** Hepatitis B vaccine (HepB), adult dosage, 3 dose schedule, for intramuscular use **90747:** Hepatitis B vaccine (HepB), dialysis or immunosuppressed patient dosage, 4 dose schedule, for intramuscular use **G0010:** Administration of Hepatitis B vaccine
Influenza*: Once per season
90630, 90672, 90674, 90682, 90685-90689, 90694, 90756: Influenza virus vaccine, quadrivalent (IIV4) **90653, 90662:** Influenza virus vaccine (IIV) **90654–90660, 90673:** Influenza virus vaccine, trivalent (IIV3), split virus, preservative-free **Q2034–Q2039:** Influenza virus vaccine, split virus **G0008:** Administration of influenza virus vaccine
Pneumococcal: An initial pneumococcal vaccine with a second pneumococcal vaccine 1 year after the first vaccine was administered
90670: Pneumococcal conjugate vaccine, 13 valent (PCV13), for intramuscular use **90732:** Pneumococcal polysaccharide vaccine, 23-valent (PPSV23), adult or immunosuppressed patient dosage, when administered to individuals 2 years or older, for subcutaneous or intramuscular use **G0009:** Administration of pneumococcal vaccine

* https://www.cms.gov/Medicare/Prevention/PrevntionGenInfo/medicare-preventive-services/MPS-QuickReferenceChart-1.html#FLU

Appendix R

COMPARISON OF CPT AND MEDICARE GLOBAL SURGICAL PACKAGES

<table>
<tr><th rowspan="2">TYPES OF SERVICES</th><th rowspan="2">CPT SURGICAL PACKAGE</th><th colspan="3">MEDICARE SURGICAL PACKAGES</th></tr>
<tr><th>MAJOR SURGERY (90 DAYS)</th><th colspan="2">MINOR SURGERY (0 OR 10 DAYS)</th></tr>
<tr><td colspan="5">Services During Preoperative Period</td></tr>
<tr><td>Pre-op days included in global package</td><td>Day of or day before surgery</td><td>Day of or day before surgery</td><td colspan="2">Day of surgery</td></tr>
<tr><td>Related E/M services</td><td>Bill ONLY if decision for surgery made during visit (modifier 57)</td><td>Bill ONLY if decision for surgery made during visit (modifier 57)</td><td colspan="2">Do not bill separately</td></tr>
<tr><td>Related or unrelated significant, separately identifiable E/M services</td><td>Bill separately (modifier 25)</td><td>Bill separately (modifier 25)</td><td colspan="2">Bill separately (modifier 25)</td></tr>
<tr><td colspan="5">Intraoperative Services</td></tr>
<tr><td>Anesthesia performed by surgeon</td><td>Bill ONLY for regional or general anesthesia</td><td>Do not bill separately for any anesthesia</td><td colspan="2">Do not bill separately for any anesthesia</td></tr>
<tr><td>Operation itself</td><td>All integral procedures included</td><td>All integral procedures included</td><td colspan="2">All integral procedures included</td></tr>
<tr><td>Complications treated by surgeon</td><td>Bill separately</td><td>Do not bill separately</td><td colspan="2">Do not bill separately</td></tr>
<tr><td colspan="5">Services During Post-Operative Period</td></tr>
<tr><td>Post-op days included in global package</td><td>Not specified</td><td>90 Days Post-op</td><td>0 day Global—Day of surgery</td><td>10 days Global—10 days Post-op</td></tr>
<tr><td>Routine E/M services</td><td>Do not bill separately</td><td>Do not bill separately</td><td>Do not bill separately</td><td>Do not bill separately</td></tr>
<tr><td>Treatment of complications</td><td>Bill separately</td><td>Bill ONLY if patient treated in operating room (Modifier 78)</td><td>Do not bill Separately</td><td>Bill ONLY if patient treated in operating room (Modifier 78)</td></tr>
<tr><td>Treatment of other conditions</td><td>Bill separately (Modifier 24, 58 or 79)</td><td>Bill separately (Modifier 24, 58 or 79)</td><td colspan="2">Bill separately (Modifier 24, 58 or 79)</td></tr>
</table>

Appendix S

SURGICAL SERVICES: PROCEDURE MODIFIERS

MODIFIER	NOTES
22 - Increased services	The work necessary to provide the service is substantially greater than typical; no other code is accurate. Submit additional documentation describing unusual service and justifying increased payment.
50 - Bilateral procedure	Same procedure provided on both sides of identical organs. Only use if procedure does not indicate laterality.
51 - Multiple procedures	Multiple services provided on same date by same physician. The highest valued code is reported without the modifier, with subsequent procedures reported with modifier.
52 - Reduced services	Physician determined to reduce or eliminate procedure; all of the components were not performed, or the procedure was attempted but unsuccessful. Another procedure was performed.
53 - Discontinued procedure	Physician terminated procedure due to well-being of the patient or extenuating circumstances. No procedure is performed. This is not used for elective cancellation.
59 - Distinct services	Procedures are separate and distinct; performed on different sites or organ systems, used separate incisions or excisions. Used for CCI edits.

SURGICAL SERVICES: MULTIPLE SURGEONS

MODIFIER	NOTES
62 - Two surgeons (co-surgeons)	Two surgeons perform distinct part(s) of the surgical procedure; documentation is separate for their procedure.
80 - Assistant surgeon	Primary surgeon reports procedure without modifier and assistant reports with modifier. Assistant does not have separate operative report.
82 - Assistant surgeon (resident unavailable)	For services provided at a teaching facility. Medicare does not reimburse for assistant surgeons at teaching facilities.
AS - Physician assistant, nurse practitioner, or clinical nurse specialist for assistance at surgery	Medicare will reimburse if the assistant surgical services are covered if provided by a physician.

SURGICAL SERVICES: DIVISION OF GLOBAL SURGICAL PACKAGE

MODIFIER	NOTES
54 – Surgical care only	Medicare recognizes modifiers when there is documentation of: a formal transfer of care, surgeons are in the same practice but different specialties, or surgeons are in different practices and do not have a covering relationship. Submit documentation with the claim to private payers to explain extenuating circumstances.
55 – Postoperative management only	
56 – Preoperative management only	

Appendix T

SURGICAL SERVICES: POSTOPERATIVE PERIOD

MODIFIER	NOTES
58 – Stage or related procedure or service by the same physician or other qualified health care professional during postoperative period	The additional service is related to but not a complication of the original surgery. Medicare rules are this service begins a new global surgical package.
76 – Repeat procedure or service by same physician or other qualified health care professional	Modifiers 76 and 77 are used to clarify the claim is not a duplicate.
77 – Repeat procedure by another physician or other qualified health care professional	
78 – Unplanned return to the operating/procedure room by the same physician or other qualified health care professional after initial procedure for a related procedure during the postoperative period	Indicates that the procedure required a return to the operating/procedure room and is therefore payable. Medicare reimburses only for the intraoperative portion of the related service. This service does not begin a new global surgical package.
79 – Unrelated procedure or service by the same physician or other qualified health care professional during the post-operative period	Treatment may or may not require a return to the operating room. This service begins a new global surgical package.

Appendix U

CODES FOR OBSTETRIC SERVICES

CPT CODE	SHORT DESCRIPTION	ANTEPARTUM SERVICES	DELIVERY SERVICES	POSTPARTUM E/M SERVICES	
				INPATIENT CARE	OUTPATIENT CARE
Appropriate E/M code	Pregnancy diagnosis	1-3 visits			
59400	Routine obstetric care	13 visits	Vaginal	2 E/M services	E/M services
59409	Vaginal delivery only		Vaginal		
59410	Vaginal delivery with postpartum care		Vaginal	2 E/M services	E/M services
59425	Antepartum care only	4-6 visits			
59426	Antepartum care only	7 or more visits			
59430	Postpartum care only				E/M services
59510	Routine obstetric care	13 visits	Cesarean	4 E/M services	E/M services
59514	Cesarean delivery only		Cesarean		
59515	Cesarean delivery with postpartum care		Cesarean	4 E/M services	E/M services
59610	Routine obstetric care	13 visits	VBAC	2 E/M services	E/M services
59612	VBAC delivery only		VBAC		
59614	VBAC delivery with postpartum care		VBAC	2 E/M services	E/M services
59618	Routine obstetric care	13 visits	Repeat cesarean	4 E/M services	E/M services
59620	Repeat cesarean only		Repeat cesarean		
59622	Repeat cesarean with postpartum care		Repeat cesarean	4 E/M services	E/M services

Appendix V

INTERRUPTION OF PREGNANCY – SURGICAL OR NON-SURGICAL ABORTION

POSSIBLE DIAGNOSIS CODES & DESCRIPTION		POSSIBLE PROCEDURE CODES & DESCRIPTIONS	
Missed Abortion/Fetal Demise (In Utero)			
O02.1 **O36.4X**	Missed abortion or early fetal death before completion of 20 weeks of gestation, with retention of dead fetus **or** Maternal care for intrauterine death	**Surgical Abortion**	
		59820	Before 14 weeks
		59821	14 weeks to 20 weeks
		Non-Surgical Abortion	
		59850-59852	*Injections* before 20 weeks
		Delivery Code	On or after 20 weeks
		59855-59857	*By suppositories* before 20 weeks
		Delivery code	On or after 20 weeks
		E/M Code	*Spontaneous/Other Medical Abortion* before 20 weeks
		Delivery code	On or after 20 weeks
		E/M code + 59414	*Spontaneous + delivery of placenta* before 20 weeks
		Delivery code	On or after 20 weeks
Induced Termination			
O04.5 **O04.6** **O04.7** **O03.8-**	Genital tract and pelvic infection after (induced) termination of pregnancy **or** Delayed or excessive hemorrhage after (induced) termination of pregnancy **or** Embolism after (induced) termination of pregnancy **or** (Induced) termination of pregnancy with other and unspecified complications	**Surgical Abortion**	
		59840	By D&C any trimester
		59841	By *D&E* 14 weeks to 20 weeks
		59841-22	20 weeks or more
		Non-Surgical Abortion	
		59850-59852	*Injections* before 20 weeks
		59855-59857	*By suppositories* before 20 weeks
		Delivery code	After 20 weeks
		E/M code	*Spontaneous/Other Medical Abortion* before 20 weeks
		Delivery codes	On or after 20 weeks
		E/M code + 59414	*Spontaneous + delivery of placenta* before 20 weeks
		Delivery code	On or after 20 weeks

Appendix W

INTERRUPTION OF PREGNANCY – SPONTANEOUS ABORTION

COMPLETE (SPONTANEOUS) ABORTION			
O03.5	Genital tract and pelvic infection after complete or unspecified spontaneous abortion **or**	E/M	Before 20 weeks 0 days
O03.6	Delayed or excessive hemorrhage after complete or unspecified spontaneous abortion **or**	Delivery code	After 20 weeks 0 days
O03.7	Embolism after complete or unspecified spontaneous abortion **or**		
O03.8-	Other and unspecified complications after complete or unspecified spontaneous abortion **or**		
O03.9	Complete or unspecified spontaneous abortion without complication		
INCOMPLETE (SPONTANEOUS) ABORTION			
O03.0	Genital tract and pelvic infection after incomplete spontaneous abortion **or**	59812	Before 20 weeks 0 days
O03.1	Delayed or excessive hemorrhage after incomplete spontaneous abortion **or**	Delivery code	20 weeks 0 days or more
O03.2	Embolism after incomplete spontaneous abortion **or**		
O03.3-	Other and unspecified complications after incomplete spontaneous abortion **or**		
O03.4	Incomplete spontaneous abortion without complication		

Appendix X

NON-OBSTETRIC ULTRASOUND CODES

CODE	SHORT DESCRIPTION	REQUIREMENTS
Transabdominal Ultrasounds		
76856	Complete transabdominal ultrasound	Description of: ▪ Uterus ▪ Adnexal structures ▪ Pelvic pathology Measurement of: ▪ Uterus ▪ Adnexal structures ▪ Endometrium ▪ Bladder (when applicable)
76857	Limited or follow-up transabdominal ultrasound	Assessment of one or more elements in 76856 and/or re-evaluation of one or more pelvic abnormalities found in a previous exam
Transvaginal Ultrasounds		
76830	Transvaginal ultrasound	Report: ▪ Uterus ▪ Tubes ▪ Ovaries ▪ Pelvic structures
76831 **58340**	Saline infusion sonohysterography Introduction of contrast material	Includes color flow Doppler with contrast

Appendix Y

COMPONENTS OF TRANSABDOMINAL OBSTETRIC ULTRASOUND CODES

OBSTETRIC ULTRASOUND CODES											
	Extent of Evaluation					Trimester			Gestation		Approach
Code	Complete Maternal/ Fetal Evaluation	Detailed Fetal Anatomic Exam	Limited	Follow-up	Specialized	1st	2nd	3rd	Single or First Gestation	Each Additional Gestation	Transabdominal, Transvaginal or Either Approach
76801	●					●			●		Transabdominal
76802	●					●				●	Transabdominal
76805	●						●	●	●		Transabdominal
76810	●						●	●		●	Transabdominal
76811	●	●					●	●	●		Transabdominal
76812	●	●					●	●		●	Transabdominal
76813					●	●			●		Either
76814					●	●				●	Either
76815			●			●	●	●	Report once for any number of fetuses		Either
76816				●		●	●	●	Report separately for each fetus		Either
76817	●					●	●	●	Report once for any number of fetuses		Transvaginal
76818					●			●	Report separately for each fetus		Transabdominal
76819					●			●	Report separately for each fetus		Transabdominal
76820					●	●	●	●	Report separately for each fetus		Either
76821					●	●	●	●	Report separately for each fetus		Either
76825					●		●		Report separately for each fetus		Either
76826				●			●		Report separately for each fetus		Either
76827					●		●		Report separately for each fetus		Either
76828				●			●		Report separately for each fetus		Either

Modifiers		Comments
26	**Professional Component**: This modifier is used when the physician component is reported separately.	Used by the *physician* to report his or her supervision and/or performance of the ultrasound examination, the interpretation, and the written report.
TC	**Technical Component**: This modifier is used when the technical component is reported separately.	Used by the *facility* to report the costs of the equipment, technician and supplies.

Appendix Z

LAPAROSCOPY PROCEDURE

PURPOSE	CPT CODE	CODE DESCRIPTION	COMMENTS
Sterilization	58661	Laparoscopy, surgical; with removal of adnexal structures (partial or total oophorectomy and/or salpingectomy)	Used when laparoscopic sterilization is performed via partial or total salpingectomy.
	58670	Laparoscopy, surgical; with fulguration of oviducts (with or without transection)	Used when traditional laparoscopic sterilization is performed via either ligation or transection, without removal of the tubes.
	58671	Laparoscopy, surgical; with occlusion of oviducts by device (eg, band, clip, or Falope ring)	Used when laparoscopic sterilization is performed with one of the devices listed or a similar device.
Treatment of Disease Process	58661	Laparoscopy, surgical; with removal of adnexal structures (partial or total oophorectomy and/or salpingectomy)	Used when an oophorectomy and/or salpingectomy is performed to address a disease process (eg, hydrosalpinx, torsion, cystic structures, etc.).
	58672	Laparoscopy, surgical; with fimbrioplasty	Used when a laparoscopic procedure is performed to treat disease or disorders of the fimbriae of the fallopian tubes—usually to repair, restore, or enhance fertility.
	58673	Laparoscopy, surgical; with salpingostomy (salpingoneostomy)	Used when an incision is made laparoscopically into the fallopian tube to address a structural issue or disease process, but the tube itself is not removed. This code is used only to address gynecologic issues—not obstetric issues.
Prophylactic	58661	Laparoscopy, surgical; with removal of adnexal structures (partial or total oophorectomy and/or salpingectomy)	Used when fallopian tubes are removed as a risk-reduction method, but no specific disease process in the tubes is present at the time of the procedure.

Appendix AA

COVID-19 LABORATORY CODES

CPT CODE	DESCRIPTION	INDICATION
	Immunology	
86318	Immunoassay for infectious agent antibody(ies), quantitative or semiquantitative, single-step method (eg, reagent strip).	To identify specific antibodies and measure the immunity level that the antibody provides using a single-step method.
86328	Immunoassay for infectious agent antibody(ies), qualitative or semiquantitative, single-step method (eg, reagent strip); severe acute respiratory syndrome coronavirus 2 (SARS-CoV-2) (coronavirus disease [COVID-19]).	To reports antibody testing for severe acute respiratory syndrome coronavirus 2 using a single-step method.
86408	Neutralizing antibody, severe acute respiratory syndrome coronavirus 2 (SARS-CoV-2) (coronavirus disease [COVID-19]); screen.	To reports a SARS-CoV-2 neutralizing antibody screen. This test is used to determine if antibodies present in a patient's specimen can directly block infection of cells from the COVID-19 virus.
86409	Neutralizing antibody, severe acute respiratory syndrome coronavirus 2 (SARS-CoV-2) (coronavirus disease [COVID-19]); titer.	To report a SARS-CoV-2 neutralizing antibody titer. This test is used to determine if antibodies present in a patient's specimen can directly block infection of cells from the COVID-19 virus.
86413	Severe acute respiratory syndrome coronavirus 2 (SARS-CoV-2) (coronavirus disease [COVID-19]) antibody, quantitative.	To provide quantitative measurements of SARS-CoV-2 antibodies to examine the patient's adaptive immune response to the virus.
86769	Antibody; severe acute respiratory syndrome coronavirus 2 (SARS-CoV-2) (coronavirus disease [COVID-19]).	To report testing to identify the presence of antibodies to the SARS-CoV-2 virus. Presence of antibodies indicate a past or current infection.
	Microbiology	
87301	Infectious agent antigen detection by immunoassay technique (eg, enzyme immunoassay [EIA], enzyme-linked immunosorbent assay [ELISA], fluorescence immunoassay [FIA], immunochemiluminometric assay [IMCA]), qualitative or semiquantitative; adenovirus enteric types 40/41.	This test detects infection by an adenovirus. Infection may affect the tonsils or other parts of the lungs or airways or the intestines.
87305	Infectious agent antigen detection by immunoassay technique (eg, enzyme immunoassay [EIA], enzyme-linked immunosorbent assay [ELISA], fluorescence immunoassay [FIA], immunochemiluminometric assay [IMCA]), qualitative or semiquantitative; *Aspergillus*.	This test detects *Aspergillus* or *Aspergillus galactomannan* antigen. Aspergillus is a life-threatening infection in patients with immune systems compromised by leukemia, organ or bone marrow transplant, or chemotherapy.

(continued)

Appendix AA: COVID-19 Laboratory Codes (continued)

CPT CODE	DESCRIPTION	INDICATION
87320	Infectious agent antigen detection by immunoassay technique (eg, enzyme immunoassay [EIA], enzyme-linked immunosorbent assay [ELISA], fluorescence immunoassay [FIA], immunochemiluminometric assay [IMCA]), qualitative or semiquantitative; *Chlamydia trachomatis*.	This test detects *Chlamydia trachomatis*, commonly transmitted through sexual contact. A sample test may be taken from the cervix, urethra, or urine.
87324	Infectious agent antigen detection by immunoassay technique (eg, enzyme immunoassay [EIA], enzyme-linked immunosorbent assay [ELISA], fluorescence immunoassay [FIA], immunochemiluminometric assay [IMCA]), qualitative or semiquantitative; *Clostridium difficile* toxin(s).	This test detects toxins produced by *Clostridium difficile* bacteria, which causes diarrhea and usually results from antibiotic use.
87327	Infectious agent antigen detection by immunoassay technique (eg, enzyme immunoassay [EIA], enzyme-linked immunosorbent assay [ELISA], fluorescence immunoassay [FIA], immunochemiluminometric assay [IMCA]), qualitative or semiquantitative; *Cryptococcus neoformans*.	This test detects *Cryptococcus* bacteria in a spinal fluid (preferred) or blood sample. This bacteria infects the brain covering in people whose immune systems are severely injured.
87328	Infectious agent antigen detection by immunoassay technique (eg, enzyme immunoassay [EIA], enzyme-linked immunosorbent assay [ELISA], fluorescence immunoassay [FIA], immunochemiluminometric assay [IMCA]), qualitative or semiquantitative; *Cryptosporidium*.	This test examines a stool sample for *Cryptosporidium*, a parasite that causes abdominal pain, cramping and diarrhea. Infection infects the gastrointestinal (GI) tract also causing weight loss and fever.
87329	Infectious agent antigen detection by immunoassay technique (eg, enzyme immunoassay [EIA], enzyme-linked immunosorbent assay [ELISA], fluorescence immunoassay [FIA], immunochemiluminometric assay [IMCA]), qualitative or semiquantitative; *Giardia*.	This test examines a stool sample for the giardia parasite. Infection causes severe diarrhea, intestinal cramping, and stomach ache that can lead to weight loss and dehydration.
87332	Infectious agent antigen detection by immunoassay technique (eg, enzyme immunoassay [EIA], enzyme-linked immunosorbent assay [ELISA], fluorescence immunoassay [FIA], immunochemiluminometric assay [IMCA]), qualitative or semiquantitative; *Cytomegalovirus*.	This test detects infection by a cytomegalovirus (CMV), part of a virus family that includes herpes zoster, Epstein-Barr, and Varicella zoster. These viruses cause a range of illnesses comprising common upper respiratory infections, hepatitis, mononucleosis, and intestinal infections.

(continued)

Appendix AA: COVID-19 Laboratory Codes (continued)

CPT CODE	DESCRIPTION	INDICATION
87335	Infectious agent antigen detection by immunoassay technique (eg, enzyme immunoassay [EIA], enzyme-linked immunosorbent assay [ELISA], fluorescence immunoassay [FIA], immunochemiluminometric assay [IMCA]), qualitative or semiquantitative; *Escherichia coli* 0157.	This test detects infection with *E. coli* bacteria that causes intestinal illness, commonly found on contaminated food. The bacteria is the causative agent of hemorrhagic colitis in food-borne epidemics.
87336	Infectious agent antigen detection by immunoassay technique (eg, enzyme immunoassay [EIA], enzyme-linked immunosorbent assay [ELISA], fluorescence immunoassay [FIA], immunochemiluminometric assay [IMCA]), qualitative or semiquantitative; *Entamoeba histolytica* dispar group.	This test detects *Entamoeba histolytica* that live in the intestines through an examination of a stool sample. Biopsies may also be performed by a separately reportable open or endoscopic procedure.
87337	Infectious agent antigen detection by immunoassay technique (eg, enzyme immunoassay [EIA], enzyme-linked immunosorbent assay [ELISA], fluorescence immunoassay [FIA], immunochemiluminometric assay [IMCA]), qualitative or semiquantitative; *Entamoeba histolytica* group	This test detects entamoeba histolytica, that live in the intestines through an examination of a *H. pylori* antibody titer, stool sample. Biopsies may also be performed by a separately reportable open or endoscopic procedure.
87338	Infectious agent antigen detection by immunoassay technique (eg, enzyme immunoassay [EIA], enzyme-linked immunosorbent assay [ELISA], fluorescence immunoassay [FIA], immunochemiluminometric assay [IMCA]), qualitative or semiquantitative; *Helicobacter pylori*, stool.	This test detects *Helicobacter pylori* infection that can cause stomach ulcers and painful inflammation.
87339	Infectious agent antigen detection by immunoassay technique (eg, enzyme immunoassay [EIA], enzyme-linked immunosorbent assay [ELISA], fluorescence immunoassay [FIA], immunochemiluminometric assay [IMCA]), qualitative or semiquantitative; *Helicobacter pylori*.	This test detects *Helicobacter pylori* infection that can cause stomach ulcers and painful inflammation.
87340	Infectious agent antigen detection by immunoassay technique (eg, enzyme immunoassay [EIA], enzyme-linked immunosorbent assay [ELISA], fluorescence immunoassay [FIA], immunochemiluminometric assay [IMCA]), qualitative or semiquantitative; hepatitis B surface antigen (HBsAg)	This test detects hepatitis B virus which is a retrovirus that can cause persistent infection leading to liver cirrhosis and hepatocellular carcinoma. Venipuncture is separately reportable if performed.

(continued)

Appendix AA: COVID-19 Laboratory Codes (continued)

CPT CODE	DESCRIPTION	INDICATION
87341	Infectious agent antigen detection by immunoassay technique (eg, enzyme immunoassay [EIA], enzyme-linked immunosorbent assay [ELISA], fluorescence immunoassay [FIA], immunochemiluminometric assay [IMCA]), qualitative or semiquantitative; hepatitis B surface antigen (HBsAg) neutralization.	This test is performed when a specimen is repeatedly reactive for Hepatitis B surface antigen. Elevated HBsAg levels past 6 months may indicate a chronic carrier (chronic hepatitis). Venipuncture is separately reportable if performed.
87350	Infectious agent antigen detection by immunoassay technique (eg, enzyme immunoassay [EIA], enzyme-linked immunosorbent assay [ELISA], fluorescence immunoassay [FIA], immunochemiluminometric assay [IMCA]), qualitative or semiquantitative; hepatitis Be antigen (HBeAg).	This test detects hepatitis B virus, and a positive result indicates active hepatitis B virus infection.
87380	Infectious agent antigen detection by immunoassay technique (eg, enzyme immunoassay [EIA], enzyme-linked immunosorbent assay [ELISA], fluorescence immunoassay [FIA], immunochemiluminometric assay [IMCA]), qualitative or semiquantitative; hepatitis, delta agent.	This test is performed only on individuals who are chronically HBsAg positive or have an exacerbation of their hepatitis. Testing is limited to individuals who carry hepatitis B or those with chronic hepatitis B that develop complication.
87385	Infectious agent antigen detection by immunoassay technique (eg, enzyme immunoassay [EIA], enzyme-linked immunosorbent assay [ELISA], fluorescence immunoassay [FIA], immunochemiluminometric assay [IMCA]), qualitative or semiquantitative; *Histoplasmosis capsulatum*.	This test detects for the presence of spores, which can be picked up from soil. *Histoplasmosis capsulatum* infection results from inhalation or ingestion of spores, and causes acute pneumonia, disseminated reticuloendothelial hyperplasia with hepatosplenomegaly and anemia, influenza-like symptoms with joint effusion, and erythema nodosum.
87389	Infectious agent antigen detection by immunoassay technique (eg, enzyme immunoassay [EIA], enzyme-linked immunosorbent assay [ELISA], fluorescence immunoassay [FIA], immunochemiluminometric assay [IMCA]), qualitative or semiquantitative; HIV-1 antigen(s), with HIV-1 and HIV-2 antibodies, single result.	This test measures the amount of HIIV genetic material present in a blood sample.

(continued)

Appendix AA: COVID-19 Laboratory Codes (continued)

CPT CODE	DESCRIPTION	INDICATION
87390	Infectious agent antigen detection by immunoassay technique (eg, enzyme immunoassay [EIA], enzyme-linked immunosorbent assay [ELISA], fluorescence immunoassay [FIA], immunochemiluminometric assay [IMCA]), qualitative or semiquantitative; HIV-1	This test measures the amount of HIIV genetic material present in a blood sample.
87391	Infectious agent antigen detection by immunoassay technique (eg, enzyme immunoassay [EIA], enzyme-linked immunosorbent assay [ELISA], fluorescence immunoassay [FIA], immunochemiluminometric assay [IMCA]), qualitative or semiquantitative; HIV-2	This test measures the amount of HIIV genetic material present in a blood sample. HIV-2 is a retrovirus related to simian AIDS.
87400	Infectious agent antigen detection by immunoassay technique (eg, enzyme immunoassay [EIA], enzyme-linked immunosorbent assay [ELISA], fluorescence immunoassay [FIA], immunochemiluminometric assay [IMCA]), qualitative or semiquantitative; influenza, A or B, each.	This test may be used to detects influenza A or B. Influenza (flu) is a viral infection of the lungs that causes fever, cough, and muscle aches. Testing may occur during the acute phase of illness, and again 10 to 14 days after start of symptoms.
87420	Infectious agent antigen detection by immunoassay technique (eg, enzyme immunoassay [EIA], enzyme-linked immunosorbent assay [ELISA], fluorescence immunoassay [FIA], immunochemiluminometric assay [IMCA]), qualitative or semiquantitative; respiratory syncytial virus.	This test detects respiratory syncytial virus (RSV), an infection that causes respiratory disease that can be severe in infants and young children.
87425	Infectious agent antigen detection by immunoassay technique (eg, enzyme immunoassay [EIA], enzyme-linked immunosorbent assay [ELISA], fluorescence immunoassay [FIA], immunochemiluminometric assay [IMCA]), qualitative or semiquantitative; rotavirus.	This test detects rotavirus through a stool sample and can cause severe infectious gastroenteritis in infants and young children.
87426	Infectious agent antigen detection by immunoassay technique (eg, enzyme immunoassay [EIA], enzyme-linked immunosorbent assay [ELISA], fluorescence immunoassay [FIA], immunochemiluminometric assay [IMCA]), qualitative or semiquantitative; severe acute respiratory syndrome coronavirus (eg, SARS-CoV, SARS-CoV-2 [COVID-19]).	This test detects viral proteins related to COVID-19 virus.

(continued)

Appendix AA: COVID-19 Laboratory Codes (continued)

CPT CODE	DESCRIPTION	INDICATION
87427	Infectious agent antigen detection by immunoassay technique (eg, enzyme immunoassay [EIA], enzyme-linked immunosorbent assay [ELISA], fluorescence immunoassay [FIA], immunochemiluminometric assay [IMCA]), qualitative or semiquantitative; Shiga-like toxin.	This test detects *Shigella* bacteria infection that causes acute gut inflammation and dysentery.
87428	Infectious agent antigen detection by immunoassay technique (eg, enzyme immunoassay [EIA], enzyme-linked immunosorbent assay [ELISA], fluorescence immunoassay [FIA], immunochemiluminometric assay [IMCA]), qualitative or semiquantitative; severe acute respiratory syndrome coronavirus (eg, SARS-CoV, SARS-CoV-2 [COVID-19]), and influenza virus types A and B.	This detects for the presence of a specific viral antigen related to coronavirus (COVID-19), influenza A, and influenza B.
87430	Infectious agent antigen detection by immunoassay technique (eg, enzyme immunoassay [EIA], enzyme-linked immunosorbent assay [ELISA], fluorescence immunoassay [FIA], immunochemiluminometric assay [IMCA]), qualitative or semiquantitative; *Streptococcus*, group A	This test detects group A *Streptococcus* (GAS) infectious antigens, that causes a wide variety of infections, including but not limited to pharyngitis, bronchitis, pneumonia, rheumatic fever, necrotizing fasciitis, and glomerulonephritis.
87449	Infectious agent antigen detection by immunoassay technique (eg, enzyme immunoassay [EIA], enzyme-linked immunosorbent assay [ELISA], fluorescence immunoassay [FIA], immunochemiluminometric assay [IMCA]), qualitative or semiquantitative; not otherwise specified, each organism.	This test detects infectious agents that are not specifically identified elsewhere, using a sample of blood, urine, stool, or spinal fluid. This test may be performed using a CLIA-waived test system.
87451	Infectious agent antigen detection by immunoassay technique (eg, enzyme immunoassay [EIA], enzyme-linked immunosorbent assay [ELISA], fluorescence immunoassay [FIA], immunochemiluminometric assay [IMCA]), qualitative or semiquantitative; polyvalent for multiple organisms; each polyvalent antiserum.	This test detects infectious agents that are not specifically identified elsewhere, using a sample of blood, urine, stool, or spinal fluid. Report once for each polyvalent antiserum. Polyvalent denotes an antibody molecule with multiple antigen binding sites.
87635	Infectious agent detection by nucleic acid (DNA or RNA); severe acute respiratory syndrome coronavirus 2 (SARS-CoV-2) (coronavirus disease [COVID-19]), amplified probe technique.	This test detects SARS-CoV and any pan-coronavirus types or subtypes. It uses specific primers and amplified probe assay to detect DNA or RNA sequences specific for the SARS-CoV-2 virus.

(continued)

Appendix AA: COVID-19 Laboratory Codes (continued)

CPT CODE	DESCRIPTION	INDICATION
87636	Infectious agent detection by nucleic acid (DNA or RNA); severe acute respiratory syndrome coronavirus 2 (SARS-CoV-2) (coronavirus disease [COVID-19]), and influenza virus types A and B, multiplex amplified probe technique.	This test detects the presence of genetic material related to COVID-19, influenza A, and influenza B. It uses specific primers and amplified probe assay to detect DNA or RNA sequences specific for the SARS-CoV-2 virus.
87637	Infectious agent detection by nucleic acid (DNA or RNA); severe acute respiratory syndrome coronavirus 2 (SARS-CoV-2) (coronavirus disease [COVID-19]), and influenza virus types A and B, and respiratory syncytial virus, multiplex amplified probe technique.	This test detects the presence of genetic material related to COVID-19, influenza A, influenza B, and respiratory syncytial virus (RSV). It uses specific primers and amplified probe assay to detect DNA or RNA sequences specific for the SARS-CoV-2 virus.
87802	Infectious agent antigen detection by immunoassay with direct optical (ie, visual) observation; *Streptococcus*, group B.	This test detects for group B strep (GBS) using a rapid antigen test. This code describes a visually read immunoassay for group B *Streptococcus* that is typically performed on pregnant women in labor or at any time during pregnancy.
87803	Infectious agent antigen detection by immunoassay with direct optical (ie, visual) observation; *Clostridium difficile* toxin A.	This test detects toxins produced by clostridium difficile bacteria that causes antibiotic-associated diarrhea, colitis, and all cases of pseudomembranous colitis (PMC)
87804	Infectious agent antigen detection by immunoassay with direct optical (ie, visual) observation; influenza	This test detects for influenza using a rapid antigen test. Influenza (flu) is a viral infection of the lungs that causes fever, cough, and muscle aches.
87806	Infectious agent antigen detection by immunoassay with direct optical (ie, visual) observation; HIV-1 antigen(s), with HIV-1 and HIV-2 antibodies.	This test detects antibodies to HIV-1 and HIV-2 infection, using a qualitative immunoassay point-of-care test.
87807	Infectious agent antigen detection by immunoassay with direct optical (ie, visual) observation; respiratory syncytial virus.	This test detects for respiratory syncytial virus using a rapid antigen test.
87808	Infectious agent antigen detection by immunoassay with direct optical (ie, visual) observation; *Trichomonas vaginalis*.	This test detects for the specific cause of vaginitis and may be performed after negative testing for yeasts or trichomonas.
87809	Infectious agent antigen detection by immunoassay with direct optical (ie, visual) observation; adenovirus.	This test detects adenovirus, a lung infection that causes lymph nodes at the back of the throat to become enlarged, which can make breathing difficult.

(continued)

Appendix AA: COVID-19 Laboratory Codes (continued)

CPT CODE	DESCRIPTION	INDICATION
87810	Infectious agent antigen detection by immunoassay with direct optical (ie, visual) observation; *Chlamydia trachomatis*.	This test detects for *Chlamydia trachomatis* infection commonly transmitted through sexual contact. It may cause nonspecific urethritis or pelvic inflammatory disease (PID), although it is commonly asymptomatic in women. Sample may be taken from the cervix, urethra, or urine.
87811	Infectious agent antigen detection by immunoassay with direct optical (ie, visual) observation; severe acute respiratory syndrome coronavirus 2 (SARS-CoV-2) (coronavirus disease [COVID-19]).	This test detects for SARS-CoV-2 or COVID-19 using a rapid antigen test. The immunoassay provides qualitative (positive or negative) detection of the nucleocapsid protein antigen from SARS-CoV-2.
87850	Infectious agent antigen detection by immunoassay with direct optical (ie, visual) observation; *Neisseria gonorrhoeae*.	This test for gonorrhea, a common sexually transmitted bacterial infection.
87880	Infectious agent antigen detection by immunoassay with direct optical (ie, visual) observation; *Streptococcus*, group A.	This test detects *Streptococcus* bacteria A which causes pharyngitis, using a rapid antigen test.
87899	Infectious agent antigen detection by immunoassay with direct optical (ie, visual) observation; not otherwise specified.	This test identifies the cause of an infection from a sample of blood, urine, stool, or spinal fluid. This code should only be reported when the infectious agent being tested does not have a more specific code.
87913	Infectious agent genotype analysis by nucleic acid (DNA or RNA); severe acute respiratory syndrome coronavirus 2 (SARS-CoV-2) (coronavirus disease [COVID-19]), mutation identification in targeted region(s).	This test detects for the presence of a mutation associated with coronavirus (COVID-19), a respiratory virus.

Appendix BB

COVID-19 VACCINE ADMINISTRATION CODES

ADMINISTRATION CODE	VACCINE CODE	PATIENT AGE	DOSING INTERVAL	MANUFACTURER
90480	91304	12 years and older	5 micrograms/0.5 mL	Novavax Inc.
	91318	6 months to 4 years	3 micrograms/0.3 mL	Pfizer-BioNTech
	91319	5–11 years	10 micrograms/0.3 mL	Pfizer-BioNTech
	91320	12 years and older	30 micrograms/0.3 mL	Pfizer-BioNTech
	91321	6 months to 11 years	25 micrograms/0.25 mL	Moderna Inc.
	91322	12 years and older	50 micrograms/0.5 mL	Moderna Inc.

Appendix CC

NEW CPT CODES IN 2025

Telemedicine

CODE	DESCRIPTION	RELATIVE VALUE UNITS (RVUs)		
		WORK RVUs	NON-FACILITY TOTAL	FACILITY TOTAL
Synchronous Audio-Video Visit: New Patient				
98000	Synchronous audio-video visit for the evaluation and management of a new patient, which requires a medically appropriate history and/or examination and straightforward medical decision making. When using total time on the date of the encounter for code selection, 15 minutes must be met or exceeded.	0.93	1.54	1.35
98001	Synchronous audio-video visit for the evaluation and management of a new patient, which requires a medically appropriate history and/or examination and low medical decision making. When using total time on the date of the encounter for code selection, 30 minutes must be met or exceeded.	1.60	2.54	2.33
98002	Synchronous audio-video visit for the evaluation and management of a new patient, which requires a medically appropriate history and/or examination and moderate medical decision making. When using total time on the date of the encounter for code selection, 45 minutes must be met or exceeded.	2.60	4.05	3.78
98003	Synchronous audio-video visit for the evaluation and management of a new patient, which requires a medically appropriate history and/or examination and high medical decision making. When using total time on the date of the encounter for code selection, 60 minutes must be met or exceeded. (For services 75 minutes or longer, use prolonged services code 99417)	3.50	5.37	5.08
Note: A medically necessary physical examination may still be required and performed remotely.				
Synchronous Audio-Video Visit: Established Patient				
98004	Synchronous audio-video visit for the evaluation and management of an established patient, which requires a medically appropriate history and/or examination and straightforward medical decision making. When using total time on the date of the encounter for code selection, 10 minutes must be met or exceeded.	0.70	1.19	1.01

(continued)

Appendix CC: New CPT Codes in 2025 – Telemedicine (continued)

CODE	DESCRIPTION	RELATIVE VALUE UNITS (RVUs)		
		WORK RVUs	NON-FACILITY TOTAL	FACILITY TOTAL
98005	Synchronous audio-video visit for the evaluation and management of an established patient, which requires a medically appropriate history and/or examination and low medical decision making. When using total time on the date of the encounter for code selection, 20 minutes must be met or exceeded.	1.30	2.08	1.88
98006	Synchronous audio-video visit for the evaluation and management of an established patient, which requires a medically appropriate history and/or examination and moderate medical decision making. When using total time on the date of the encounter for code selection, 30 minutes must be met or exceeded.	1.92	3.07	2.80
98007	Synchronous audio-video visit for the evaluation and management of an established patient, which requires a medically appropriate history and/or examination and high medical decision making. When using total time on the date of the encounter for code selection, 40 minutes must be met or exceeded.	2.60	4.07	3.78
Synchronous Audio-Only Visit: New Patient				
98008	Synchronous audio-only visit for the evaluation and management of a new patient, which requires a medically appropriate history and/or examination, straightforward medical decision making, and more than 10 minutes of medical discussion. When using total time on the date of the encounter for code selection, 15 minutes must be met or exceeded.	0.90	1.46	1.29
98009	Synchronous audio-only visit for the evaluation and management of a new patient, which requires a medically appropriate history and/or examination, low medical decision making, and more than 10 minutes of medical discussion. When using total time on the date of the encounter for code selection, 30 minutes must be met or exceeded.	1.55	2.42	2.24
98010	Synchronous audio-only visit for the evaluation and management of a new patient, which requires a medically appropriate history and/or examination, moderate medical decision making, and more than 10 minutes of medical discussion. When using total time on the date of the encounter for code selection, 45 minutes must be met or exceeded.	2.42	3.77	3.53
98011	Synchronous audio-only visit for the evaluation and management of a new patient, which requires a medically appropriate history and/or examination, high medical decision making, and more than 10 minutes of medical discussion. When using total time on the date of the encounter for code selection, 60 minutes must be met or exceeded. (For services 75 minutes or longer, use prolonged services code 99417)	3.20	4.90	4.64

(continued)

Appendix CC: New CPT Codes in 2025 – Telemedicine (continued)

CODE	DESCRIPTION	RELATIVE VALUE UNITS (RVUs)		
		WORK RVUs	NON-FACILITY TOTAL	FACILITY TOTAL
Synchronous Audio-Only Visit: Established Patient				
98012	Synchronous audio-only visit for the evaluation and management of an established patient, which requires a medically appropriate history and/or examination, straightforward medical decision making, and more than 10 minutes of medical discussion. When using total time on the date of the encounter for code selection, 10 minutes must be exceeded.	0.65	1.09	0.95
98013	Synchronous audio-only visit for the evaluation and management of an established patient, which requires a medically appropriate history and/or examination, low medical decision making, and more than 10 minutes of medical discussion. When using total time on the date of the encounter for code selection, 20 minutes must be met or exceeded.	1.20	1.90	1.73
98014	Synchronous audio-only visit for the evaluation and management of an established patient, which requires a medically appropriate history and/or examination, moderate medical decision making, and more than 10 minutes of medical discussion. When using total time on the date of the encounter for code selection, 30 minutes must be met or exceeded.	1.75	2.78	2.56
98015	Synchronous audio-only visit for the evaluation and management of an established patient, which requires a medically appropriate history and/or examination, high medical decision making, and more than 10 minutes of medical discussion. When using total time on the date of the encounter for code selection, 40 minutes must be met or exceeded. (For services 55 minutes or longer, use prolonged services code 99417)	2.60	4.04	3.78
Brief Synchronous Communication Technology (Virtual Check-In)				
98016	Brief communication technology-based service (e.g., virtual check-in) by a physician or other qualified health care professional who can report evaluation and management services provided to an established patient, not originating from a related evaluation and management service provided within the previous 7 days nor leading to an evaluation and management service or procedure within the next 24 hours or the soonest available appointment, 5-10 minutes of medical discussion	0.30	0.49	0.45

Surgery

CODE	DESCRIPTION	RELATIVE VALUE UNITS (RVUs)		
		WORK RVUs	NON-FACILITY TOTAL	FACILITY TOTAL
Intra-abdominal Tumor Excision or Destruction				
49186	Excision or destruction, open, intra-abdominal (ie, peritoneal, mesenteric, retroperitoneal), primary or secondary tumor(s) or cyst(s), sum of the maximum length of tumor(s) or cyst(s); 5 cm or less	22.00	N/A	39.50
49187	Excision or destruction, open, intra-abdominal (ie, peritoneal, mesenteric, retroperitoneal), primary or secondary tumor(s) or cyst(s), sum of the maximum length of tumor(s) or cyst(s); 5.1 to 10 cm	28.65	N/A	50.48
49188	Excision or destruction, open, intra-abdominal (ie, peritoneal, mesenteric, retroperitoneal), primary or secondary tumor(s) or cyst(s), sum of the maximum length of tumor(s) or cyst(s); 10.1 to 20 cm	34.00	N/A	60.32
49189	Excision or destruction, open, intra-abdominal (ie, peritoneal, mesenteric, retroperitoneal), primary or secondary tumor(s) or cyst(s), sum of the maximum length of tumor(s) or cyst(s); 20.1 to 30 cm	40.00	N/A	70.17
49190	Excision or destruction, open, intra-abdominal (ie, peritoneal, mesenteric, retroperitoneal), primary or secondary tumor(s) or cyst(s), sum of the maximum length of tumor(s) or cyst(s); greater than 30 cm	50.00	N/A	86.50

Appendix DD

CATEGORY III CODES*

CPT CODE	CPT DESCRIPTION
0786T	Insertion or replacement of percutaneous electrode array, sacral, with integrated neurostimulator, including imaging guidance when performed
0787T	Revision or removal of neurostimulator electrode array, sacral, with integrated neurostimulator
0788T	Electronic analysis with simple programming of implanted integrated neurostimulation system (eg, electrode array and receiver), including contact group(s), amplitude, pulse width, frequency (Hz), on/off cycling, burst, dose lockout, patient-selectable parameters, responsive neurostimulation, detection algorithms, closed-loop parameters, and passive parameters, when performed by physician or other qualified health care professional, spinal cord, or sacral nerve, 1-3 parameters (Do not report X005T in conjunction with 43647, 43648, 43881, 43882, 61850-61888, 63650, 63655, 63661, 63662, 63663, 63664, 63685, 63688, 64553-64595, 64XX2, 64XX4, 95970, 95971, 95972, 95976, 95977, 95983, 95984, 0587T, 0588T, 0589T, 0590T, X004T, 0X43T, 0X44T, 0X46T, 0X48T.)
0789T	Electronic analysis with complex programming of implanted integrated neurostimulation system (eg, electrode array and receiver), including contact group(s), amplitude, pulse width, frequency (Hz), on/off cycling, burst, dose lockout, patient-selectable parameters, responsive neurostimulation, detection algorithms, closed-loop parameters, and passive parameters, when performed by physician or other qualified health care professional, spinal cord or sacral nerve), 4 or more parameters (Do not report 0X48T in conjunction with 43647, 43648, 43881, 43882, 61850-61888, 63650, 63655, 63661, 63662, 63663, 63664, 63685, 63688, 64553-64595, 64XX2, 64XX4, 95970, 95971, 95972, 95976, 95977, 95983, 95984, 0587T, 0588T, 0589T, 0590T, X004T, X005T, 0X43T, 0X44T, 0X46T.)
0587T	Percutaneous implantation or replacement of integrated single device neurostimulation system for bladder dysfunction including electrode array and receiver or pulse generator, including analysis, programming, and imaging guidance when performed, posterior tibial nerve (Do not report 0587T in conjunction with 64555, 64566, 64575, 64590, 64XX2, 95970, 95971, 95972, 0588T, 0589T, 0590T.)
0588T	Revision or removal of integrated single device neurostimulation system for bladder dysfunction including electrode array and receiver or pulse generator, including analysis, programming, and imaging guidance when performed, posterior tibial nerve (Do not report 0588T in conjunction with 64555, 64566, 64575, 64590, 64XX4, 95970, 95971, 95972, 0587T, 0589T, 0590T.)
0589T	Electronic analysis with simple programming of implanted integrated neurostimulation system for bladder dysfunction (eg, electrode array and receiver), including contact group(s), amplitude, pulse width, frequency (Hz), on/off cycling, burst, dose lockout, patient-selectable parameters, responsive neurostimulation, detection algorithms, closed-loop parameters, and passive parameters, when performed by physician or other qualified health care professional, posterior tibial nerve, 1-3 parameters (Do not report 0589T in conjunction with 43647, 43648, 43881, 43882, 61850-61888, 63650, 63655, 63661, 63662, 63663, 63664, 63685, 63688, 64553-64595, 95970, 95971, 95972, 95976, 95977, 95983, 95984, 0587T, 0588T, 0590T, X005T.)

(continued)

*These codes were added in 2024.

Appendix DD: Category III Codes (continued)

CPT CODE	CPT DESCRIPTION
0590T	Electronic analysis with complex programming of implanted integrated neurostimulation system for bladder dysfunction (eg, electrode array and receiver), including contact group(s), amplitude, pulse width, frequency (Hz), on/off cycling, burst, dose lockout, patient-selectable parameters, responsive neurostimulation, detection algorithms, closed-loop parameters, and passive parameters, when performed by physician or other qualified health care professional, posterior tibial nerve, 4 or more parameters (Do not report 0590T in conjunction with 43647, 43648, 43881, 43882, 61850-61888, 63650, 63655, 63661, 63662, 63663, 63664, 63685, 63688, 64553-64595, 95970, 95971, 95972, 95976, 95977, 95983, 95984, 0587T, 0588T, 0589T, X005T.)

ACOG | 2025 Coding Resources

Guidance you need to help code your claims.

Coding Quick Reference Guides

ACOG's Coding Quick Reference Guides have been revised to provide obstetrician–gynecologists and their staffs quick access to the most up-to-date, commonly used diagnosis and procedural codes for billing ob-gyn services at their fingertips.

OB/GYN Evaluation & Management (E/M) Services Coding Quick Reference Guide

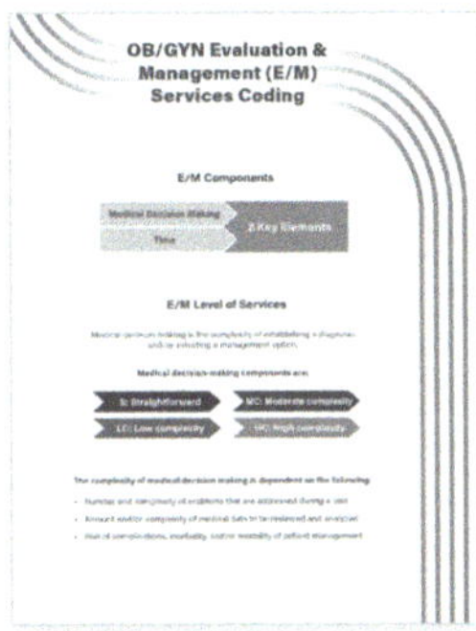

Revised to provide quick reference to current and newly updated CPT codes for inpatient, outpatient, observation, consultation, emergency department visits, elements of medical decision-making, and modifiers.

Item No.: AA677S, Single copy
2022 / 6-page foldout / folds to 8.5″ x 11″
Price: $15.95, Members: $12.76
ISBN: 978-1-948258-83-8

Item No.: AA677, Pack of 10
Price: $120.00, Members: $96.00
ISBN: 978-1-948258-84-5

OB/GYN Diagnostic Coding Quick Reference Guide

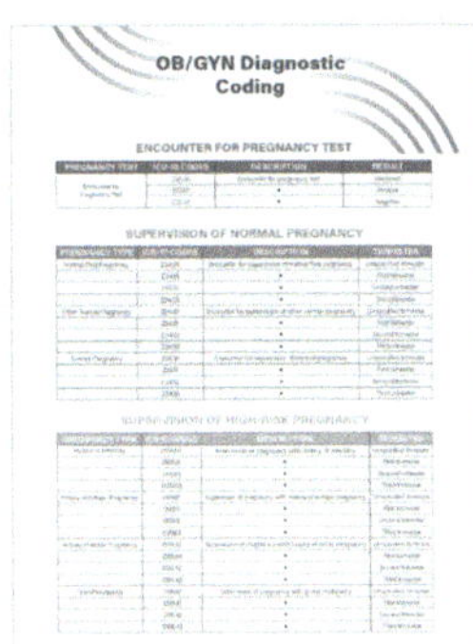

Features various ICD-10-CM codes for coding and billing obstetric and gynecologic services.

Item No.: AA674S, Single copy
2022 / 4-page foldout /
folds to 8.5″ x 11″
Price: $12.95, Members: $10.00
ISBN: 978-1-948258-77-7

Item No.: AA674, Pack of 10
Price: $110.00, Members: $80.00
ISBN: 978-1-948258-78-4

OB/GYN Preventive Services Coding Quick Reference Guide

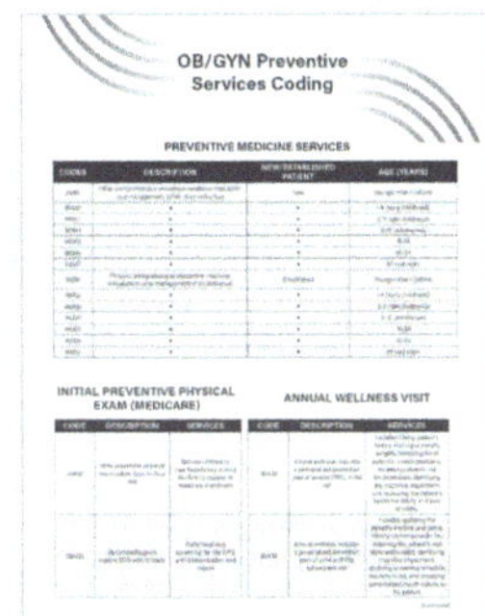

This guide provides users with quick reference to CPT codes for billing preventive medicine services performed during ob-gyn visits.

Item No.: AA676S, Single copy
2022 / 4-page foldout /
folds to 8.5″ x 11″
Price: $12.95, Members: $10.00
ISBN: 978-1-948258-81-4

Item No.: AA676, Pack of 10
Price: $110.00, Members: $80.00
ISBN: 978-1-948258-82-1

OB/GYN Surgical Coding Quick Reference Guide

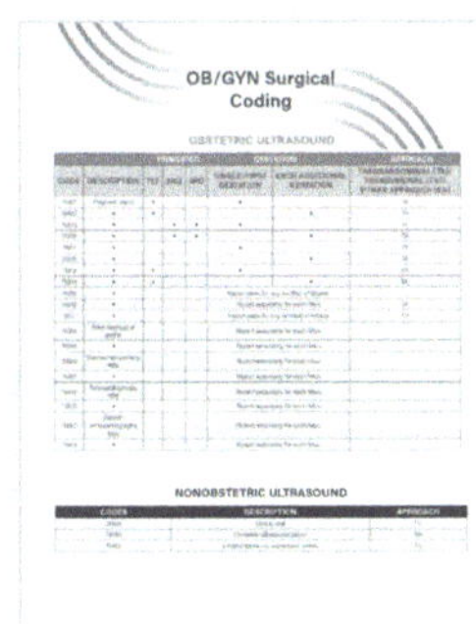

This guide provides up-to-date and quick reference to surgical CPT codes for billing obstetric delivery, ob-gyn ultrasound, gynecologic embolization, laparoscopy, and radiofrequency ablation procedures, and applicable surgical modifiers.

Item No.: AA675S, Single copy
2022 / 4-page foldout / folds to 8.5″ x 11″
Price: $12.95, Members: $10.00
ISBN: 978-1-948258-79-1

Item No.: AA675, Pack of 10
Price: $110.00, Members: $80.00
ISBN: 978-1-948258-80-7

TO ORDER CALL 800-762-2264